Praise for the first edition

"Yes! An easy-to-read, fascinating review of the science behind new parents' biggest health questions. Many of these issues—infant sleep, breastfeeding, vaccines—will hit your 'Should I panic?' button. With gentle guidance, Alice Callahan puts your fears to rest."

—Tracy Cutchlow, author of *Zero to Five:
70 Essential Parenting Tips Based on Science
(and What I've Learned So Far)*

"Name a complex or controversial topic and Callahan provides the science on both sides of the arguments to help parents make wise choices."

—*Psychology Today*

"[Callahan's] compassion and empathy for the difficulties of parenting shine through in every chapter, from breastfeeding to vaccines to feeding to sleeping."

—*Forbes*

"Alice Callahan, PhD, combines the critical eye of a scientist with the heart of a mother to create a helpful resource for all people interested in evidence-based infant care and parenting."

—*Science & Sensibility* (Lamaze International)

"[Callahan] takes a compassionate, non-preachy approach with a goal of not telling the reader what to do but rather how to seek wise advice and make smart decisions and to enjoy having a baby, which is what it is all about."

—*Live Science*

"Alice Callahan has written a breakthrough book, combining the compassion, warmth, and angst of a mother with the measured reasoning of a scientist. She helps parents not only understand how science works but how they can access that science to answer their questions. She's found a way to access the scientist in all of us."

—Paul A. Offit, MD, The Children's Hospital of Philadelphia, author of *Overkill: When Modern Medicine Goes Too Far*

"A timely and necessary book for parents . . . It will help both moms and dads work together to choose the right parenting methods for them and give them a research-based approach to raising a child."

—*Patheos*

"Finally, someone has brought some science—and some sense—to the mommy wars. Should be required reading for all new (and old) parents."

—Emily Oster, Brown University, author of *Cribsheet: A Data-Driven Guide to Better, More Relaxed Parenting, from Birth to Preschool*

"A rare gem in the parenting canon—smart, sensitive, and a lifesaver for a generation of parents caught in the nebulous spider's web of Internet 'wisdom.'"

—Suzanne Barston, author of *Bottled Up: How the Way We Feed Babies Has Come to Define Motherhood, and Why It Shouldn't*

"Families routinely search for health information. *The Science of Mom* makes it easy, collecting evidence for health decisions and putting it into perspective with a mom-to-mom connection. Callahan's advice is thoughtful, backed by science, and feels fueled by love. She is willing to provide powerful advice when detailing the science and safety of vaccines. Keep this book in arm's reach as you support your infant for calm and direction."

—Wendy Sue Swanson, MD, MBE, FAAP, Seattle Children's Hospital, author of *Mama Doc Medicine: Finding Calm and Confidence in Parenting, Child Health, and Work-Life Balance*

"Think of all the controversial, hot-button topics that parents obsess about in a child's first year—from vaccines to feeding, bed-sharing to sleep training. Weighing the scientific evidence, Callahan offers balanced insights and in-depth answers—a far cry from the oversimplified advice prescribed by many 'parenting experts.' The result: a must-have guide that's substantive and extremely engaging."

—Jena Pincott, author of *Do Chocolate Lovers Have Sweeter Babies? The Surprising Science of Pregnancy*

"[S]hould be required reading for all new parents. [Callahan] calms fears and provides parents with real facts. She doesn't make the decisions for you, but she makes it a lot easier to make sound decisions."

—*MomSense*

"A fresh and enlightening approach. I'd highly recommend this book to any mom expecting her first child or her fourth."

—*Uncommon Motherhood*

"Dr. Callahan isn't bossy, and isn't out to tell you what she thinks. Her book tells you what the science says, and explains how we know what we know, and what things we still need to learn more about. There's humility and warmth here, which I think parents of newborns will find reassuring."

—*The Pediatric Insider*

"This is science-based medicine writing at its best. Callahan doesn't cherry-pick. She knows how to evaluate the entire body of research and put it into perspective along with practical parenting considerations. She enhances her message with a personal touch, including anecdotes about her own experiences as a new mother and about the experiences of her friends and family. If I had three thumbs, I would give this book a three-thumbs-up recommendation."

—*Science-Based Medicine*

"[A] solid resource for any new parent or parent to be. Callahan does the work of sorting through the science of baby's first year, so you don't have to."

—*Raise Healthy Eaters*

"A book long-overdue in the parenting literature."

—*Momma Data*

"*The Science of Mom* stands out from the crowd . . . an easy-to-read, certifiable resource."

—*American Reference Books Annual*

The Science of Mom

THE
SCIENCE OF
MOM

A Research-Based Guide to Your Baby's First Year

SECOND EDITION

Alice Callahan, PhD

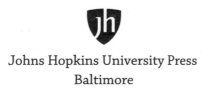

Johns Hopkins University Press
Baltimore

Johns Hopkins University Press
2715 North Charles Street
Baltimore, Maryland 21218-4363
www.press.jhu.edu

Library of Congress Cataloging-in-Publication Data

Names: Callahan, Alice, 1980– author.
Title: The science of mom : a research-based guide to your baby's
    first year / Alice Callahan, PhD.
Description: Second edition. | Baltimore : Johns Hopkins
    University Press, 2021. | Includes bibliographical references and
    index.
Identifiers: LCCN 2020051671 | ISBN 9781421441993 (paperback)
    | ISBN 9781421442006 (ebook)
Subjects: LCSH: Infants—Care. | Infants—Health and hygiene.
Classification: LCC RJ61 .C23 2021 | DDC 618.92/02—dc23
LC record available at https://lccn.loc.gov/2020051671

A catalog record for this book is available from the British Library.

Special discounts are available for bulk purchases of
this book. For more information, please contact Special Sales
at specialsales@jh.edu

For my two Charlottes:
the one who brought me into the world
and
the one who brought me into motherhood

CONTENTS

CONTENTS

PREFACE

I write this today having just finished months of editing and updating this book for the second edition. This was a process of sifting through the research published in the past six or seven years to ensure that the science in this book is up to date, and because science is always moving us forward, that meant reading hundreds more papers. I shouldn't have been surprised, but I found much more new science to incorporate than I had anticipated. Updating this book also meant poring over the words I wrote as many years ago and letting them draw me back to the questions of new parenthood, remembering all the worry and wonder of that time. Cee, my first child, recently celebrated her tenth birthday, which means I've closed out my first decade as a parent. Max, my second and last child, started kindergarten this fall—albeit from home, as we're in the midst of a global pandemic. It feels like the end of an era. I'm glad to have this book as part of the record of my children's first years (and my early years as a parent) and for the opportunity to ensure it continues to be a current and relevant resource for today's new parents.

The COVID-19 pandemic has turned our lives upside down in a year also marked by tumultuous politics, a long-overdue reckoning with systemic racism, and terrifying wildfires, which enveloped my town in smoke last month as the forests we love burned. Some days, it was difficult to focus on the research and writing required to update this book. What motivated me to sit down with it each day were the memories of those early days and nights of parenthood: the fatigue of constant caregiving, the anxiety that we might be doing it all wrong, and the late-night internet searching for answers, or at least some reassurance. Even in the best, most normal of times (although I'm not sure what "normal" means anymore), parenting is hard. However, it can also infuse your life with sweetness and give you hope for the future. My sincere wish is that this book can relieve some of your mental load—the worries and questions of new parenthood—and tip your balance toward enjoying the sweetness of a new baby.

I believe, now more than ever, that science can be a light that leads us forward. I'm counting on it to lead us out of this pandemic and to help us solve the climate crisis, but also, to shed a little light on the everyday tasks of raising children. For although much has changed over the last decade, my trust in science has not.

ACKNOWLEDGMENTS

Before I became a parent, I had no idea how much work it would be, how much I had to learn, and how radically it would change my life. I can say the same about writing this, my first book. And just like raising a child, writing a book, I now know, takes lots of help. I couldn't have done it on my own.

This book would never have happened without the gracious support of the readers of my blog, *Science of Mom*. They convinced me that there are other parents who, like me, want and need evidence-based information on parenting. They inspired me to get started, encouraged me to keep going, and were patient when my blog grew quiet so that I could focus on finishing the book.

Writing this book gave me a good reason to fully immerse myself in stacks of fun and interesting parenting science. I'm grateful to all the scientists who have trained and mentored me over the years. They probably had no idea how I might apply this skill set, but I think I've put it to good use.

Most of the science in this book came from my digging through the published literature, but conversations with researchers and clinicians also helped clarify and illuminate the data for me and sometimes revealed fascinating stories behind the science. For this, my thanks to Drs. Thomas Anders, Helen Ball, Peter Blair, Martin Blaser, Camila Chaparro, Leita Dzubay, Jeffrey Ecker, Anne Estes, David Fleischer, Penny Glass, Frank Greer, Margaret Hammerschlag, Douglas Leonard, Maria Mascola, Lauren Marcewicz, Jodi Mindell, Rachel Moon, Paul Offit, Tonse Raju, Henry Redel, Robert Sidonio, Paul Slovic, Douglas Teti, Carina Venter, and Kristi Watterberg. In the years between the first and second editions of this book, my journalistic work has given me the privilege of interviewing countless more researchers and clinicians, who have also informed the updates in this book.

Just as much, I am grateful to all of the parents who generously shared their real life stories, helping me to put the science in context: Suzanne Barston, Eve F., Cheryl Green, Jordan Green, Stefani Leavitt, Esmee McKee, Janie Oyakawa, Leah R., and Valerie Wheat. In addition, my late grandmother, Margaret Green, opened an old wound in her heart to tell me the story of the death of her young son. I think with gratitude about the couple of days I spent with her in 2013, my voice recorder running, as I asked the questions I wouldn't have had the courage to ask without a book deadline looming, and she answered in hopes that her story would be meaningful to today's parents.

Thank you to Vincent Burke, my first editor at Johns Hopkins University Press, for recognizing the potential in this book, and to him and the staff at the Press for expertly guiding me through the process of publishing the first edition. For the second edition, I was honored to work with the indefatigable Tiffany Gasbarrini, whose support and patience with me never wavered, pandemic and all. Thanks also to Juliana McCarthy, Esther Rodriguez, Hilary Jacqmin, and the many others at the Press who worked their magic in the long process between my manuscript submission and publication day. And thank you to my copyeditor, Joanne Haines.

I am forever indebted to my mother, Charlotte Green, for many reasons. She was my first example of gentle and respectful parenting, and she raised me to be a reader and a writer. She was also my best editor throughout the process of writing this book. She let my preoccupation with the book take over our long weekly phone conversations, and she thoughtfully read and critiqued chapter after chapter.

Many other friends and family members also read chapters and provided valuable feedback: Rob Callahan, Sarah Holexa, Dorit Reiss, Sarah Ruttan, Jessica Smock, Gregory Stanton, Miya Tokumitsu, and Robin White. Thanks also to the anonymous peer reviewers who provided honest and insightful comments on the manuscript.

Thank you to Rob, my husband, friend, and partner in parenting, for his constant encouragement, unwavering support, and for all of the days he took on more than his fair share of childcare and told me to go back to my desk and keep writing. And finally, thank you to my children, Cee and Max, for being my inspiration, keeping me humble, and growing my heart.

The Science of Mom

INTRODUCTION

I was a scientist first. I started working in research labs as a college student, then as a lab technician, and then went on to graduate school for a PhD in nutritional biology. By the time my husband and I decided we were ready for a baby, I was a postdoctoral fellow studying fetal physiology. For the previous decade of my life, I had been working to understand the world through the lens of science. I asked questions and sought answers by designing and conducting experiments in the lab. I pored over journal articles, trying to make sense of my data and figure out what important questions to ask next. My job was to measure, analyze, and explain. If I felt lost, then the way out of darkness was always to learn more, maybe by repeating an experiment or immersing myself in the scientific literature until things started to look a little clearer.

It should come as no surprise, then, that when I didn't get pregnant in the first couple of months of trying, I tackled it in the best way I knew how: with science. I measured my basal body temperature and tracked my cervical mucus. I recorded my bodily data in a spreadsheet and searched for patterns in color-coded graphs. I pulled out my reproductive physiology textbook to brush up on ovulation and how to optimize our chances at fertilization. It's hard to say whether any of this helped me to get pregnant any faster, but it did at least give me a feeling of control, though perhaps at the expense of romance.

1

When I eventually did get pregnant and became a mother, this same story played out again and again, with different details. Pregnancy and childbirth were just the beginning. Caring for my first child, Cee, brought lots more questions. Where should she sleep, and when could I expect her to sleep through the night? When should she start solid foods, and what should I feed her? Should I be worried about vaccine safety? Between feeding and rocking, changing and bouncing, and soothing and singing, I found myself digging into the science of parenting.

At about the same time, I left the research lab so that I could spend more time with Cee and explore other career paths, but I missed talking about science with like-minded colleagues. I started the *Science of Mom* blog as a place to share and discuss what I was learning about parenting, and I was thrilled to find a community of equally inquisitive parents looking for solid science. My blog readers were fascinated by the complexities of the science and always ready with new questions, which inspired me to keep researching and writing. At some point, I wanted to be able to develop these topics in a more cohesive manner, and that journey became this book.

Why do we look to science for answers to parenting questions? For most of human history, how we cared for our babies was passed quietly from generation to generation, one mother to the next. It varied around the world, and it changed over time, but it was informed by culture, environment, and necessity—not science. But for our generation, new parenthood means making a huge number of decisions with little familial or cultural guidance. Most of us live far away from the parents and grandparents, aunts and uncles, and brothers and sisters who might have guided us into parenthood in generations past. Instead, we have unlimited advice from the internet, a resource that empowers us to find our own answers but at the same time overwhelms us with confusing information. If our babies won't nap or we're struggling with breastfeeding, we can ask Google for answers or solicit opinions from our vast networks on social media. Very quickly, we find ourselves in a minefield of conflicting information and opinions, often paired with a little judgment from all sides.

Science is a tool that can help us get closer to the truth in the midst of all this confusion. It can help us to sidestep the opinions and philosophies and anecdotes that fuel parenting debates. We look to science, not to confirm what we want to believe or to prove others wrong, but rather to make the best decisions we can as parents.

It isn't that science has all the answers. For some parenting questions, like those that are medical in nature, science can be a great guide. For others, like parenting practices, it can often only give us clues, and then we have to figure out how they might (or might not) apply to our own families. The truth is, from a scientific standpoint, parenting is an immensely complicated thing to study. How do we sort through and quantify so many variables—along with all the differences between babies and families—and, statistically, make some sense of it all? Something so complex can rarely be reduced to a right way and a wrong way. What science can do is zoom out to look at large numbers of babies and families to reveal patterns and averages and ranges of normal. It can give us a broader perspective that can be hard to find during the day-to-day tasks of caring for a baby. It can reveal risks and benefits that we may not have considered, allowing us to approach decisions in an objective way. Science may not offer a protocol for parenting, like the procedures that I perfected in my research lab, but it can help us make smart decisions for our families.

Science can also help us rise above parenting controversies. In many cases, if you carefully study the data, as I did in my research for this book, you see that there's rarely a strong case for everyone doing things in the same way. There's plenty of room for parents to make different choices about how their baby eats and sleeps, for example. When you understand the limitations of the science, you are empowered to follow your heart and your child's lead. And in cases where the science gives us a clearer answer, it can help us make decisions more confidently. We don't have to waste our energy arguing or defending ourselves, because we've looked at the evidence, and we're comfortable with our choices. This frees up valuable time and energy to focus on our babies, do the work or hobbies that bring us fulfillment and satisfaction, or even take a much-needed nap.

I begin this book, in chapter 1, with a sort of crash course in evidence-based parenting. If we want to examine parenting decisions in a scientific way, then we must first understand how science works, how to parse through many studies to find the most relevant ones, and how to interpret research in a meaningful way. Chapter 1 will give you an idea of how I approached each topic in this book, and it should also prepare you to tackle your own questions with science as your guide.

In chapters 2 and 3, I zoom in on a few medical questions important to newborn babies, including when we should cut the umbilical cord, whether babies born by cesarean should be "seeded" with their mothers' microbes, when and how they should receive their first bath, and why they get an injection of vitamin K and a smear of antibiotics in their eyes. These may be small questions in the scheme of a baby's first year of life, but they each provide a fascinating case study in the history and science of newborn medicine. In chapter 4, I step away from decision making and appreciate new babies as scientists do, for their incredible abilities to sense and explore their new world with touch, sound, sight, and smell. Understanding our newborns sets the stage for how we care for them responsively and how the parent-child relationship develops over time.

In the rest of the book, I examine some of the biggest questions and sources of angst for parents: vaccine safety (chapter 5), sleep safety and bed sharing (chapter 6), baby sleep patterns (chapter 7), breast milk and formula feeding (chapter 8), starting solid foods (chapter 9), and healthy nutrition for the older baby (chapter 10). As I researched and wrote each chapter of the book, I read hundreds of scientific papers, talked to scientists, and interviewed parents about their experiences. I looked for answers, but I also wasn't afraid to investigate and question the parts of science where things are still uncertain, and that is often where I found some of the most interesting stories.

I didn't write this book pretending to be a parenting expert. I wrote it as a parent with questions, probably similar to your own, and I had the scientific training and the curiosity to dig for the answers. I didn't set out to argue one side or the other on controversial topics. Instead, I've tried to be honest about what the science does and doesn't tell us, even when that might be different from the simplified recommendations handed down to us from parenting authority figures. I loved delving into labyrinthine literature searches, trying to find some kind of truth that could be useful to you and me. Thanks for coming along on this journey with me. I hope it makes your job as a parent a little easier—and maybe more interesting, too.

1

SHOW ME THE SCIENCE

A Crash Course in Evidence-Based Parenting

Until I became pregnant, my science life and my home life rarely converged. I spent long hours conducting experiments in the lab and reading and writing scientific papers in my office and at my kitchen table. But for the most part, when my work was done for the day, I set the science aside. I saw the scientific process as a way for me to understand my little corner of research, not as a helpful tool in making everyday decisions. If I had a question about gardening, cooking, or training our dog, I'd do a quick internet search and read advice from a few different sites, but I had neither the time nor the inclination to dive into the scientific literature for answers.

All of that changed when I became pregnant. Suddenly I had a lot of questions, and these felt more important than any I'd previously faced. I realized that, as a parent, I was tasked with the responsibility of making decisions for another person, and I wanted to get this right. I needed to figure out what chemicals and procedures in my research lab might pose a health risk to me or my baby. I wanted to eat well and exercise appropriately for an optimal pregnancy, and plan and prepare for birth in the same detail-oriented way that I mapped out a protocol in the lab. And science, I recognized, was a tool that could help me do all this. Best of all: I knew how to use it. As a scientist, surely I could make this an evidence-based pregnancy and an evidence-based baby. Good data could soothe my anxieties and insecurities about becoming a parent.

If only it was that simple. Science did help me to make some decisions, and that's what this book is all about. But I also found that the reality often deviated from the plan. No amount of planning could prepare me for how a labor contraction would feel as it screamed through my body, or for how I would cope when my baby had been up for hours, needing me, in the middle of the night. I learned that part of parenting is accepting that it usually won't go as planned and that we can't control every variable. We have to learn as we go. We adjust and adapt and then go back to the science with new questions, wanting to learn more.

Many of the areas of research that I investigated for this book were much more complex than any scientific question I had tackled before. I was accustomed to studying lab animals or isolated cells, grown in a test tube or petri dish, where I could control nearly every variable, tweaking the one in question to determine its importance or to get my experimental conditions just right. But parenting questions have so many more variables. For example, most of us, at some point, wonder how we can help our babies to sleep better at night. How can we answer that with science? We can't put babies in a laboratory and control every variable that might affect their sleep. Babies are born to different parents, who have different philosophies and cultural traditions that they carry with them into parenting. Our homes are different, with varying amounts of light, noise, and activity. And of course, the babies themselves are different, born with their own unique personalities and needs. Even if we could control these variables, would we want to? I don't think so. Human variation is part of what makes life beautiful.

All this natural variation between babies and families makes parenting research difficult to do and even harder to interpret. A major task of science is to describe variation quantitatively and then try to understand the patterns that emerge from the data. With enough data points and studies, we can see which patterns are consistent and repeatable, and we can start to tease out truths that can help us make sense of the everyday challenges of parenting—like how to help a baby sleep well at night.

But taking an evidence-based approach to parenting also means being aware of the limitations of science and approaching the data with curiosity and skepticism. We need to be able to find relevant studies, judge their quality, interpret their results, and then figure out whether they can inform our own approaches to parenting. Science can be such a valuable tool, but only if we understand how it works.

In this book, I explore what I think are some of the most interesting parenting decisions in a baby's first year, but it isn't a complete guide, and it won't answer all your questions by any means. However, my hope is that this book will give you the tools you need to search the science for your own answers. To help you understand my approach to interpreting science for this book and how you can apply it yourself, let's walk through some of the most important concepts for understanding science.

1. SCIENCE IS A PROCESS

The scientific method allows us to observe the world in a systematic, objective way. It is simple enough that children begin practicing it in elementary school, if not sooner. I have fond memories of conducting science fair experiments and preparing my trifold poster displays with big, stenciled letters for each of the major steps—question, hypothesis, prediction, experimental method, analysis, and conclusion—not so different from the headings I used when I wrote journal articles years later. We now know that even babies and toddlers practice their own version of the scientific method as they make observations about the world, form their own predictions, and test them in experiments.[1]

The scientific method is a simple framework for inquiry, and it is exactly this simplicity that makes it so valuable. It means that other scientists can repeat the experiment to verify the results, or change one or two variables to determine how they affect the outcomes. What makes it meaningful is that we all use the same process, and over time, it helps us to better understand the world. Good science takes lots of experiments (repeated, checked, and challenged, over and over), time, and people with diverse perspectives and backgrounds to build a body of knowledge. But it always starts in the same place: with a question, and the desire to answer it.

2. GOOD SCIENCE IS PEER-REVIEWED

A critical part of the scientific process is peer review and publication of results. Even the most exciting research is essentially meaningless if it exists only in lab notebooks or in digital files stored on the lab's server. Publication is a permanent record of scientific discovery. To be considered credible and to add to scientific knowledge, studies need to be published so that other researchers can check the work and build on it.

When scientists are ready to publish their results, they write them up in the form of a research paper and then submit it to a scientific journal. Journals, especially the best ones, receive many more papers than they publish, and they're selective about what they accept. If the editor thinks a paper could be a good fit for the journal, it will be subjected to peer review. This means that several experts in that specific area of research will read and critique the paper. They'll check to see whether the researchers used appropriate experimental and statistical methods to test the hypothesis and whether the interpretation of the results is reasonable. Peer reviewers aren't paid to do this job, but they take the responsibility seriously, knowing that the legitimacy of their field of research rests on good peer review. They're also usually anonymous, so they can freely offer their opinions and concerns without fear of damaging relationships with other scientists.

The peer review system is a quality control filter for science. It's designed to catch and reject papers that don't meet certain standards (although this means they're often resubmitted to a lower quality journal). For those that do meet standards of publication for the journal, peer review often increases the quality of research before it's published. Peer reviewers may ask authors to collect more data, analyze it in a different way, or consider alternative explanations for the results. The purpose of peer review is to keep everyone honest and to keep the standards of scientific publication high.

So, if you're looking to science for answers to your parenting questions, be sure you're looking at peer-reviewed science. Most papers published in scientific journals are peer-reviewed, but you can check journal web pages to be sure. Letters to the editor and commentaries published in journals aren't usually peer-reviewed, although they can make for interesting reading. Most books are not peer-reviewed, except those published by university presses (including this one), which usually have a formal peer review process. Nonprofit organizations and for-profit companies sometimes publish reports or "white papers" that are intentionally made to look like scientific papers, but they're most likely not peer-reviewed. They may or may not be based on solid science, but they're almost certainly published because they fit a narrative that benefits the organization or company, so approach them with a healthy dose of skepticism.

3. ONE STUDY IS NEVER ALL THAT MEANINGFUL ON ITS OWN; WHAT MATTERS IS SCIENTIFIC CONSENSUS

Scientific knowledge has to start somewhere, but one study is never worth much on its own, even after peer review. Scientists can and do make mistakes, use flawed methodology, or simply misinterpret their data, so we like to see studies repeated and hypotheses tested in different ways before we get too excited about results.

For an example of the pitfalls of putting too much weight on one study, look no further than Andrew Wakefield's 1998 paper attempting to link the measles, mumps, and rubella (MMR) vaccine to autism. Wakefield's study used methodology that was weak and ethically problematic, and it didn't even provide evidence that MMR caused autism. Somehow, it got through the standard process of review by some of his peers and was published in the *Lancet*, a prestigious medical journal. After the problems with Wakefield's paper came to light, the *Lancet* retracted it in 2010, essentially removing it from the archives of reputable science.[2] And the story didn't end there; Wakefield's hypothesis was investigated by many more scientists, looking at it from different angles and using better methods, and their results haven't supported any link between the MMR vaccine and autism. We now have a huge amount of science showing that Wakefield was wrong (more details on this story can be found in appendix D).

Wakefield's MMR study is a dramatic example. It reached an unusual level of infamy because it damaged public trust in vaccines, and the article had so many problems that it was eventually retracted—the journal's way of disowning the research. However, studies are published every day with results that are later refuted by other studies. A 2017 analysis estimated that about half of study results covered by newspapers turn out to be wrong when they're revisited in follow-up research.[3] That may happen for any number of reasons: because of errors, too small of a sample size, a rush to publish exciting results, or researchers missing an alternative explanation for their observations. As I write this in the midst of the COVID-19 pandemic, it often feels as if the studies reported in the news this week contradict the ones that made last week's headlines. This isn't a failure of science. Rather, it's all part of the testing and replicating, trying and failing, revising and revisiting that make up the scientific process. The problem comes when we put too much stock in the findings of any one study. If you're looking for answers to a parenting question—or any personal question for that matter—it's best to wait and see what other studies find rather than making your decision based on one study alone. The system of science isn't foolproof, but it is usually self-correcting, over time.

One study can't tell us much on its own, but when multiple studies and lines of scientific evidence point in the same direction, we begin to reach scientific consensus. If you put a bunch of scientists together in a room, what do 95 percent of them agree on? If only a couple of studies have been conducted on the topic, you're likely to hear a lot of debate and disagreement in the room. Scientists are skeptical by nature, and it's their job to ask questions and consider different explanations. But over time, as different scientists using different methodologies conduct more and more studies, a consensus emerges. For example, there is a strong scientific consensus that evolution explains the diversity of life, that the climate is changing because of human activity, and that the benefits of vaccines far outweigh the risks. Our understanding of these fields will continue to grow and evolve, but they're unlikely to change radically, because they're already backed by so many studies.

Other areas of science have less certainty. Some examples discussed in this book are how babies' resident microbiota affect their health and when to introduce solid foods to babies. These questions are hotly debated in scientific communities. That's a sign to us that there are some aspects of these topics that science hasn't yet explained very well. The debate drives the field forward and inspires better studies. And it tells us that there's room within evidence-based parenting to make different choices.

4. SOME TYPES OF STUDIES ARE MORE VALUABLE THAN OTHERS

With a few clicks of your keyboard and in less than a second, the internet can dump truckloads of science on your doorstep. Databases like PubMed or Google Scholar give us access to millions of scientific abstracts (summaries of research papers), and often, full text papers. But access to millions of articles is useful only if you can make sense of them.

Let's say you're wondering if you should give your baby a probiotic (live bacteria taken in supplement form), so you search PubMed for "infant probiotic." You get 2,808 results. Most citations listed in PubMed are peer-reviewed journal articles, so they've passed a certain degree of scrutiny already. But is each of these 2,808 articles equally important? How do you figure out which are most relevant and helpful?

The type of study design is one key piece of information that can help you sift through published research and judge its quality and relevancy. Here's a quick guide to study types, listed roughly in or-

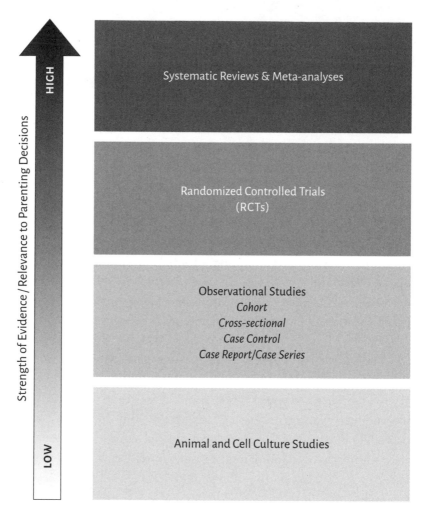

A rough guide to scientific study designs and their relevance to parenting decisions, ranked, from top to bottom, as most useful to least useful.

der from most to least relevant for answering health and parenting questions.[4]

- *Systematic reviews and meta-analyses*: A *systematic review* is a survey of studies meant to summarize what the research says, collectively, about a specific topic or question. The authors systematically search scientific databases for studies of the topic, and then they whittle down their results to include only those studies that meet their prespecified criteria for quality and study design. Following their methods, if you searched the same scientific databases, you should be able to end up with the same collection of studies. The authors then report the overall findings, giving you a summary of the field, including where results are conflicting. This type of paper is useful because it interprets a lot of studies and puts them in context with each other. You will also find review papers that aren't systematic, sometimes called "narrative reviews." These can be helpful but are considered less reliable because the authors may have cherry-picked certain studies and left others out to support their preferred narrative.

A *meta-analysis* is a systematic review that goes one step further by combining the quantitative data from each of the relevant studies and conducting a statistical analysis of these combined data.

A well-known and reliable source for systematic reviews and meta-analyses is Cochrane, a nonprofit organization made up of an international network of researchers that conduct research reviews to inform evidence-based medicine. If you're looking for information about probiotics for infants, for example, you're in luck. A 2019 Cochrane review summarized the evidence on whether probiotics are helpful for infants with colic, defined as "full-force crying for at least three hours per day, on at least three days per week, for at least three weeks."[5] (Just reading that very clinical definition makes me shudder at how torturous it must be to live with all that crying, and I can completely understand the desire to look toward something like a probiotic for help.) At the time of their search, the authors found six studies, including a total of 1,886 infants, that met their criteria for quality and relevancy. When they pooled the data from those studies, they found that probiotics didn't prevent colic but did decrease crying by about half an hour per day, with no major side effects noted. However, the authors noted that they had a low degree of certainty in their conclusions because of the relatively small number of studies, variability in the data, and the risk that the studies were biased by funding from formula or supplement companies that could benefit from positive results. You can see how reading that review would give you a better understanding of what we know—and don't know—about probiotics for colicky babies than any one study alone. Cochrane also does a nice job of including a "plain language summary" for every paper, so you don't have to be a scientist familiar with the jargon of the field to understand the authors' findings. Cochrane is one of the first places I check when I want to get the lay of the scientific landscape for a health question, but there are also excellent systematic reviews and meta-analyses published in other journals.

- *Randomized controlled trials*: Randomized controlled trials are considered the gold standard for clinical trials, with the highest quality study design. For these studies, researchers recruit a group of people who agree to participate in the study and are then randomly allocated to two or more groups, one of which is a control group and the other of which is subjected to some type of change or intervention. For example, one of the most impactful studies on babies in the last decade was the Learning Early About Peanut Allergy (LEAP) trial, with results published in the *New England Journal of Medicine* in 2015. The researchers recruited 640 infants whose parents agreed to their participation and who had severe eczema or an egg allergy, making them high risk for developing a peanut allergy. Half of the infants' parents were told that they should strictly avoid exposing their babies to peanut protein for the first 5 years of life (the control group), and the other half were told that they should feed their babies peanut (in a baby-safe form) beginning as early as 4 months of age (the intervention group). Because they were randomly assigned, these two groups should have been very similar in every way except for their early exposure to peanut. Therefore, when the researchers found that the group of children with early peanut exposure were much less likely to have a peanut allergy at age 5, they had a high degree of certainty that it was the early peanut exposure that caused that benefit, and not some other factor.[6]

Randomized controlled trials are incredibly valuable, but they are also difficult and sometimes unethical to do in parenting research. For example, researchers couldn't conduct a randomized controlled trial to test whether parents cosleeping, or bed sharing, with their babies increases the risk of sudden infant death syndrome (SIDS). For one thing, it would be unethical to ask or encourage parents to bed-share when we already have significant data showing that bed sharing is associated with a greater risk of infant death. In addition, many parents wouldn't want a scientist to dictate how they should raise their babies, and many other factors, like a babies' personality and the parents' parenting philosophy, affect decisions like where a baby sleeps. For this reason, we often depend on observational studies in parenting science.

- *Observational human studies*: Unlike randomized controlled trials, observational studies don't include interventions. Rather, they simply collect observations about people, such as their behavior, what they eat, how they sleep, or the supplements or medications they choose to take—whatever factors the researchers want to investigate. Then the researchers check for correlations between their observations and the outcomes of interest. For example, Gideon Lack, a professor of pediatric allergy at King's College London and the lead researcher for the LEAP trial, published an observational study in 2008 reporting that the prevalence of peanut allergy was much higher in the United Kingdom than in Israel, where infants are routinely offered peanut protein earlier in life.[7] This type of study design couldn't show that early peanut exposure directly caused the reduced incidence of peanut allergy because there could have been other differences between the children in the UK and Israel that affected their allergy risk. Still, it was an intriguing observation, and it led to Lack's hypothesis that early exposure to peanut may protect children from developing peanut allergy, which he and his colleagues tested in the LEAP trial.[8] (We'll learn much more about the research on food introduction and allergies in chapter 9).

Most studies related to parenting are observational. They generally require less funding and time and are less likely to be limited by ethical issues than randomized controlled trials. They can also often describe larger, more diverse groups of families and capture a greater array of real-life variables. But observational studies have a major limitation: they can only show correlations. They can't provide evidence for causation, just as Lack and colleagues' observation about children in Israel couldn't prove that early peanut exposure prevented peanut allergy. Because they don't start with randomized groups of people, the observed differences between groups could be explained by other factors. For example, Lack's observation about children in Israel might also be explained by differences in genetics, breast- or formula-feeding, or exposure to pets—all factors that can influence allergy risk. These factors that complicate the interpretation of observational studies are called *confounding factors*.

There are also different types of observational study designs. In a *cohort study*, people are followed longitudinally, over a period of time, as researchers collect observations about them. For example, a cohort study might enroll a group of babies to study how parents introduced solid foods to them and whether they developed food allergies. As you can imagine, this type of study is more powerful if it is prospective and follows the babies from early infancy into childhood, assessing their eating habits and signs of allergies along the way, than if it is retrospective and asks parents to try and re-member what and how much their babies ate several months or years ago. There are also *cross-sectional studies*, in which researchers look at people at one point in time. For exam-ple, a cross-sectional study might survey groups of parents in several countries to determine how common food allergies are among children of different ages in different places. These types of studies are useful in their own way, but cohort stud-ies give us more information about how variables interact and change as children grow.

Another type of observational study is a *case-control study*, in which subjects who have something in common, usually a medical condition or outcome, are compared with controls who don't have that condition. Case-control studies are dis-cussed in detail in chapter 6, on sleep safety and SIDS.

The least useful type of observational study is a *case report*, a description of a single medical occurrence. For example, a pediatrician might publish a case report about a baby who was allergic to rice cereal. This tells you that this allergy can occur and how it appeared in that one baby—useful informa-tion—but it doesn't tell you anything about how common a rice allergy is or what might increase or decrease the risk of it happening. A *case series* is simply a group of similar case reports published together.

- *Animal and cell culture studies*: A lot of important science starts in petri dishes containing cells (i.e., cell cultures), is then test-ed in animals, and if it looks promising, may be tested in hu-mans. Cell culture and live animal studies are vital, because they can help us to understand mechanisms for how things work and lay the foundation for well-designed, safe studies on humans. However, cell culture and animal studies are of little use in answering parenting questions. Human babies aren't mice, and they're much more complex than cells grown in a petri dish.

5. CORRELATION IS NOT CAUSATION

We've already established this as one of the major limitations of observational studies, but it's so important that it bears repeating. If your baby stayed up an hour past her bedtime and then took her first unassisted steps the next day, would you infer that slight sleep deprivation is good for gross motor development? Of course not. There is a correlation between these two events—staying up late and achieving a new milestone—but you can recognize that this is most likely a coincidence.

The same caution is needed when looking at large data sets. An example is the strong correlation between organic food consumption and autism diagnoses.[9] Would you conclude from the graph shown here that organic food causes autism? Or that autism makes people buy more organic food? Neither is a likely explanation for the data in the graph. What is more likely is that the two variables are completely unrelated to each other. (There is also good evidence that the main explanation for the rising rates of autism diagnoses is increased awareness and screening and broader diagnostic criteria, not a true epidemic of the condition.)[10]

This is not to say that correlations are never useful. Sometimes a correlation is a clue that encourages scientists to look closer, leading them to an important finding. For example, case-control studies in the 1980s found that babies who died of SIDS were more likely to be sleeping on their tummies than control babies, who survived. At the time, researchers didn't know if tummy sleeping *caused* SIDS, and they didn't understand the mechanism, or explanation, for why this might be. However, the correlation between the two factors was a consistent finding in multiple studies, and health organizations started recommending that babies be put "Back to Sleep." This campaign was followed by a dramatic drop in SIDS rates.[11] Later studies showed that babies sleeping on their tummies sleep more deeply and have a harder time arousing from sleep, providing a possible mechanism for tummy sleeping caus-

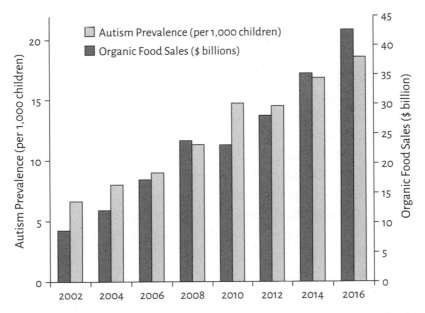

There is a strong *correlation* between autism diagnoses and organic food sales, but it is unlikely that organic food causes autism (or vice versa).

Sources: Organic Trade Association, *2011 Organic Industry Overview* (Washington, DC: OTA, 2011); Organic Trade Association, "COVID-19 Will Shape Organic Industry in 2020 after Banner Year in 2019," press release, June 9, 2020, https://ota.com/news/press -releases/21328; Centers for Disease Control and Prevention, "Data and Statistics on Autism Spectrum Disorder," accessed October 6, 2020, https://www.cdc.gov/ncbddd /autism/data.html.

ing SIDS.[12] While this began as just a correlation in observational studies, scientists now feel pretty certain that this relationship also represents causation. And the hypothesis that tummy sleeping causes SIDS could never be tested in a randomized controlled trial, because it would be unethical to ask parents to put their babies to sleep on their tummies knowing that it might increase their chances of death. Thus, our understanding of SIDS is very dependent on observational studies, but we always want to stay alert to the distinction between correlation and causation and be open-minded to alternative explanations.

21

6. NUMBERS MATTER

Larger studies, those that include a greater number of participants, usually give us better evidence than smaller studies. It's hard to give a rule of thumb here, but I'll try. For most of the parenting questions in this book, the best studies include hundreds of babies. For some of the biggest questions, like effects of breastfeeding, we find studies with hundreds to thousands of babies. For something as important as vaccine safety, we expect studies to include thousands to tens of thousands of children. Scientists usually work to ensure that their studies have enough "power," meaning that they include an adequate number of subjects to test their hypothesis, but if you're comparing two studies of the same question with a similar design, the one with the larger sample size will usually provide stronger evidence.

7. CONSIDER THE FUNDING SOURCE

When I pull up a scientific paper for the first time, one of the first things I check is the affiliation of the authors, to see if they are from an academic institution or employed by a corporation, such as in the pharmaceutical, baby food, or formula industries. Then, I scroll down to read the fine print, usually at the bottom of the first page or at the end of the paper, to see who funded the study. I have more trust in studies that are funded by government or academic institutions than those funded by corporate sponsors. Industry funding of studies represents a potential conflict of interest and can introduce bias, intentional or not, as the results can be leveraged to sell more products. In fact, there's a Cochrane review on this topic. Published in 2017, the review combined the results of 75 studies on drugs or medical devices and found that industry-sponsored studies were more likely to report results that favor the sponsor than those without industry funding.[13] Not surprising. These may be great studies, carefully designed and conducted by smart people with good intentions, but funding source is always worth keeping in mind.

Industry funding is especially prevalent in nutrition, the field in which I earned my PhD. Nutrition science, including research that could help us understand how to best nourish infants, has been chronically underfunded by public sources, and industry has willingly stepped in to fill that gap. For example, much of the research on the molecules found in breast milk is funded by infant formula companies seeking to improve the quality—and sales—of their products. While it may be good science and may help us to better understand breast milk, that funding source is problematic, because formula companies stand to benefit from more babies consuming their product. Not surprisingly, they'll cite their research to justify adding new ingredients to their products and marketing them as "brain-boosting" or "tummy-soothing" to give them an edge in a competitive marketplace.[14]

A corporate funding source raises my level of skepticism and scrutiny, but it doesn't mean I dismiss every study funded by industry as junk science. There are excellent studies funded by formula companies, for example, and for scientists working in this area with so little public funding, it may be hard for them to fund their research without accepting some grants from industry. Likewise, large clinical trials of vaccines are usually funded by the companies developing them; new vaccines require a huge amount of investment, and it makes sense that the company that will profit from their development should foot at least part of that bill. Those studies are also subjected to a high degree of scrutiny by public agencies and medical organizations, who know it is in everyone's best interests to ensure the science is solid before a new vaccine is recommended to the public.

8. DON'T BELIEVE EVERYTHING YOU READ ON THE INTERNET

You can use the tools I just described to sift through the research literature, but this is a ton of work. In my research for this book, I read hundreds of studies, trying to judge their quality and draw meaningful conclusions from them, but this took me a lot of time. Meanwhile, I had my own questions as my daughter turned from baby to toddler to preschooler, and because I was working on this book, I had to find quicker answers. Those questions haven't stopped as my children have grown, and I usually don't have time or energy for a literature search for each new parenting dilemma.

Like most of us, I often turn to the internet, hoping that someone else can summarize the research for me. However, I have high standards for who I trust when it comes to parenting or health information. I definitely steer clear of websites trying to sell me something or those with sensationalist claims, personal attacks, or conspiracy theories. Instead, I look for information from university, governmental, and medical institutions or organizations as good starting points. I look for websites that are current and written by someone with formal training in the field and/or include input from experts and cite peer-reviewed studies. I check at least some of those studies to see whether they actually support what the article is saying. If I think I have found a reliable source, then I cross-check it against another one. For reporting on a recent study, I look toward major news organizations with experienced science journalists and fact-checkers, who I know don't just repeat what they read in the press release but dig into the details of the study and ask other researchers for their views on its importance and limitations.

This parsing of what's true and what's not on the internet isn't easy, and the influence of social media on our lives makes it even harder. A 2017 study published in the journal *Science* analyzed 126,000 claims posted to Twitter between 2006 and 2017, tweeted by 3 million people more than 4.5 million times. False claims were 70 percent more likely to be tweeted or retweeted on the social network, and falsehoods spread much more quickly than did true information.[15] And it's not just people who are misinformed who are spreading false information. Twitter and other social networks are full of bots and Russian trolls, and these bad actors intentionally use divisive issues such as vaccines to attract attention and sow discord.[16] It's easy to be misled or pulled down a rabbit hole of misinformation on social media, so always keep your BS detector running in the background as you scroll your social media feeds.

Finally, if you read something that doesn't sound quite right, fact check it. Go out of your way to search for information that may contradict what you'd like to believe, that offers a more nuanced view, and that comes from true experts in the field. We all have cognitive biases and blind spots, but a little curiosity and skepticism can go a long way toward keeping them in check.

9. FIND SMART ALLIES

I consider myself savvy about science, but I am easily paralyzed by decisions, in part because I care so much about making the right ones. And parenting brings so many decisions! Approaching them from an evidence-based perspective can seem to require a crash course in pediatrics, epidemiology, immunology, statistics, nutrition, physiology, and psychology. But let's face it: we're kidding ourselves if we think we can become experts in all these areas. We can't know everything, and sometimes we need help to make evidence-based choices.

Accepting the limits of my knowledge, I seek out health care providers who are committed to practicing evidence-based medicine and are willing to look at the science with me and help me make good decisions. I expect them to listen to my concerns and questions, but then I listen to their advice and value their training and expertise. For new parents, a trusted pediatrician can be an indispensable resource.

10. KNOW THAT WE CAN'T ELIMINATE RISK

Everything we do carries some risk. When we feed our children, we risk choking, food allergies, and food-borne pathogens. When we tuck in our babies at bedtime, there is a terrifying, though very small, risk of SIDS. And yet, clearly, the advantages of eating and sleeping outweigh these small risks. Our job, as parents, is to do our best to minimize the risks within the context of our daily lives, but this means considering all sources of risk, some of which may be personal to us and not considered in the scientific studies or the policy statements that advise us to do things one way or the other.

Take breastfeeding, for example. We know that formula-fed babies, on average, are more likely to have gastrointestinal and respiratory infections than breastfed babies. We all want our babies to be as healthy as possible, so all else being equal, most parents would choose the option associated with the lowest infection risk. But what about the mother who, to safely breastfeed, must stop taking the medication that normally helps her manage her mental illness? Or the one for whom breastfeeding is a struggle, and continuing it is causing stress or pain or severe sleep deprivation? In these situations, there is also a risk that breastfeeding is jeopardizing the mother's health and her relationship with her baby. Risks and benefits are personal. Science can give us some understanding of risks and benefits in a population of study subjects, but we also have to trust that each family does its best to balance the risks and benefits that are personal to them.

11. FORGET ABOUT PERFECTION, AND PAY ATTENTION TO *YOUR* BABY

No amount of science will mean that you'll make the right decisions all the time. So much of parenting is trial and error; it's part of how we learn about our children and ourselves. Do your best to keep an open mind and admit when something isn't working well. Be willing to adjust course if needed or if new science emerges. Science is a process, and so is parenting.

The most important work we do as parents is difficult to measure and quantify in a scientific study. It's in our daily, mundane interactions with our kids. It's in the way we show up every day to care for them and the way we give them space to become their own people. It's in the way we talk to them, read to them, play with them, and let them explore the world. These are the things that make our kids who they are, not to mention each child's innate temperament and personality. Use science to the extent that it helps you make choices with confidence or to the extent that it just plain fascinates you, but recognize that it is just one of many tools in your parenting kit.

2

BIRTH DAY, FIRST DAY

Easing Your Newborn's Transition into the World

I think of my transition to parenthood as the roughly 30 hours that I was in labor with Cee: starting at midnight on a Sunday and ending on a sunny Tuesday morning. It was a wild and surreal time, marked not by the clock but by contractions, and at some point, a welcome epidural that let me rest for a few hours. Once I started pushing, there was no measure of time but the nurse's counting me through pushes, over and over and over, for several hours, until finally, I pushed my child into the world.

Just like that, she was here. As transformative as that moment may have felt for me, it was even more so for my daughter, as she had to quickly adapt to a vastly different world. She left behind the dark, protective uterus and entered a place of bright lights, loud sounds, and dry air, in which she'd have to obtain oxygen and nutrients more independently. At first, she was a little blue and limp, but within a minute or so, she took her first breath. Her lungs—which had been compressed throughout her fetal life—expanded with air, and her blood flowed into an intricate network of pulmonary vessels. As she cried for the first time and then settled onto my chest and opened her eyes toward my voice, she began to get to know the people who would take care of her. But at the same time, she was also getting to know the ubiquitous microbes that far outnumber us in this world. They are mostly helpful or at least harmless, but there are a few dangerous ones.

I am fascinated by these first moments, and as parents, I think it's worth considering what we can do to ease this transition for our newborns. In this chapter, we cover three aspects of the newborn's transition: cutting the umbilical cord, seeding the microbiome, and giving the baby's first bath.

CUTTING THE UMBILICAL CORD

Before birth, Cee had relied on the placenta as her source of life and building blocks for her growth and development. The placenta was the interface between my blood and her blood. Here, our two blood supplies sidled up next to each other, not mixing, but passing close enough that substances could exchange across a few layers of cells. The umbilical cord was Cee's lifeline to the placenta. Through the cord and across the placenta, nutrients and oxygen passed from me to Cee, and carbon dioxide and waste products were handed off from Cee to me.

To a new baby, part of a healthy birth transition means making the switch from getting oxygen from blood circulating through the placenta to getting oxygen from air, through the lungs. But this switch doesn't have to be abrupt. At birth, whether vaginal or by cesarean, the umbilical cord is still attached to the placenta, which will be delivered shortly after the baby. ("You're not done yet, Alice," I remember my obstetrician gently reminding me before asking me to push yet again.) If the cord isn't cut right away, circulation continues to and from the placenta for a few minutes, even as the baby breathes. Over the course of those minutes, much of the blood in the placenta will flow toward the baby, before the cord naturally stops pulsating. Cut the cord immediately, and that blood stays with the placenta, which is usually thrown out with the rest of the hospital's waste. Waiting to cut the cord for two to three minutes after a vaginal birth can give around 80 to 100 milliliters of additional blood (about one-third of a cup) to the average full-term newborn, amounting to 20 to 40 percent of an infant's blood volume at birth.[1] This short delay must have happened throughout most of human history, and it is certainly what occurs after the birth of most mammals.

When to cut the cord has been a topic of discussion for at least the past few centuries. Erasmus Darwin, a physician, and grandfather to Charles Darwin, wrote in his 1796 medical text, *Zoonomia*: "Another thing very injurious to the child, is the tying and cutting [of] the navel-string too soon; which should always be left till the child has not only repeatedly breathed, but till all pulsation in the cord ceases. As otherwise the child is much weaker than it ought to be; a part of the blood being left in the placenta, which ought to have been in the child."[2]

Despite grandfather Darwin's admonition, there was a shift in the early to mid-1900s to cutting the cord within 10 to 15 seconds of birth. This practice became very common, and not just in Western developed nations. International surveys—published in the early 2000s and including countries such as Bangladesh, China, Egypt, Ethiopia, and Tanzania—revealed that most babies had their cords cut immediately.[3] This change in routine procedure probably came with the shift of childbirth from the realm of midwives in the home to that of doctors in the hospital, where efficiency became a goal and the umbilical cord was, quite literally, the dividing line between the specialties of obstetrics and pediatrics. But this was a practice of convenience; there was never any evidence that cutting the cord immediately was beneficial.

Over the past few decades, timing of cord clamping has again come under scrutiny, with researchers asking how immediate cord clamping affects the baby. And although this is just one small decision among many that we make as caregivers of infants, this story is a fascinating case study in the history and science behind childbirth choices.

An Inside Look at Cord Clamping Research

In the early 2000s, Camila Chaparro was a young graduate student of nutrition at the University of California, Davis, working under Dr. Kay Dewey. I was a grad student in the same program around the same time, but our experiences were vastly different. While I toiled away in a tedious research lab on campus, Chaparro spent several years in a large obstetrics hospital in Mexico City, conducting a randomized controlled trial of early versus delayed cord clamping.

In her mid-twenties, having seen only a video of childbirth, Chaparro found herself signing up study participants in the hospital's large labor rooms. "I knew basically nothing," Chaparro told me, and this was an interesting place to begin an education in childbirth. There were usually around six women laboring in one room, with no family members allowed. There was no privacy for these mothers; in addition to Chaparro and the study staff, the wards were crowded with obstetricians, anesthesiologists, and medical and nursing students.[4]

For each of the 476 women who agreed to participate in the study, Chaparro or another member of the study staff randomly drew a sealed envelope that assigned the laboring mother to either early or delayed cord clamping. This is what made the study a randomized controlled trial, the highest quality study design. Because the two groups were randomly assigned, the only thing that should have been different about them was the timing of cord clamping. As the baby was born, Chaparro or an assistant would stand with a stopwatch and give the obstetrician the okay to cut the cord after 10 seconds for the early group or after 2 minutes for the late group. They then took a range of measurements in the babies, beginning on the first day of life and following up until they were 6 months old, to see whether timing of cord clamping made a difference to their health.

Chaparro and her colleagues found that timing did matter a great deal, and they published their findings in 2006 in the prestigious medical journal the *Lancet*.[5] It was one of the most careful studies in this field, and it was followed by studies from other researchers confirming the benefits of delayed cord clamping.

What a Difference Two Minutes Makes

Delayed cord clamping gives a baby more blood at birth, carrying with it approximately 40 to 75 milligrams (mg) of additional iron. Iron is an essential part of the protein hemoglobin, found in red blood cells and responsible for transporting oxygen around the body. In the first weeks after birth, old red blood cells break down, and the iron is recycled and stored in the body, to be used as needed by the baby in the coming months.[6]

Iron stores are like a nutritional savings account that the baby will spend down as he grows and develops. In addition to its role in hemoglobin, iron is also needed for muscle growth, as well as brain function and development. It's required for the synthesis of neurotransmitters like serotonin and dopamine and for the myelination of nerve tissue, which allows rapid delivery of nerve signals around the body.[7]

With delayed cord clamping, a baby starts life with more iron, and this comes in handy several months after birth. This was evident in Chaparro's study. At 6 months of age, the babies with delayed cord clamping had 88 percent more iron stored than the babies whose cords had been clamped immediately.[8] Other studies have found that babies with delayed cord clamping are less likely to be anemic at 2 to 3 months of age and have higher iron stores at 4 to 6 months of age.[9] In one recent randomized controlled trial conducted in Nepal, infants whose cords were clamped three minutes or later after birth had a lower prevalence of iron deficiency and iron-deficiency anemia even as old as 8 months of age, compared with infants whose cords were clamped at less than a minute after birth.[10]

Early trials of delayed cord clamping, like that of Chaparro and her colleagues, were conducted in low- and middle-income countries with a higher prevalence of iron deficiency. For a time, obstetricians in the developed world were hesitant to change their practice until studies in higher income countries demonstrated both benefits and safety. In fact, when I wrote the first edition of this book in 2014, the American College of Obstetricians and Gynecologists (ACOG) had not yet recommended delayed cord clamping for infants born full-term. (In 2012, they recommended delayed cord clamping for preterm infants because, as we'll discuss shortly, there was stronger evidence of benefits for these more vulnerable babies.)[11] ACOG shifted their stance on delayed cord clamping in 2017, when they officially endorsed a delay in cord clamping of at least 30 to 60 seconds for all newborns, a policy change that I covered for the *New York Times*. "As more and more evidence accumulated, I think our comfort level with saying this looks like the right thing for all babies, term and preterm, seemed the right thing to do," Dr. Maria Mascola, lead author of ACOG's policy statement, told me.[12]

Key to the shift in policy was a randomized controlled trial conducted in Sweden that compared outcomes in 400 full-term infants randomized to early (less than 10 seconds after birth) and late clamping (at least 3 minutes after birth). The delayed clamping group was less likely to be anemic at birth, and at 4 months, they had a lower incidence of iron deficiency (0.6 percent compared with 5.7 percent in the early clamping group).[13] At 4 years old, the children with early cord clamping had modestly lower scores in social and fine motor skills. For example, in one test, the children were asked to trace between two lines and scored based on how well they could stay within the "bicycle trail"; 13 percent of the children in the early clamping group failed this test compared to just 4 percent of the children in the delayed clamping group. Similarly, 26 percent of children in the early clamping group had an immature pencil grip at 4 years old, compared with 13 percent of children in the delayed clamping group. This difference in development was especially pronounced in boys, who are more prone to iron deficiency than girls.[14]

As I'm updating this chapter in 2020, my children are home from school due to the global COVID-19 pandemic, and my role in their lives has expanded to include teacher as well as parent. My 5-year-old son, Max, struggles with his pencil grip, and his efforts to make the shapes of letters are jerky and barely legible. He's behind in these skills, and while I have confidence that we can help him catch up, I also can't help but think about those results in the

Swedish children. Max's cord was cut within seconds of his birth, and I wonder if he might have benefitted from the extra iron endowed during a delay in cord clamping.

We have no way of knowing if the rush to cut Max's cord somehow affected his development. That's the trouble with an anecdotal experience like mine and even observational studies; a correlation is not the same as causation. However, the Swedish randomized controlled trial does provide compelling evidence that immediate cord clamping can hinder normal neurodevelopment, if in subtle ways. Further evidence comes from a recent randomized controlled trial conducted in Rhode Island and published in 2018, which found that at 4 months, infants given a 5-minute delay in cord clamping had both higher iron levels and greater brain myelination, which is essential for brain processing speed, compared with those with immediate cord clamping.[15]

There is a large body of literature documenting the effects of iron-deficiency anemia, which occurs when iron deficiency is severe enough to result in low blood hemoglobin. These studies showed that, on average, children with iron-deficiency anemia had lower scores on cognitive, motor, and behavioral tests. In children older than 2 years of age, giving iron supplements to correct an iron deficiency usually resulted in improved test scores. However, children who had iron-deficiency anemia at 6 months of age and then received an iron supplement to correct the deficiency still had slower activation of nerve pathways as toddlers and preschoolers, suggesting that some setbacks during the early years may be irreversible. (Correcting a deficiency is still important to prevent further deficits, however.) Moderate iron deficiency without anemia, which is more common in developed countries, was also associated with cognitive and motor deficits, though the results were subtler and less conclusive.[16]

Iron stores are especially critical for breastfed babies because there is little iron in breast milk. (Formula is fortified with iron, so iron deficiency is unusual in formula-fed babies.) The iron in breast milk is well absorbed, but the amount is so small that it can provide only a fraction of the baby's needs. A breastfed baby thus relies on the savings account of iron stores from birth to provide most of what is needed for growth and development until she starts eating solid foods. With early cord clamping, iron stores can dwindle by 3 to 4 months of age. Late cord clamping adds several months' worth of iron, making it last until 6 to 8 months.[17] Other factors, including maternal anemia, diabetes, and premature birth, can also reduce the iron stores present at birth and increase the risk of iron deficiency.[18]

The iron bump from delayed cord clamping can make a big difference, because most babies aren't ready to eat an appreciable amount of solid foods until around 6 months of age, and some take longer to get the hang of solids. To cover this gap in iron supply, the American Academy of Pediatrics (AAP) Committee on Nutrition recommends that, beginning at 4 months, breastfed babies take a liquid iron supplement.[19] But this advice is controversial. The AAP's own Section on Breastfeeding responded to this recommendation with major concerns and, along with other researchers in this field, worried that supplementing all breastfed infants could be risky.[20] For example, one study of Swedish and Honduran infants found that iron supplementation was helpful to babies that had low iron, but for babies that already had sufficient iron, the supplement slowed growth and increased the incidence of diarrhea.[21] Citing similar concerns about risks and a lack of high quality evidence of benefit, the European Society for Paediatric Gastroenterology, Hepatology, and Nutrition Committee on Nutrition recommended in 2014 against universal iron supplementation of breastfed infants in populations with a low prevalence of iron-deficiency anemia, as in Europe.[22] There's also the very real problem that iron supplements literally taste like rust, and some babies flat out reject them. I tried giving one to Cee for a while, but she invariably spat it back at me, staining whatever clothes we were both wearing.

It's estimated that between 5 and 20 percent of toddlers in Europe and the United States are iron deficient. The prevalence of iron-deficiency anemia is lower, around 2 percent of toddlers in the United States and between 3 and 9 percent in Europe.[23] Importantly, babies in the United States aren't routinely screened for anemia until around 12 months of age. In other words, an older baby, particularly an exclusively breastfed baby whose cord was clamped early and who isn't yet getting good dietary sources of iron, could easily have a moderate iron deficiency go unnoticed in a critical period of development. (I discuss good options for iron-rich solid foods in chapter 10.)

Delayed cord clamping is helpful to full-term babies, but it is even more beneficial for preterm infants. A 2019 Cochrane review combined the results of 40 studies with 4,884 preterm infants, mostly conducted in high-income countries, and found that those with delayed cord clamping were less likely to die in the hospital. The authors estimated that 74 per 1,000 preemies died with immediate cord clamping compared with 54 per 1,000 infants with delayed cord clamping. They also found that delayed cord clamping reduced the incidence of intraventricular hemorrhage, or bleeding in the brain, a life-threatening complication of preterm birth.[24] In another study, babies born preterm with delayed cord clamping were less likely to have motor development delays at 18 to 22 months old compared to those whose cords were clamped immediately.[25] Many of the studies of preterm babies used only a 30- to 45-second delay in cord clamping because of the rush to get medical attention to these fragile babies, but benefits were observed even with this short delay.

Risks of Delayed Cord Clamping

Because immediate cord clamping was the norm for several generations, health care providers wanted to be sure that changing to delayed cord clamping wouldn't inadvertently cause harm to infants or their mothers. One concern was that infants with delayed cord clamping might end up with a condition called polycythemia, in which they simply have too many red blood cells. Another is that they could have a greater risk of jaundice, caused by a buildup of bilirubin, a normal breakdown product of red blood cells. All newborns are breaking down red blood cells, but in some babies, the liver can't filter bilirubin quickly enough and jaundice develops. If bilirubin levels get too high, this can be treated with phototherapy—placing the baby under special lights that help metabolize bilirubin. Without treatment, bilirubin can damage the brain, so monitoring and timely treatment are important.

It makes sense that babies with delayed cord clamping could be at higher risk for polycythemia or jaundice, since they end up with more blood and hence more red blood cells to break down after birth. However, while some studies have found that infants with delayed cord clamping may have slightly higher hematocrit (indicating more red blood cells) and bilirubin levels, others have not. And looking at those studies together, infants with delayed cord clamping don't seem to have a greater incidence of jaundice or other complications. These higher blood values may in fact be physiologically normal—just different from the norms established in infants with immediate cord clamping.[26]

Obstetricians have also worried that delayed cord clamping might increase the mother's risk of postpartum hemorrhage, but

Summary of benefits and risks of delayed cord clamping

BENEFITS	
In preterm infants	Decreased risk of newborn death
	Reduced need for blood transfusions
	Reduced incidence of intraventricular hemorrhage
In preterm and full-term infants	Higher iron stores and reduced risk of iron deficiency and anemia in infancy
	Improved social and motor skills in early childhood

RISKS	
In preterm and full-term infants	Could interfere with timely medical attention in complicated births

studies show that whether the cord is clamped immediately or several minutes after birth doesn't affect maternal bleeding or the time it takes to pass the placenta, including in cesarean deliveries.[27]

As more studies showed that delayed cord clamping was beneficial to babies, medical organizations have increasingly endorsed it. The World Health Organization (WHO) and the UK's National Institute for Health and Care Excellence (NICE) both recommend that cord clamping be delayed for at least one minute after birth.[28] ACOG recommends waiting at least 30 to 60 seconds.[29] But changing practice takes time, and surveys of obstetricians reveal that delayed cord clamping hasn't been universally adopted, so it's worth talking with your birth provider about their approach to cord clamping ahead of time.

The Resuscitation Question

In 2012—by this time armed with a PhD in nutrition and her experience in the crowded Mexico City hospital—Camila Chaparro gave birth to her first child, Peter. Throughout her pregnancy, and on the day of her delivery, Chaparro was cared for by a certified nurse midwife practice in a university hospital in Washington, DC. The midwives were on board with everything that Chaparro and her husband wanted for their son's first moments, including delayed cord clamping, all written down in their birth plan.[30]

Despite their planning and preparation, Peter's first moments in the world were scary, and things didn't go according to plan. Peter was born with his umbilical cord wrapped tightly around his neck (called a nuchal cord), and he didn't breathe right away after birth. Chaparro held her limp baby on her chest and watched as the midwife quickly clamped and cut the cord. "And all of a sudden, there were, like, fifteen people in the room, and they immediately transferred him over to the warmer," she told me. Nurses and neonatologists swarmed around her son, trying everything to help him breathe, and eventually deciding to intubate him to get air to his lungs. "He didn't really start breathing on his own for the first ten to fifteen minutes, which was incredibly scary," Chaparro remembered.

37

Chaparro wondered, in retrospect, whether it might have helped Peter to leave the cord attached a bit longer. After all, it was pulsing with oxygenated blood. But at the time, she told me, this was the last thing on her mind. She just wanted to see her baby's chest rise and fall as air filled his lungs. (It did, and by the time she recounted her experience to me, Peter was a healthy, happy toddler.)

Chaparro's experience illustrates one of the most controversial points of the cord clamping debate and the area where we most need more research. Delayed cord clamping throws a wrench into protocols for caring for newborn babies in trouble. And doctors love protocols—not because doctors are inflexible, but because protocols give everyone a job, increase speed when a quick response is critical, and prevent mistakes. And in most hospital delivery rooms, cutting the cord immediately is part of the protocol for helping babies in trouble, so that they can be moved to a warmer to receive expert care. How does delayed cord clamping fit into that picture?

Some doctors and midwives argue that if a baby needs help breathing, that help should be given with the cord still attached.[31] In the case of a nuchal cord, like Peter had, by the time the baby is born, blood volume and oxygen supply may already be very low. Waiting to cut the cord can help the baby recover some blood and oxygen, perhaps giving the baby a chance to breathe on his own or helping the resuscitation. Neonatologist Tonse Raju described it to me like this: "People forget that the placenta actually continues to breathe for the baby even after the baby is born, as long as the umbilical cord is not severed. When the baby is in the mother's womb, it is the placenta that is doing gas exchange, and it will continue to do its job after the baby is born, even if the baby has not started breathing through his lungs . . . Therefore, in babies who require resuscitation, getting the extra blood may make the doctor's job of resuscitation much easier."[32]

But the way most hospital delivery rooms are set up, both spatially and in terms of their protocols, means that the infants who could most benefit from the transfusion of blood from the placenta at birth—including those who are born preterm or with difficulty with breathing—are the least likely to receive delayed cord clamping. Experimenting with the logistics of leaving the cord intact while also tending to the very time-sensitive needs of a fragile infant is the next frontier of cord clamping research. Several groups around the world have developed rolling resuscitation carts or portable platforms that can be placed right next to the mother and have all the equipment needed for neonatal resuscitation. Early trials have shown that obstetric and pediatric providers can coordinate their dance of care in a small space to care for babies in this way, and they've hinted at benefits such as higher oxygen levels for infants resuscitated with the cord attached. Large clinical trials are underway; these will be big enough to determine if leaving the cord intact until an infant begins to breathe affects the most important outcomes, such as the incidence of intraventricular hemorrhage and death.[33]

SEEDING THE MICROBIOME

At birth, cutting the umbilical cord may be the most obvious transition, but there's another shift happening—one much less visible but just as dramatic. In the squeeze through the birth canal or during the emergence from a cesarean section, a newborn crosses the threshold from a relatively sterile womb into a world teeming with microbes, many eager to take up residence on and within the youngest members of the human species. Over the last couple of decades, our appreciation for these microbes as friends and partners in our physiology has grown. We now understand that our bodies hold just as many, if not more, bacterial cells as human cells.[34] This population of microbes, collectively making up our microbiomes, lives mostly in symbiosis with us. We provide them with a habitat and steady food supply, and they help us digest food and manufacture vitamins. Of particular importance to infants, our bacterial friends also seem to help guide the development of the gut and the immune system. An essential immune function is to be able to differentiate the self from an intruder, and friends from foes, and early bacterial exposure teaches infants which bacteria are friendly and which warrant an immune response.

A constellation of factors affects which microbial settlers will come to call your baby home, but whether your baby is born vaginally or by cesarean is among the first determinants. Although there's some evidence of microbes in the placenta and uterus, this area of research is controversial, and most scientists agree that a baby is not extensively colonized by microbes at least until the fetal membranes are broken.[35] At this point, a baby born vaginally descends through the birth canal, bathing in and swallowing microbes along the way. Thus, a mother's vaginal microbes are among the first to have the chance to colonize a vaginally born infant. Those born by cesarean, on the other hand, are first exposed to microbes found on the skin of the people who hold them and in the hospital environment.[36]

Does it matter whether your baby gets this "bacterial baptism" conferred by vaginal birth? Maybe. Researchers tracking the development of babies' gut microbiomes have found detectable differences in those born vaginally or by cesarean as far out as 4 years of age, although another recent study found no effect of birth mode by 6 weeks of age, so there's some disagreement on this point.[37] Epidemiological studies have consistently found that children born by cesarean have a greater incidence of obesity and chronic conditions such as asthma, food allergies, and inflammatory bowel disease.[38] These studies are observational, so they can only indicate correlations; they can't show that cesarean birth *causes* these outcomes or that microbial exposure during vaginal birth would have prevented them. There are numerous potential confounding factors that could also affect the development of a child's microbiome and later health, including early exposure to antibiotics, maternal obesity, formula feeding, preterm labor, and time spent in the NICU—all of which are more common among children born by cesarean. Still, it's becoming increasingly clear that our microbes matter, so it seems worth paying attention to those that first colonize infants.[39]

What does this mean if your baby is born by cesarean? First, keep in mind that the science of the microbiome is still in its infancy—a frustrating fact for parents today, who understandably may worry that their decisions now could affect their children's health for years to come, all because of miniscule microbes that scientists are only just beginning to understand. Second, let's acknowledge that most people don't choose a cesarean birth out of convenience or preference; most happen because they're recommended by a health care provider after what is ideally a careful assessment of risks and benefits. In the United States, 32 percent of all births are by cesarean, but just 2.5 percent of these are cesareans requested by the mother.[40] And while it's widely accepted that rates of cesarean birth are now far higher than they should be in much of the world, the procedure is also life-saving and often needed to bring a baby into the world safely.[41]

That said, if you do end up with a cesarean birth, you may wonder if it's possible to seed your baby with vaginal microbes to try to replicate the same exposure your baby would have seen in the birth canal. This idea has gained popularity, probably because it's been covered in mainstream media publications and suggested in several recent books and documentaries.[42]

As I write this in 2020, there has only been one published study of vaginal seeding in the research literature, and it was small and short-term. The study, published in 2016 in the journal *Nature Medicine*, was led by Dr. Maria Dominguez-Bello (now at Rutgers University) and included 18 mothers giving birth in a hospital affiliated with the University of Puerto Rico. Seven of the mothers gave birth vaginally, and of the 11 infants born by planned cesarean, four were gifted with what the study authors called "microbial restoration." The procedure involved moistening a square of sterile gauze with saline solution, folding it like a fan, and inserting it into the mother's vagina for an hour before the surgery. As soon as the baby was delivered and moved to a warming table, the gauze was wiped over the baby's lips, face, chest, arms, legs, genitals, anus, and back, in that order.[43] Welcome to the world, baby—time to meet your mother's microbes!

Dominguez-Bello and colleagues followed these babies and the development of their microbiota for one month after birth, periodically checking to see which microbes established themselves and where. As expected, the infants born vaginally had microbes matching those found in their mothers' vaginas, such as *Lactobacillus,* all over their bodies on the first day of life. These same microbes were also found on the babies that had the vaginal seeding procedure, but not on the other cesarean-born infants. In the first week of life, the microbial populations on the seeded infants' skin and in their mouths were more like the vaginal-born infants than the other cesarean-born infants. However, when the researchers analyzed the babies' gut bacteria, they found that the seeded infants looked more like the other cesarean infants than those born vaginally. The failure of the vaginal seeding procedure to alter the gut microbiome is notable, as the microbes that settle in the gut are thought to be especially important for immune and digestive development. And while all the babies' skin and mouth microbes started to resemble adults by 1 month of age, their gut microbiota remained distinct. So, while the study showed that vaginal seeding could at least temporarily shift the skin and mouth bacteria to look more like those found on vaginal-born infants, it also showed little effect on the bacteria residing in the babies' intestines.

There were some important limitations to this study. "We stress that our work represents a proof of principle on a small cohort and with limited follow up time," the authors acknowledge in their paper. Because the study ended after one month, it couldn't show how long the seeded bacteria remained in residence or whether they affected the babies' health or development. These are open questions, and Dominguez-Bello and other researchers are continuing to study them in larger trials that will track babies for at least the first year of life, looking at outcomes such as obesity and food allergies.[44]

Until those studies are published, it's unknown whether vaginal seeding is beneficial to babies. And medical professionals are quick to point out that the procedure does come with some possible risks. ACOG, the Danish Society of Obstetrics and Gynaecology, and physicians from the UK and Australia have all published statements saying that, although they're increasingly receiving requests for vaginal seeding from patients, they recommend against the procedure, unless it's done as part of an approved research study.[45] They warn that vaginal seeding could not only inoculate newborns with desirable bacteria but also infect them with pathogens, such as herpes simplex virus, human papillomavirus (HPV), group B *Streptococcus*, or *Neisseria gonorrhoeae*, the bacteria that causes gonorrhea. In the United States, women are often tested for at least some of these pathogens at some point in pregnancy, but this screening doesn't guarantee that they're not infected at the time of delivery, and screening is less routine in other countries.

There's at least one example of such an infection, described in a 2018 case report from Australia of a newborn who developed an eye infection after vaginal seeding following a cesarean birth.[46] The infection was caused by herpes simplex virus, carried unknowingly by the baby's mother, who wasn't tested before giving birth. A case like this can't prove with certainty that it was vaginal seeding that caused the infection, but it's a reasonable hypothesis. And while the baby's infection was limited to her eyes, she needed 14 days of intravenous antibiotics to treat it. This and other pathogens can manifest as far more serious infections, causing sepsis and meningitis.[47] Given this risk and no data supporting benefits of vaginal seeding, it's understandable that medical groups aren't endorsing it. If a handful of parents here and there choose seeding, then infections caused by it will be rare, limited to an occasional case report, like the infant in Australia. But if seeding is widely adopted, you could imagine that infections could be a much bigger problem, requiring more vigilant testing protocols and perhaps even increasing antibiotic use in newborns, which would be counter to the goal of healthy microbiome development. Even Dominguez-Bello and her colleagues have stated publicly that parents shouldn't try vaginal seeding on their own, only as part of a clinical trial.[48]

Still, you don't have to look far to find well-informed people choosing to vaginally seed their newborns. Rob Knight, a well-known microbiome researcher at the University of California, San Diego, tells the story of seeding his cesarean-born daughter with vaginal microbes in *Dirt is Good*, a book for parents about the microbiome that he coauthored.[49] And a 2016 article about vaginal seeding published in the *New York Times* included a quote from a maternal-fetal medicine specialist who noted that the procedure wasn't recommended by medical societies, but she had arranged to have her own newborn swabbed with her vaginal fluids at birth.[50] Talk about mixed messages.

You could argue that this exposure is natural, and had your baby been born vaginally, he would have had the same risk of infection. As UK obstetrician Dr. Amali Lokugamage and coauthor wrote in a 2019 commentary, "To unintentionally infer that the average human vagina is dangerous could provoke feminist consternation."[51] It's a valid point. However, the fact remains that the seeding procedure could directly cause an infection that would otherwise have been avoided in a cesarean birth, so the choice to seed your baby with vaginal fluids is not entirely risk-free.

There's also reason to question whether vaginal seeding could be a magic bullet for our microbial woes. For one thing, there's the reality that initial exposure to microbes is far from the only difference between babies born vaginally or by cesarean. There are all those pesky confounding factors already mentioned, like exposure to antibiotics and formula feeding, which are more common for babies born by cesarean. There are also all the factors that led to the cesarean, and the fact that the labor process involves hormonal and inflammatory changes in both the mother and baby, which could influence the baby's developing microbiome in a way that can't be replicated by a quick wipe-down with vaginal fluids.[52]

Then there's the question of whether the microbes colonizing the mother's vagina are truly important to a newborn's developing microbiome, as they're not necessarily well-adapted to the gut and don't seem to set up shop there for the long-term.[53] However, there's another common and potent source of microbes that often accompanies vaginal birth: poop. It's one of the realities of birth that people don't like to talk about, but between the baby's head pushing down on the mother's colon and the intense contractions and pushing, it's common for the mother to pass some stool during labor. The microbes therein are already well-adapted to the gut environment and readily colonize the newborn, described in one paper as "a quintessential fecal-oral transfer."[54] Recent studies have shown that in infants born vaginally, vaginal microbes were present in their gut for the first few days of life, but they were transient inhabitants and faded from the gut community, probably because they prefer a more acidic environment. Microbes traceable to the mother's stool, on the other hand, remained more abundant and persistent in the infant's gut.[55] If a mother's fecal microbes are a vital component of the microbial experience of vaginal birth, the vaginal swab used in the seeding procedure would probably miss them.

However, feeding a cesarean-born newborn some of his mother's fecal microbes might do the trick, and this idea was tested in a small "proof-of-concept" study published in the journal *Cell* in October 2020, just as I was wrapping up the second edition of this book.[56] In the study, Finnish women donated a fresh fecal sample three weeks before their planned cesarean births. Through blood and fecal tests, they were carefully screened for a range of pathogens. If they cleared these tests, their cesarean-born infants were fed a dose of their mothers' stored feces, mixed into breast milk, at their first feeding. Unlike vaginal seeding, this fecal transplant procedure did seem to result in the infants' gut microbiomes looking very similar to those found in a comparison group of vaginally born babies. However, this study ended up with only seven mother-infant pairs, in part because 29 percent of those screened were positive for pathogenic microbes. This fact underscores the reality that a fecal transplant carries significant risk and definitely shouldn't be attempted unless you're participating in a trial. And while the results of this small study are promising, they should be considered preliminary; much larger clinical trials are needed, and at least one is underway.[57] With better understanding of which microbes are most important for new babies, we can hope that someday we'll have an oral probiotic, formulated just for cesarean newborns, to give them the right mix of beneficial microbes without the risk of infection by pathogens, but we need much more research to know what that mix would be.[58]

So, dear readers, when it comes to fecal transplants for newborn babies, please don't try this at home. Vaginal seeding is a bit more of a gray area. As with any decision, we weigh the risks and benefits, but that's difficult with so little data available. On the one hand, vaginal seeding is such an alluring idea—a simple, natural antidote for the microbial deficits of the modern world—purportedly offering lifelong health benefits to children. On the other, there's no evidence for these benefits yet, and seeding comes with some amount of risk, however small. If you do choose to seed your newborn, keep an eye out for any signs of infection in the first few weeks of life, and please be sure to let your baby's medical provider know right away that vaginal seeding was part of your baby's early life exposures. That could inform the provider's thinking about possible causes of your baby's symptoms, the tests they run, and the treatments they offer.

BABY'S FIRST BATH

I've seen the evolution of baby bath protocols firsthand with my children. Cee, born in 2010, spent her first hour or two of life on my chest, breastfeeding and resting. Then a nurse took her to the newborn nursery, and Cee must have had her first bath during that time. When I awoke from a much-needed nap, a nurse handed me a clean, expertly swaddled, soft-skinned newborn baby, and it didn't even occur to me to ask when she'd had her first bath, or how it went.

46

Max was born in 2014 at a different hospital, where the default was for babies to stay with their parents and all procedures to be done in their presence. He received his first bath in the delivery room after a couple of hours of breastfeeding and skin-to-skin time. Our nurse deftly held him in one hand over the sink, warm water running, using her other hand to gently rinse him off. With both babies, our first awkward attempts at bathing them ourselves came after we brought them home.

As I write this in 2020, both of our baby bathing experiences are now out of date based on current recommendations. Today, more hospitals are delaying the baby's first bath until at least 24 hours after birth, a policy recommended by the WHO and the Association of Women's Health, Obstetric and Neonatal Nurses.[59] (The WHO says that if there are cultural reasons for bathing sooner, you should wait at least six hours for temperature stability.) Hospitals are also more likely to bathe babies in a warm tub instead of using running water or sponge bath methods, and many are encouraging parents to take the lead on giving their babies their first baths, with guidance from hospital staff, so that they go home with a little more confidence in caring for their baby.

Birth is a messy affair, and babies are born coated with a variety of fluids, which can include blood, amniotic and vaginal fluids, the mother's stool, and sometimes a bit of meconium. It's understandable to want to clean these fluids from your sweet baby (though we just discussed intentional vaginal seeding!), and in some cases, such as if the mother is infected with HIV or hepatitis viruses, babies may need to be cleaned sooner. But for most, it's enough to simply pat them dry and wait a day before thinking about a bath.

One reason to wait on the bath is to leave the protective layer of vernix intact on your baby's skin. White in color and cheesy in texture, vernix is made by your baby and secreted from hair shafts during the third trimester. This substance—composed of about 80 percent water, 10 percent protein, and 10 percent fat—forms a protective barrier on newborns' delicate skin, helping to ease the transition of birth. Vernix helps to keep newborns' delicate skin hydrated and promotes a slightly acidic pH, which protects against infection. In addition, vernix contains many proteins with antimicrobial and wound-healing functions.[60]

There's also some evidence that delaying the first bath can support breastfeeding. Several studies have reported that as hospitals adopted a protocol of delayed newborn bathing, the rates of exclusive breastfeeding in the hospital increased.[61] For example, a study conducted at a Cleveland Clinic hospital and published in 2019 found that their in-hospital exclusive breastfeeding rates increased from 60 percent under their old protocol of bathing newborns two hours after birth to 68 percent when they started delaying the first bath until 18 hours after birth.[62] This type of observational study can't prove that delaying the bath directly causes more breastfeeding, as there could have been other changes around the same time that influenced breastfeeding rates. But you can imagine that delaying the bath could help babies get a good start with breastfeeding, simply by taking the bath off the postpartum to-do list. That eliminates one of the reasons why newborns might be taken from their parents, even for a short amount of time, and frees up more time for skin-to-skin and breastfeeding attempts. However, several studies haven't noted any improvement in breastfeeding rates in hospitals adopting delayed bathing, although these were conducted in hospitals that already had high breastfeeding rates and so had less room for improvement.[63]

Some studies also show that delaying the first bath reduces the incidence of hypothermia (low body temperature) and hypoglycemia (low blood glucose) in newborns, who have thin, delicate skin and relatively little body fat so can lose heat quickly. Whether it happens soon after birth or the next day, a bath almost always results in a drop in body temperature for a newborn, and rewarming requires them to ramp up their metabolic rate, using more glucose and oxygen. Some studies show that babies regain normal temperature more quickly, and fewer babies drop into the hypothermic and hypoglycemic range, if their bath is delayed until the next day.[64] In one study, newborns were also subjected to fewer heel sticks to check their blood glucose when their baths were delayed. It makes sense to avoid the temperature stress of the first bath for at least a day; newborns have enough to adapt to on that first day of life without adding the chilliness of emerging from a bath to the mix.

Delaying your newborn's bath also means you're more likely to be ready to bathe your baby yourself the next day, ideally with some guidance from hospital staff. That brings us to the next question: how do you bathe a newborn, anyway? A sponge bath used to be standard hospital protocol, in part because it was thought that keeping the umbilical cord stump dry would help it heal and reduce the risk of infection. However, a small randomized controlled trial conducted in a Canadian hospital and published in 2004 found that newborns lost less heat when they were given a full immersion bath in a warm tub of water rather than a sponge bath, with no difference in cord healing.[65] A 2012 study at Brigham and Women's Hospital in Boston replicated this finding in late preterm infants (born at 35 to 37 weeks), whose immaturity and smaller size made them more susceptible to cold stress than full-term infants.[66] Not surprisingly, in the Canadian study, the babies given the tub baths were also much happier with the process—some of them so relaxed that they fell asleep—whereas a majority of the sponge-bathed babies cried during their baths.[67]

The goal of the baby's first bath is to quickly wash off undesirable substances, keeping it as short as possible to avoid temperature stress. A gentle bath can even leave some of the vernix intact. After the bath, resting skin-to-skin is an excellent way to help warm up your baby.[68]

MY BABIES' BIRTH TRANSITIONS

I love digging into the science of infancy and thinking about how we can apply our knowledge of babies' physiology to help give them the gentlest transition on their birth days. But then I remember that while I can describe this ideal to you—delayed cord clamping, a "natural" microbial inoculation, and delayed bathing—it doesn't fully represent either of my babies' first days. That's because they were born into the real world, where things don't always go as planned, and practice doesn't always keep up with the latest science. Both of my babies had immediate cord clamping because the obstetricians attending their births were concerned about their well-being, and neither were comfortable tending to those concerns with the cord attached. Both times, I trusted their clinical judgement and just wanted to be sure my babies were healthy. (They were fine, but perhaps they wouldn't have been if my doctors hadn't acted quickly.) Both of my babies were born vaginally, but they were bathed within a couple of hours of birth. At the end of the day, they were healthy and in my arms, and I let go of whatever ideal I'd had in mind. I tend to over-research and overanalyze decisions, which is part of what qualifies me to write this book. But I also try to not attach too much importance to any one decision, because flexibility and looking at the big picture is essential to parenting survival. Plus, there will be more decisions to research and analyze tomorrow.

SPLISH SPLASH: BATHING YOUR BABY

Many infants and parents enjoy the routine of a bath before bedtime, but it's not necessary to bathe your baby daily. In fact, daily bathing can dry out your baby's skin. The American Academy of Pediatrics recommends bathing your baby with soap about three times per week, and I'll be honest: I bathed my babies less frequently than this with no ill effect (except perhaps a pungent sour milk smell). Pediatricians recommend using a mild, neutral pH cleanser, choosing one that is fragrance-free to avoid unnecessary exposure to phthalate chemicals, which may act as hormone disruptors. Use caution with natural and herbal cleansers, as these may not have been tested on infants. Some herbs have been shown to cause or exacerbate eczema; these include chamomile, calendula, aloe, goldenseal, tea tree oil, yarrow, and arnica.

Source: J. M. Kuller, Update on Newborn Bathing, *Newborn and Infant Nursing Reviews* 14, no. 4 (2014): 166–70; D. Navsaria, "Bathing Your Baby," Healthy Children.org, last updated March 3, 2020, https://www.healthychildren.org/English/ages-stages/baby/bathing-skin-care/Pages/Bathing-Your-Newborn.aspx.

3

OF INJECTIONS AND EYE GOOP

Newborn Medical Procedures

When I think back to the moments after Cee's birth, there are a few clear memories that I hope I can hold in my mind forever: the quiet on her face as we gazed at each other, her confidence in her first breastfeed, and the exhilaration of being on the other side of childbirth. But a lot of other things were going on during that time, and they're mostly a blur. There was the placenta to deliver and a few stitches for me, and for Cee, a bunch of routine medical procedures that happened in the first hours and days of her life—a quick succession of heel sticks, screening tests, injections, and eye goop. These procedures can feel a little intrusive during this time when you're trying to get to know your new baby, and it's understandable if you wonder about their risks and benefits, and whether they're truly necessary. In this chapter, I explore in depth the science of two recommended newborn procedures—the vitamin K shot and erythromycin eye ointment—and summarize a few others at the end of the chapter. Know that with all these newborn procedures, you can ask that they be delayed for at least the first hour after birth so that your getting-to-know-you time is uninterrupted.

THE VITAMIN K SHOT

One Baby's Story

Olive Eloise Leavitt slid into the world early one morning in January 2014 at a birth center in Washington State. Her mother, Stefani, had labored without medication through the night. When it was time to push, Stefani climbed into the birthing tub, pushed through three contractions, and then had her healthy little girl in her arms. Olive's first month was a sweet blur of sleeping and breastfeeding, while her parents and big sister got used to being a family of four.[1]

But a month later, on Valentine's Day, Stefani started to worry about Olive. They'd been up for most of the night, struggling to breastfeed, and now Olive seemed sleepy and completely uninterested in eating. By the afternoon, she was so lethargic that she was barely able to open her eyes. Stefani took her to the emergency room.[2]

What happened next is a parent's worst nightmare. What at first seemed like a minor concern was suddenly a life-threatening emergency. A lumbar puncture (spinal tap) showed blood in Olive's spinal fluid, and she was rushed to a better-equipped hospital. It took many attempts to get an IV placed because Olive's fragile veins kept rupturing. Finally, a CT scan revealed the biggest problem of all: a huge mass of blood filled Olive's skull, pushing her brain to one side. The doctors told Stefani and her husband that Olive had an intracranial hemorrhage, and if she survived, there was a good chance that her brain would be severely damaged.

At some point, as the doctors worked on Olive, one of them asked Stefani if her baby had received a vitamin K shot at birth. The answer was no, and this explained everything. Like all newborn babies, Olive was born with very little vitamin K in her body. Vitamin K is essential for the formation of blood clots, and Olive didn't have enough of it. This was why it was hard to establish an IV, and it was why she had an intracranial hemorrhage. A simple injection of vitamin K at birth would have prevented Olive's pain and suffering, the fear and anxiety of her parents, and the medical expense of her treatment.

Olive needed brain surgery, but first, she needed to be able to clot her blood; otherwise, the surgery would cause even more bleeding. She received an IV infusion of vitamin K, and after about an hour, her blood began to clot. Doctors worked through the night to remove the mass of blood from her brain.

In the days that followed, Olive's parents sat by her side and watched, not knowing how much damage might have been done before the doctors relieved the pressure on Olive's brain. They watched as she moved her leg for the first time, as she opened her eyes, and finally, after her breathing tube was removed four days later, as she cried. "I have never been happier to hear a baby cry," Stefani wrote on her blog.[3]

Two weeks later, Olive was discharged from the hospital. Her paperwork included a long list of diagnoses: "Hemorrhagic Disease of the Newborn Due to Vitamin K Deficiency, Subdural Hematoma, Acute Respiratory Failure, Increased Intracranial Pressure, Ischemic Brain Damage, Seizure, Cerebral Infarction of the Left Hemisphere, and Cholestatic Jaundice." In the months and years since, Olive's parents and doctors have watched her closely for signs of lasting brain damage. But at age 6, she's now taking gymnastics and learning to read. "Olive is doing wonderfully right now, especially considering her rocky start. She's in occupational therapy for some sensory issues and possible ADHD, but it's really up in the air as to whether that was caused by the brain injury or just Olive being Olive," Stefani wrote in her most recent email to me.[4] Olive is incredibly lucky.

That Olive didn't get her vitamin K shot seems to have been an unfortunate oversight at the birth center where she was born. Some parents, however, intentionally decline the vitamin K shot for their newborns, and doctors say they're seeing this more and more often.[5] Parents worry about the pain of the injection and think that the shot is an unnatural and unnecessary intervention. Some may have heard that the vitamin K shot can cause cancer.[6] There is a ton of misinformation about vitamin K online to fuel these concerns, and at the very least, it leaves parents confused. When I dug into the science on this topic, I found a fascinating history, intriguing physiology, and a clearer understanding of the benefits and risks of the vitamin K shot.

The History and Science of Vitamin K

Boston doctor Charles W. Townsend published a description of 50 cases of strange bleeding in newborns, many of them fatal, in 1894.[7] The cause was unknown, and all that doctors could do was try to control the bleeding, hoping that the blood would eventually start to clot. At that time, nobody knew what vitamin K was, much less that it could stop these babies from bleeding.

The discovery of vitamin K was an accident. In the 1930s, a Danish biochemist named Henrik Dam was feeding baby chicks low-fat diets as part of his work on cholesterol metabolism. He noticed that some of the chicks were bleeding in their muscle and under their skin.[8] In a series of careful experiments, Dam substituted different types of foods in the chicks' diets. He found that the bleeding occurred when he fed them only foods such as rice, sunflower seeds, corn, and rye, but it was completely prevented by kale, hemp seed, and pig liver. Dam eventually isolated the protective factor from alfalfa leaves, and he and other researchers showed that it could stop hemorrhaging not just in baby chicks but also in newborn infants. Dam named this fat-soluble compound vitamin K, for "Koagulations."[9] For their work on vitamin K, Dam shared the 1943 Nobel Prize in Physiology or Medicine with Edward Doisy, an American biochemist.[10]

The ability of blood to clot is essential to mammalian life. Our bodies are full of blood, pumping through the vast network of the circulatory system, but this system works only if the blood stays within the walls of the blood vessels. If one of these vessels is damaged—not hard to do, since their walls are thin and fragile—immediate clotting of the blood is what prevents hemorrhage.

Vitamin K is required for the liver's synthesis of four proteins that contribute to blood clotting.[11] Some of the richest sources of vitamin K_1, also called phylloquinone, in the human diet are foods such as leafy green vegetables (kale, Swiss chard, collard greens), cruciferous vegetables (Brussels sprouts, cabbage, broccoli), and soybean and canola oils. Vitamin K_2, a group of similar compounds called menaquinones, is made by bacteria, including gut microbes in humans. It isn't clear what role menaquinones play in human nutrition because they are not well absorbed from the gut.[12]

When it comes to vitamin K, babies are born at a disadvantage. During pregnancy, very little vitamin K crosses the placenta from mom to baby; cord blood levels of the vitamin are so low that they're often undetectable.[13] Even if a mother takes large amounts of oral or injected vitamin K before giving birth, her baby is still born with negligible amounts.[14] After birth, there's not much improvement in this situation. Breast milk is very low in vitamin K, and the nascent bacterial population in a newborn's gut doesn't contribute much in the way of vitamin K_2.[15] The intestinal bacteria most prevalent in breastfed babies, *Bifidobacterium* and *Lactobacillus*, protect them from diarrheal illness but do not produce vitamin K.[16]

Most newborn babies do okay despite these low vitamin K levels, but some develop one of three types of vitamin K deficiency bleeding (VKDB).[17]

- Early VKDB occurs within the first 24 hours after birth. It is rare, and when it does occur, it's almost always in babies whose mothers were taking medications like blood thinners or anticonvulsants during pregnancy.

- Classical VKDB occurs between 2 and 7 days of age. Bleeding is often seen from the umbilical cord, skin, nose, gastrointestinal tract, or site of circumcision. Estimates suggest that, without receiving vitamin K at birth, as many as 1 in 59 babies would have classical VKDB.[18] So long as medical care is available, most babies will fully recover.

- Late VKDB, the type that affected Olive, occurs between 8 days and 6 months of age. Although rare, with an estimated incidence of 35 in 100,000 babies not receiving vitamin K, late VKDB can be devastating.[19] In one analysis of published cases, 63 percent had severe brain hemorrhage and 14 percent died. Among those that survived, 40 percent had lasting neurological damage.[20]

Classical and late VKDB are completely prevented by a dose of 1 mg of vitamin K given as an intramuscular injection at birth, as recommended by the AAP since 1961.[21] And while the statistics on VKDB make it seem relatively rare, without the vitamin K shot at birth, we could expect more than 70,000 infants in the United States to have unnecessary bleeding and hemorrhage each year, pediatrician Phoebe Danziger pointed out in a 2020 editorial published in the *New York Times*.[22]

Exclusively breastfed babies are most susceptible to VKDB. Human milk has just 1 to 2 micrograms (µg, or one-thousandth of a milligram) vitamin K per liter, lower than that of other animal species. Infant formula is supplemented with at least 55 µg per liter, enough to prevent VKDB in infants who are at least partially formula-fed.[23] Without the vitamin K shot, breastfed newborns, especially those with early feeding difficulties (or if the mother's milk is slow to come in), can rapidly deplete their small vitamin K reserves, leaving them susceptible to classical VKDB. Late VKDB almost always occurs in apparently healthy, exclusively breastfed babies.[24] Note that the incidence of VKDB given above reflects the data for entire populations of babies, many of whom received formula. Since late VKDB usually only affects exclusively breastfed babies, the true incidence in these babies is probably much higher. (Once infants begin eating solid foods, they get usually enough vitamin K from dietary sources to prevent VKDB.)

Babies born with liver diseases that impair the secretion of bile, necessary for the absorption of fat-soluble vitamins like vitamin K, are at especially high risk for late VKDB. This turned out to be the case with Olive, although her liver disease wasn't discovered until more than a month after her brain hemorrhage.[25] Unfortunately,

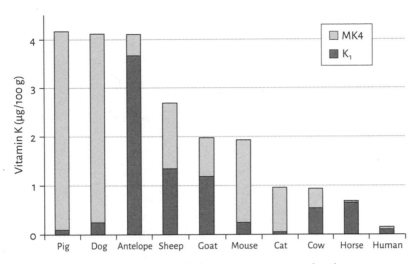

Vitamin K concentrations in milk from various mammals. The two major types of vitamin K found in milk are phylloquinone (K_1) and menaquinone-4 (MK4, a type of K_2).

Source: H. E. Indyk and D. C. Woollard, "Vitamin K in Milk and Infant Formulas: Determination and Distribution of Phylloquinone and Menaquinone-4," *Analyst* 122, no. 5 (1997): 465–69.

there often aren't any signs of underlying liver disease before VKDB happens. Vitamin K at birth spares these most vulnerable babies from the severe effects of late VKDB.[26]

There is some evidence that we're seeing more cases of VKDB because more parents are declining the vitamin K shot, and perhaps in part because more babies are exclusively breastfed. During just eight months in 2013, pediatricians at Vanderbilt University Medical Center were alarmed to see five babies with late VKDB, including four with brain hemorrhages, after at least five years of no late VKDB cases at their hospital.[27] In all five cases, these were healthy breastfed infants who had not received the vitamin K shot at birth. That same year, 3 percent of babies born at the Vanderbilt hospital did not receive vitamin K at birth, but 28 percent of those born at local birth centers missed the shot.[28] Mothers who give birth at birth centers are often more interested in minimizing interventions and in breastfeeding, and it's a cruel irony that the same babies who may not receive vitamin K at birth are also the most vulnerable to VKDB. After a media campaign and collaborative efforts among midwives, nurses, doulas, childbirth educators, and pediatricians in central Tennessee, the rate of vitamin K refusal dropped significantly. As of 2016, there had been no additional cases of VKDB in the region.[29]

The Vitamin K and Cancer Scare

One of the reasons parents give for declining the vitamin K shot is that they've heard it might cause cancer, and there's an interesting history behind this concern. In 1992, British epidemiologist Jean Golding and colleagues published a retrospective observational study in the *British Medical Journal* reporting a correlation between childhood leukemia and the vitamin K injection, but not oral vitamin K (commonly used in the United Kingdom at the time).[30] In response, the journal was flooded with letters to the editor from doctors and researchers, most criticizing the study.[31] They pointed out flaws in the study design, including issues of bias and possible inaccuracies of the data. Researchers from the United Kingdom and the United States also noted that cancer rates had not increased over time, even as vitamin K administration had become more common.[32] These limitations put the study's conclusions on shaky ground, but the media reports focused on the scary cancer connection, not the problems with the science. Understandably, parents were afraid.

Golding's study showed a *correlation* between two variables, but it could not prove that vitamin K *caused* cancer—the classic limitation of observational studies. And so, more studies were done. At least 12 more studies were conducted to look at this question—many larger and with better experimental designs—and together they found no good evidence for a link between cancer and vitamin K.[33] Meanwhile, there is a known outcome for not giving vitamin K: babies can die or become severely disabled because of VKDB.

This story illustrates several points about scientific evidence mentioned in chapter 1: correlation is not the same as causation, and one study is rarely enough to be conclusive. What's important is the consensus of multiple studies, conducted by different researchers, in different places, using different methodology. Golding's study has since been overshadowed by many more finding no link between cancer and vitamin K. However, we can still find scary articles on the internet claiming that the vitamin K shot causes cancer, complete with peer-reviewed research from a well-respected journal. But if we're savvy consumers of information, and we look at all of the research together, we find a strong scientific consensus that vitamin K doesn't cause cancer. Anyone who claims otherwise is cherry-picking from the evidence, choosing one study that supports the claim and completely ignoring the rest.

The Scoop on Oral Vitamin K

Everyone agrees that a single intramuscular vitamin K shot at birth prevents both classical and late VKDB. However, because of the cancer scare and because nobody wants to poke a newborn baby unless it's necessary, many countries have tried various methods of oral dosing.

Since VKDB is so rare, it isn't practical to conduct randomized controlled trials to determine the most effective dosing protocols. Instead, countries that use oral dosing have just tried different plans—like one dose at birth or multiple doses during the first months of life—and then tracked the number of VKDB cases. This gives us surveillance data, and when we compare the results from different countries using different plans, we can see what worked and what didn't.[34]

Together, these data clearly show that intramuscular vitamin K is most effective at preventing VKDB.[35] Oral dosing plans, on the other hand, have had mixed success, often preventing classical but not late VKDB. For example, in the Netherlands, the standard practice between 1990 and 2011 was to give 1 mg of vitamin K at birth followed by 25 µg per day. However, this resulted in a higher incidence of late VKDB relative to other European countries, so the Dutch increased the daily dose to 150 μg in 2011. This helped some, but the incidence of VKDB remained unacceptably high, and in 2017, the Dutch Health Council recommended that all babies receive the vitamin K shot at birth rather than an oral regimen.[36]

More success was reported with a few other oral dosing schemes. In Switzerland, late VKDB was prevented by a 2 mg dose at 4 hours, 4 days, and 4 weeks after birth (a protocol chosen in part because it is easy to remember).[37] Under this plan, there were just four cases of late VKDB between 2005 and 2011, and in all of these, the parents had either refused vitamin K or forgotten to complete the doses. In Denmark, giving 2 mg orally at birth, followed by a weekly 1 mg dose for 3 months, prevented late VKDB, even in babies with liver disease.[38] However, Denmark now recommends the vitamin K shot as the best way to prevent VKDB, as does Canada, the UK, and the European Society for Paediatric Gastroenterology.[39] If parents refuse the shot, organizations from these countries recommend oral dosing plans similar to those studied in Switzerland and Denmark.

Oral doses are tricky for a few reasons. First, oral dosing assumes that the baby will actually swallow all of the liquid vitamin solution, which can apparently have a foul taste and is frequently spit back out by infants, causing them to run the additional risk of aspirating the liquid.[40] Second, absorption of an oral dose from the digestive tract into the body is highly variable even among healthy babies and especially among babies with liver disease. Third, unlike other fat-soluble vitamins, vitamin K doesn't stick around in the body very long. In adults, the body's vitamin K supply turns over in a matter of a day or two.[41] This is why multiple oral doses are necessary, but it's not surprising that parents could forget a dose or two in the haze of early parenting. On the other hand, when vitamin K is injected, it seems to be stored in the muscle and slowly absorbed into the blood over time, providing a continuous

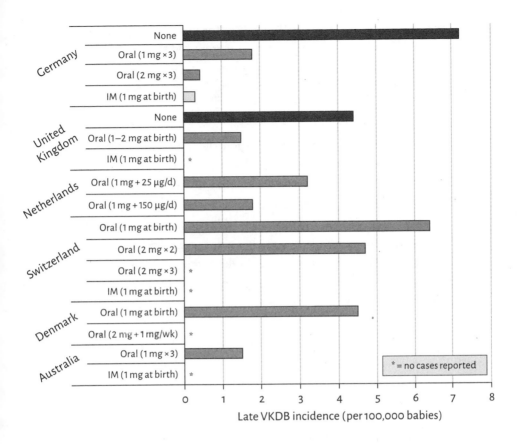

Late VKDB incidence (per 100,000 babies)

Incidence of late vitamin K deficiency bleeding (VKDB) with different vitamin K dosing protocols. Values do not include cases where parents refused vitamin K or did not complete the dosing series. An intramuscular (IM) injection of 1 mg of vitamin K at birth offers complete or near-complete protection from VKDB, whereas protection by oral doses varies. For oral dosing protocols, "x2" indicates that doses were given at birth and again in the first week, and "x3" means a third dose was given after about a month.

Sources: M. Cornelissen et al., "Prevention of Vitamin K Deficiency Bleeding: Efficacy of Different Multiple Oral Dose Schedules of Vitamin K," *European Journal of Pediatrics* 156 (1997): 126; B. Laubscher, O. Bänziger, and G. Schubiger, "Prevention of Vitamin K Deficiency Bleeding with Three Oral Mixed Micellar Phylloquinone Doses: Results of a 6-Year (2005–2011) Surveillance in Switzerland," *European Journal of Pediatrics* 172, no. 3 (2013): 357–60; Y. N. Löwensteyn et al., "Increasing the Dose of Oral Vitamin K Prophylaxis and Its Effect on Bleeding Risk," *European Journal of Pediatrics* 178, no. 7 (2019): 1003–42; M. J. Shearer, "Vitamin K Deficiency Bleeding (VKDB) in Early Infancy," *Blood Reviews* 23, no. 2 (2009): 49–59.

supply for the first few months of life.[42] It's also worth pointing out that in European countries with documented success with oral dosing, new parents often have the advantage of home visits from midwives or health visitors, who can administer doses or remind parents to do so.

Some hospitals in the United States may offer to give vitamin K orally if parents refuse to allow their newborns to receive the shot.[43] This means using the injectable vitamin K preparation off-label, since there currently isn't a vitamin K product licensed by the US Food and Drug Administration (FDA) for oral use in babies. Products marketed for babies are available to purchase online, but it's important to remember that the supplement industry in the United States is poorly regulated. Unlike the process for approval of prescription or over-the-counter drugs, the FDA doesn't review supplements to determine if they're safe or effective before going to market.[44]

Among the misinformation about vitamin K that you can find online is the suggestion that eating lots of kale or taking vitamin K supplements while pregnant and breastfeeding can prevent VKDB. Remember that vitamin K barely crosses the placenta in pregnancy, even if you take large amounts of supplements.[45] As for breast milk, eating a diet rich in food sources of vitamin K or taking a normal supplement results in little to no increase in the vitamin in breast milk.[46] In one study, mothers took a very large vitamin K supplement (5 mg/day), and though that dose raised breast milk concentrations to levels similar to infant formulas, their infants still had plasma vitamin K levels lower than those of formula-fed infants.[47] Five milligrams is also a lot of vitamin K; standard supplements contain just 0.1 mg, and obtaining 5 mg through diet would mean eating more than 50 cups of chopped kale daily.[48] This method could also fail if either the mom or the baby has low vitamin K absorption. In other words, trying to prevent VKDB through your diet might be possible, but it's a roll of the dice compared with the certainty of the vitamin K shot.

What Ingredients Are Found in the
Vitamin K Shot? Are They Safe?

As in any medication and many foods, the ingredients in the newborn vitamin K shot can seem intimidating at first glance. In addition to vitamin K, the shot also includes several "inactive" ingredients. These have unfamiliar chemical names, and you might feel worried about injecting them into your newborn.

To make matters worse, if you read the package insert for the vitamin K shot, you'll see lots of dire warnings about the ingredients. This makes great fodder for scary internet articles, which is exactly what you'll find if you search online for information about the vitamin K shot. However, the package insert is required to include warnings about *any* cases of toxicity linked to any ingredient in the shot, even if they occurred in different drugs, doses, or types of patients. For example, most of the warnings listed on the vitamin K label refer to critically ill patients or premature babies receiving much larger doses of these ingredients intravenously, over many days. The package insert ensures that you're fully informed of every possible risk, but most of it is irrelevant to you and your baby. (The same is true of vaccine package inserts.)

Knowing that the package insert wasn't of much use, I started digging through the toxicology literature to find more information about the ingredients. I found that every ingredient is there for a reason. Some ensure that the vitamin K stays in the solution, rather than separating out. Vitamin K is fat-soluble, so just as oil and water don't mix, it can't simply be dissolved in water or saline for the injection. Other ingredients are used to keep the pH of the solution in a neutral range or to prevent bacterial growth, important aspects of safety of the shot. Any chemical can be toxic in a high enough dose, which is why the package insert for vitamin K is a scary read. But when I looked at the amounts of each ingredient used, it was clear that there is no reason to fear that the shot, given as a one-time intramuscular dose, is toxic to newborns. For those who want to learn more, I have included a detailed description of each ingredient and relevant toxicological data in appendix A.

There are just a few possible side effects of the vitamin K shot. The most immediate is the pain of the injection. However, this is brief, and you can help ease it by holding your newborn skin-to-skin and breastfeeding or giving a sugar solution on a pacifier during the shot.[49] Among the millions of doses of vitamin K given to newborns, only one case of anaphylaxis due to an intramuscular vitamin K injection has been reported. This baby was treated and fully recovered.[50]

Is There an Evolutionary Explanation for Vitamin K Deficiency?

It's tempting to look at the relative vitamin K deficiency in human babies and wonder whether there is an evolutionary explanation for the poor placental transport, low breast milk concentration, and limited production by gut bacteria in breastfed babies. Could there have been an evolutionary advantage to low vitamin K in our ancestors, even if it also increased infants' risk of hemorrhage?

"There probably was, but whatever it was, it doesn't exist anymore." That's what Dr. Frank Greer, a neonatologist and professor of pediatrics at the University of Wisconsin School of Medicine and Public Health told me when I posed this question to him.[51] He's been doing research on infant nutrition, including vitamin K, for over 30 years, and he hasn't figured out this mystery. He wonders whether low vitamin K might have protected babies with severe birth trauma and asphyxiation, who today would probably be born by C-section, from developing disordered blood clotting. "But I'm just wildly speculating," he said. "Whatever it is isn't an advantage anymore, because nobody has observed any harm from the vitamin K shot."

Other researchers speculate that perhaps ancestral babies did have a bit more vitamin K, maybe because their moms ate more leafy greens and had more vitamin K–producing gut bacteria.[52]

Although it's unlikely that these factors could completely prevent VKDB, they may have reduced the incidence. It's also important to remember that VKDB is rare, and among all the other dangers facing early human babies, it likely couldn't have exerted much evolutionary pressure. It's interesting to think about evolution and vitamin K, but it doesn't change what modern science has clearly revealed: giving your baby a shot of vitamin K at birth safely and effectively prevents a potentially devastating bleeding disorder.

NEWBORN EYE OINTMENT

Why the Goop?

I adore newborn photos. Whenever a close friend goes into labor, I wait and wait, with anticipation and a bit of anxiety, for the ding of a text with a photo attached. Even though each of these babies brings to the world unique genetics, facial features, and personality, their photos look remarkably similar. They're almost always wrapped in a gender-neutral pink and blue flannel blanket, and their eyes are shiny with a thin layer of ointment. What is up with that eye goop?

To understand why we put ointment on the eyes of newborn babies, we have to turn back to the maternity hospitals of nineteenth-century Europe. One of the major threats to newborn health during this time was an eye infection called neonatal ophthalmia, which developed soon after birth. It was usually caused by gonorrhea, a sexually transmitted disease carried by 35 percent of women giving birth in hospitals at the time and passed from mother to baby during childbirth. Newborn eye infections were such a problem that hospitals had separate wards for babies showing signs of infection. If a woman had gonorrhea, her baby was placed in a crib that was out of reach of the mother's bed, and it was only when a nurse brought the baby to the mother for feeding that the two were allowed to be together.[53] This was before the discovery of antibiotics, so there wasn't an effective treatment for these infections. Gonococcal eye infections (caused by gonorrhea) left nearly a quarter of infected babies with lasting vision damage.

It was the largest cause of blindness in infancy at the time; half of the children in European schools for the blind were there because of gonorrhea.[54]

Dr. Carl Credé, a German obstetrician and director of a maternity hospital in Leipzig where nearly 14 percent of newborn babies developed neonatal ophthalmia, was determined to improve this situation. Recognizing that babies were being infected during labor, Credé's first idea was to attempt to disinfect the vaginas of infected women, and he went so far as to apply douches of carbolic or salicylic acid every 30 minutes while women were in labor. Credé called the results of this experiment "poor and unsatisfactory," and I can only imagine how the laboring women felt about this treatment.[55]

Next Credé tried treating the babies' eyes at birth. He put a single drop of an antiseptic, silver nitrate, in each eye, and he found that it almost completely prevented neonatal infections in babies whose mothers had gonorrhea. Knowing that many women had asymptomatic infections, he began applying silver nitrate drops to the eyes of every baby born in his hospital, and he thankfully retired the douching protocol. In 1883, he reported that of 1,160 babies treated with silver nitrate under his care, there were only two cases of neonatal ophthalmia. He urged other obstetricians and midwives to try this prophylaxis (a medical treatment meant to prevent disease), and it was adopted around the world, saving countless babies from lifelong blindness.[56]

Newborn Eye Prophylaxis in the Modern Era

More than a century later, newborns around the world are still given eye prophylaxis soon after birth, in much the same way that Credé treated the infants in his hospital. Because silver nitrate had the unfortunate side effect of causing eye inflammation, or chemical conjunctivitis, in 50 percent to 60 percent of infants, an antibiotic ointment called erythromycin is now commonly used in many parts of the world and is currently the only drug approved in the United States for newborn eye prophylaxis. In the US, eye prophylaxis has long been considered such an important part of routine newborn care that it is mandated by law in most states.[57]

Not surprisingly, much has changed since Credé's time, so it's fair to consider whether eye prophylaxis still makes sense for today's newborns. Most importantly, the incidence of gonorrhea in the general population has dropped significantly.[58] Less than 1 percent of cases of neonatal ophthalmia are caused by gonorrhea today, although its rarity is in part because of prophylaxis. Most cases are instead caused by chlamydia or other types of bacteria, which are not effectively prevented by erythromycin ointment, and which cause less severe infections than gonorrhea and generally don't cause blindness.[59] We also now have antibiotics, so unlike in Credé's day, infections can be treated (at least until antibiotic resistance renders those medicines ineffective). Nobody wants to see a new baby get an eye infection, but the outcomes aren't nearly as scary as they used to be.

Another thing that has changed is that we have excellent tests to screen for gonorrhea and chlamydia. Ideally, pregnant people who are at risk for these diseases are tested, and if positive, they and their sexual partners are treated before the baby is born. This approach improves the health of both the mother and her partner, decreases the risk of pregnancy complications caused by sexually transmitted diseases, and minimizes the risk to the baby.[60]

Eye prophylaxis was a slam dunk for public health in the time of Credé. Today, it isn't so clear. The problem is not as grave, and with the availability of good screening tests and antibiotics, we have other ways to prevent and treat these infections. Does it still make sense to treat every baby with eye prophylaxis at birth?

The WHO and US Preventive Services Task Force (USPSTF) still maintain that all newborns should receive eye prophylaxis.[61] The USPSTF notes that cases of gonorrhea in the United States have surged over the last decade, increasing from 98 cases per 100,000 people in 2009 to 179 cases per 100,000 in 2018.[62] This is likely an underestimate; the real incidence is thought to be twice this since many people with gonorrhea have no symptoms and don't realize that they're infected.[63] And while universal screening in pregnancy might be a better way to prevent transmission of gonorrhea and chlamydia from mother to baby, the reality is that 15 percent of pregnant people receive no or inadequate prenatal care in the United States and so might not have the opportunity to be tested.[64] Among those who do have prenatal care, some might not be tested because they don't seem to fit the risk profile for sexually transmitted diseases (i.e., new or multiple sex partners, sex partners with other concurrent partners).[65] It's also possible for a person who tested negative early in pregnancy to be infected later on (for example, if either partner is having sex with someone else), and that's not the kind of information that is usually shared at the birth of a baby. These realities leave some babies vulnerable to gonococcal infection at birth.

If a woman has gonorrhea at the time of childbirth, her baby has a 30 percent to 40 percent chance of developing an eye infection caused by the disease.[66] This usually occurs during a vaginal birth, but it can also happen to a baby born by C-section if the fetal membranes were broken before the surgery.[67] Although rare, a gonorrhea infection can be very serious to a baby, and it isn't a fair way to start life. Treatment requires hospitalization and injected or IV antibiotics, and the disease can not only cause permanent vision damage but also serve as an entry point for a systemic infection, which can cause septicemia, arthritis, and/or meningitis.[68]

Universal eye prophylaxis is a public health strategy. It's understood that most babies aren't at risk for gonococcal eye infections. "We are treating a lot of babies so that we don't miss one or two who might otherwise get a devastating disease," Dr. Kristi Watterberg, former chairperson of the AAP's Committee on Fetus and Newborn, told me.[69] The case for eye prophylaxis is that it's an inexpensive, simple treatment, most likely to protect babies born into the least fortunate situations and with limited access to medical care.

However, in 2015, the Canadian Paediatric Society, having previously recommended universal eye prophylaxis for newborns, took the position that it should no longer be required by law. They noted that *Neisseria gonorrhoeae*, the bacteria that causes gonorrhea, is showing increasing resistance to many antibiotics, including erythromycin, so the standard eye goop may be losing efficacy at preventing infections. They also pointed out that newborn eye pro-phylaxis was abandoned in Denmark, Norway, Sweden, and the UK decades ago. Instead of prophylaxis, the Canadian group advocates for universal prenatal testing for gonorrhea and chlamydia, testing and treatment at delivery if necessary, and educating parents about the importance of seeking medical care for any infants with signs of an eye infection.[70]

Medical opinions about eye prophylaxis are also evolving in the United States. In 2018, the AAP's Committee on Infectious Diseas-es said that it's time to reevaluate legal mandates for eye prophy-laxis and focus on prenatal screening as in Canada. However, this opinion is counter to that of the USPSTF and not yet reflected in the recommendations from the Centers for Disease Control and Prevention (CDC). It's also worth noting that public health strat-egies are customized to the public that they serve, and the United States has a higher incidence of gonorrhea and less-coordinated system of maternity care with greater disparities compared with Europe and Canada. For example, in 2018, the incidence of gonor-rhea (in cases per 100,000) was 26 in the European Union and 96 in Canada, compared with 179 in the United States.[71]

Are There Risks to Using Erythromycin Eye Ointment?

Erythromycin eye ointment occasionally causes chemical con-junctivitis, but this resolves on its own within a day or two. I was unable to find an estimate for how common this is, but Dr. Margaret Hammerschlag, director of pediatric infectious diseases at SUNY Downstate Health Sciences University, told me that it's so rare that "it's a non-issue."[72] A local neonatologist told me that he couldn't recall ever seeing a case of it in more than 10 years of practice.[73]

One concern about eye prophylaxis is that it might affect a new baby's vision, perhaps compromising bonding with parents after birth. Studies done in the late 1970s and early 1980s in Colorado observed the behavior of babies and their parents with and without silver nitrate eye drops.[74] Compared with babies who got silver nitrate soon after birth, those who hadn't yet received it had their eyes more wide open and were more likely to visually follow a shape that was passed across their field of vision. What was more interesting, however, was the behavior of the parents. When their baby's eyes were wide open (without silver nitrate), mothers smiled at their babies more, and the dads spent more time looking at their babies, affectionately touching them, picking them up, and talking to them. Eye prophylaxis might not matter much to the baby, because babies can't see that well at birth anyway, and they're using their other senses to get to know us (see chapter 5). But whether a baby's eyes are open may matter to parents. Eyes are a meaningful way of connecting with another person, including a newborn baby, and wide-open eyes seem to invite more of a connection.

Unfortunately, these studies were done using silver nitrate, and there isn't any research to tell us whether these same effects are seen in newborns treated with erythromycin. Regardless, you can ask that your baby's application of eye ointment be delayed until after your first hour and first feeding together. By this time, your baby may be getting sleepy and will have had enough interaction for a while anyway. The AAP supports a one-hour delay in eye prophylaxis.[75]

There are a couple of possible big-picture risks of newborn eye prophylaxis. One is that this widespread use of erythromycin might contribute to the evolution and proliferation of microbes with resistance to these drugs. There is one published report of an outbreak of erythromycin-resistant eye infections (caused by *Staphylococcus aureus*) in a newborn nursery, occurring in Minnesota in the late 1980s.[76] However, I haven't been able to find more recent reports of this problem, and there isn't any direct evidence that use of erythromycin ointment is contributing to the problem of antimicrobial resistance.

Another concern with the prophylactic use of erythromycin eye ointment in newborns is that it might affect the development of their microbiomes. In a newborn baby, the skin and gastrointestinal tract are rapidly colonized with microbes, and antibiotic use at birth or soon after can certainly alter their developing microbiome.[77] However, whether a very small amount of antibiotic ointment applied once to a baby's eyes could affect microbes in the gut would depend on whether it is absorbed systemically (i.e., into the blood) in a sufficient quantity. There is a bit of evidence to suggest that this is plausible. For one thing, research on other eye medications shows that they can be absorbed systemically, though I wasn't able to find reports specific to erythromycin ointment.[78] However, a study conducted in Texas and published in 2000 found that newborns who received erythromycin eye ointment had their first poopy diaper more than two hours earlier than those who received silver nitrate.[79] Erythromycin is known to increase intestinal motility, or contractions of the intestine, including in infants.[80] The finding that erythromycin ointment appeared to speed up the babies' first bowel movement supports the idea that enough of the antibiotic might be absorbed to affect the gut. However, this was an observational study, and as far as I know, it hasn't been replicated.

The idea that erythromycin eye ointment might affect the microbiome is just a hypothesis, and so far we have little evidence to support it. There is interest in this question among microbiome experts,[81] and the only way to resolve it is to study it. I will certainly be watching for more data to be published.

But What About My Baby?

Newborn eye prophylaxis might make sense as a public health measure in some settings, but you're probably more concerned with your own very special baby. If you know you don't have gonorrhea because you were tested in pregnancy, and you're in a trusted, monogamous, long-term relationship, then your baby has little risk of being infected during childbirth. Does it make sense for your newborn to get erythromycin ointment?

I think you could argue this either way, and how you feel about it probably comes down to how you weigh risk and your comfort level with medications. On the one hand, erythromycin ointment is most likely harmless to your baby, and there's a chance, however miniscule, that it might prevent a dangerous eye infection. On the other hand, if you know your baby has a very low risk for infection, it would also be reasonable to opt out of routine eye ointment and treat your baby only if an infection does arise.

There's just one problem with this choice as I've presented it. In many states in the US, it isn't a choice. Eye prophylaxis is often mandated by state law, and it can be difficult to opt out. In my opinion, this is too bad, if only because it makes parents feel powerless at a particularly tender and overwhelming time. If you're interested in declining the erythromycin, you'll want to talk with your obstetrician, pediatrician, and the birthing facility before giving birth so that you know what to expect.

OTHER COMMON NEWBORN PROCEDURES

There are a few other recommended medical procedures that your baby will experience in the first day or two of life:

- *Screening for inherited diseases*: Between 24 and 48 hours after birth, your newborn's heel will be pricked with a needle to collect a few drops of blood. From this small sample, signs of up to 50 inherited or congenital disorders can be detected, including metabolic, hormonal, blood, immune, and enzyme disorders. These are serious diseases that can cause cognitive impairment, slowed growth, seizures, and even death, but early treatment allows children to lead longer and healthier lives.[82]
- *Hearing test*: One to two newborns per 1,000 are born with hearing loss. Hearing is an important way for babies to learn, and hearing loss can get in the way of normal language and cognitive development. With early intervention, such as speech therapy, sign language, and/or cochlear implants, babies can develop normal language skills. The hearing test takes about 5 to 15 minutes, is noninvasive, and can even be completed while your baby is asleep.[83]

- *Congenital heart disease screening*: An astonishing 1 in 100 infants are born with congenital heart disease, and the sooner it is identified, the better the prognosis for treatment. This test is very simple: a painless sensor is placed on the baby's hand or foot to measure heart rate and blood oxygen level. The test should be done at least 24 hours after birth and before discharge from the hospital.[84]

The hepatitis B vaccine is also recommended for newborns within the first day of birth. The rationale behind this vaccine is discussed in detail in appendix B. The newborn screening tests and hepatitis B vaccine detect or prevent rare, but potentially catastrophic, diseases or disorders. Their rarity can sometimes make parents think these procedures are unnecessary interventions, but there's no question that skipping them puts your newborn at greater risk for serious outcomes. Weighing the risks and benefits, the brief discomfort or inconvenience of these procedures is easily outweighed by the peace of mind of knowing that your baby is protected.

RECOMMENDED INFANT HEALTH RESOURCES

Beginning during pregnancy, new parents-to-be have lots of questions about infant health, from the common medical interventions and tests discussed in this chapter to late-night worries about your baby's first cold. Your pediatrician's office is an invaluable resource, especially if it offers an after-hours phone line allowing you to talk with a nurse about your concerns. In addition, I recommend having one of these pediatrician-authored books on hand as a trusted source of information to save yourself from falling into the rabbit hole of internet searching when what you need is a quick and clear answer. And because I know that it's easier to hold a crying baby and a phone than a crying baby and a big reference book, I've also listed some reliable websites for health information.

Books
- *Baby 411: Your Baby, Birth to Age 1* by Dr. Ari Brown and Denise Fields (9th edition, 2019)

- *Caring for Your Baby and Young Child: Birth to Age 5* by the American Academy of Pediatrics (7th edition, 2019)
- *Heading Home with Your Newborn: From Birth to Reality* by Dr. Jennifer Shu and Dr. Laura A. Jana (4th edition, 2020)
- *Mayo Clinic Guide to Your Baby's First Year: From Doctors Who Are Parents, Too!* (2nd edition, 2020)

Websites

- About Kids Health (from The Hospital for Sick Children, Canada): aboutkidshealth.ca
- After the Baby Arrives (from the CDC): cdc.gov/pregnancy/after .html
- Evidence Based Birth: evidencebasedbirth.com
- HealthyChildren (from the AAP): healthychildren.org
- Mayo Clinic: mayoclinic.org
- National Health Service (UK): nhs.uk

4

GETTING TO KNOW YOU

How Newborns Explore, Communicate, and Connect

Baby Isla was born in a Toronto hospital in 2012. Like all human babies—the most neurologically immature of primates at birth—Isla was born with only 30 percent of her adult brain size.[1] In the coming months, she would depend on her parents and other caring adults to meet nearly all her needs. But beginning in the moments after her birth, she also demonstrated an extraordinary ability to explore her new world and connect with the people in it.

The doctor placed Isla on her mother's chest, and Isla looked up brightly at her face. "I kissed her and gave her the welcome-to-the-world speech I had prepared, and all the while she was making kissy lips at me," remembered Isla's mother, Leah. "Then she started wriggling, found my nipple and started nursing. It was amazing. She knew just what to do."[2]

Newborn babies make an incredible transition on their birth days. They pass from a dark uterine home, the only one they've ever known, into a new world. Their senses are bombarded with new sights, sounds, and smells. How do they navigate through this unfamiliar environment and begin to build relationships with the people who will care for them? What makes them ready for this task?

This chapter was not part of my original plan for this book. But I was interested in the science behind practices like holding newborns skin-to-skin, and as I poked around in the literature, I stumbled upon a rich body of scientific research seeking to understand how infants sense the world. I realized that when Cee was an infant, I was so focused on meeting her basic needs (which, honestly, felt like a huge and overwhelming task) and researching the next decision on the horizon that I rarely slowed down enough just to watch her and appreciate how she might be experiencing the world. Learning about the research on infant senses before Max's birth helped me to go about the tasks of meeting his basic needs with a greater sense of ease and calm, mostly because I started from a place of observation and appreciation for him as a full person who was actually pretty good at communicating what he needed. Of course, part of that ease came from the fact that Max was our second baby, and my husband and I were more confident and less likely to second-guess our decisions. But I wish that I'd been able to observe Cee with more wonder and less anxiety, and I think that a better understanding of the science of infant senses would have helped.

Much of the research on babies' senses is centered on how they connect with their mothers. That's in part because mothers are a bridge between babies' intrauterine and postnatal lives, and they are often a primary source of caregiving in the early days. However, the gender bias in this literature also exists because some of these studies are several decades old, when few researchers were paying attention to diverse family structures and how infants connect with fathers or other parent figures. The studies still hold up, and I think they can tell us how newborns connect with any parent, or for that matter, any caring person in their lives.

THE BREAST CRAWL

Leah had watched in awe as her newborn daughter wriggled to her breast, but her behavior was not unusual. The "breast crawl" has been carefully documented in research papers, including a 2011 study led by Swedish researcher Ann-Marie Widström.[3] The paper describes the behavior of 28 newborns placed on their mothers' chests, skin-to-skin, just after birth. In places, it reads like the narration of a wildlife documentary, recording the movements of newborn humans in their native habitat. "Gradually, the reflexes come to life," the story begins.

At birth, the babies in Widström's study cried for a couple of minutes as they were dried off and then placed on their mothers' chests. The mothers were encouraged to talk to their babies and to stroke them, but they were asked not to interfere with their movements. Instead, they watched as their brand-new babies did the work. The babies soon grew quiet and began a characteristic sequence of behaviors:

> In the relaxation phase, the baby did not move any parts of the body, not even the mouth. Soon thereafter, the infant entered an awakening phase and started to make small thrusts with its head and small movements with its shoulders and arms. The awakening phase was followed by an active phase, when the infant showed more distinct activity. Most of the behaviors described . . . (e.g. looking at the breast, looking at the mother's face, rooting movements, hand-to-mouth activity, soliciting sounds) occurred during the active phase . . . During the crawling phase, the infant approached the areola [the darkly pigmented area surrounding the nipple], and during the familiarization phase, the baby became acquainted with the areola by licking and touching the nipple before eventually entering the suckling phase, in which the baby started suckling the breast without help.[4]

Watch a baby working on the breast crawl, and you'll usually see a serene, focused face and deliberate movements. Kym, another mother who told me about her daughter's breast crawl, recalled, "There was no struggling or crying. I have pictures where the look on her face is just really intense and alert."[5] Indeed, among the careful research notations about babies attempting the breast crawl, there is no mention of babies getting fussy or frustrated in the process, although it was noted that some of them fell asleep on the job.

Widström and her colleagues believe that the breast crawl is a chance for babies to gradually, in their own time, become familiar with their environments and to naturally zero in on their evolutionary source of nutrients: their mothers' breasts. "We hypothesize that the full-term healthy infant when skin-to-skin with its mother immediately after birth optimizes its ability to reach self-regulation within the first period of wakefulness when going through the inborn biological program to find the mother's breast," they write.[6]

But not all the babies in Widström's breast crawl study began nursing on their own. All 28 babies actively looked for a maternal breast, but only about two-thirds of them found one. Just over half began nursing on their own, on average an hour after birth. Infants who made more "soliciting sounds" (short, affirmative noises—not cries) and more hand movements from their mothers' breast to their own mouth were more likely to zero in on the areola and begin nursing.

A lot of meaning and magic are attached to the breast crawl, and the internet hosts plenty of claims that it is a requisite part of the natural birth transition, as if actual childbirth isn't enough of a rite of passage for a newborn baby.[7] Although this makes a nice story, I couldn't find any evidence that babies who complete the breast crawl are better off than those simply cradled to their mother's chest and guided to the breast. No breast crawl study has followed babies for more than a day or so to see whether the successful crawlers end up as better feeders or with stronger bonds to their mothers.

But for Leah, watching baby Isla wiggle her way to the breast to begin her first feed gave her a huge sense of relief. She had been anxious about how breastfeeding would go, and seeing Isla take the lead in that first latch was reassuring. For my part, I didn't know about the breast crawl before Cee was born, so I simply held her and helped her latch on, which felt completely natural to me. But by the time Max was born, I'd written the first edition of this book and was so intrigued with the breast crawl that I looked forward to watching him try it. At first, he was quiet and still, his skin still a blue-gray color after being born with his umbilical cord wrapped around his neck. After a few moments and a stimulating rub-down from the nurse, his skin began to pink up, and he looked more alert. Slowly, he started to lift his head, bob it around, and wriggle his body toward my left breast. He opened his mouth wide and latched on to my nipple. Not only did he demonstrate resilience after the trauma of birth, but he also asserted a bit of personal aptitude, and all of this happened within a few minutes. (Had I been more scientific, I would have timed it. For better or worse, I was too busy marveling and breathing a sigh of relief.)

Your baby might be different, and please, if you let your baby try the breast crawl, try not to think of it as some kind of pass-or-fail test. Your baby might just rest, fumble around as if looking for something that is always out of reach, or clumsily bob up and down on the nipple. Your baby might very well need some help getting started with feeding, and that's totally fine. And for any number of reasons, you might not be able to hold your baby skin-to-skin after birth, and that's okay, too. You and your baby are in this together for the long haul; you'll both play a part in getting to know each other in your own way.

Whether you try the breast crawl with your baby, and regardless of how it goes, the fact that babies are born with a drive to search and find their source of nutrition within minutes of birth is impressive. Human infants can't stand up after a few minutes and wobble around to follow their mothers like newborn foals, or physically cling to their mothers for protection like the newborns of many other primate species.[8] And yet, they do have the ability to sleuth out a breast and to move toward it. What I love about the breast crawl is that it highlights how much newborn babies know at birth, and how quickly they collect and process information about their worlds. And if we take the time to observe them, then we get to appreciate just how tuned into their worlds they are, through all their senses.

A NEWBORN'S SENSE OF TOUCH

Of all the senses, touch is the earliest to develop in fetal life. Beginning at around 8.5 weeks of gestation, touch receptors appear around the fetus's mouth, and then, between 10.5 and 12 weeks, on the palms of the hands and soles of the feet. Finally, by 20 weeks, touch receptors spread throughout the surface of the skin. In newborns, a light touch in the palm of the hand activates more parts of the brain than a flash of light, the sound of a woman's voice, or a Chopin piano piece.[9] Touch is powerful.

Newborn babies exhibit a characteristic set of motor reflexes—involuntary movements that occur either spontaneously or in response to certain stimuli.[10] Many of these are dependent on touch receptors, and they're evaluated at birth to test for normal nerve and brain activity. For example, if you stroke a baby's cheek, she'll turn toward your touch. If you touch the roof of her mouth, she'll begin sucking. Both of these reflexes are essential to helping her find the nipple and begin feeding. Another reflex is grasping: stroke the palm of a baby's hand, and she will close her fingers around yours. The grasp reflex appears around 16 weeks of gestation, but the sucking reflex does not begin until week 32. This is why a very premature baby might be able to tightly grasp your finger but be unable to feed effectively on her own.[11]

The newborn reflexes may occur involuntarily, but they're not empty actions. For example, newborns seem to be able to differentiate their own touch from that of another person, because the rooting reflex is much stronger when someone else touches a baby's cheek than when a baby brushes her own cheek.[12]

Newborns are also able to collect information about an object's shape and texture by exploring it with their hands and mouth. In one study, researchers found that if they placed a small wooden cylinder in the palms of 2- to 4-day-old infants, they grasped it tightly. If they presented the same cylinder to them repeatedly, they held it for less and less time, presumably because they lost interest in it (or got tired!). But then, they placed a small wooden prism—with hard edges instead of rounded ones—in the babies' hands, and they held

Newborn reflexes

REFLEX NAME	HOW TO ELICIT THE REFLEX
Rooting reflex	Stroke the corner of the baby's mouth, and she will turn her head toward your touch, with mouth open.
Sucking reflex	Touch the roof of the baby's mouth, and she will begin sucking.
Moro reflex	Hold the baby facing up, supporting her head. Let the head drop slightly (1–2 cm) but suddenly. The baby will startle, arms and legs extending and fingers spreading, and then she'll pull her limbs back in. You may also observe this reflex (even in a sleeping baby) in response to a loud noise, sudden movement, or even the baby's own cry.
Grasping reflex (palmar and plantar)	Stroke the palm of the baby's hand, and she will close her fingers around yours (palmar grasp). Likewise, if you stroke the middle of the foot, from heel to toe, her toes will curl around your finger (plantar grasp).
Stepping reflex	Hold the baby upright with her feet touching a solid surface. She will move her feet in an alternating stepping motion.

Note: All of these reflexes indicate normal neurological development and are tested as part of the newborn exam.

it for much longer, exploring the new shape with their sense of touch.[13] (This works both ways: whether you start with a cylinder or a prism, a baby will spend more time with the less familiar object.) This experiment has been repeated in premature babies as young as 28 weeks of gestation.[14] Even at this age, though underdeveloped in so many ways, babies are able to collect information about the world with their hands.

In another experiment, newborn babies were presented with two objects identical in size, shape, and texture. Both were small cylinders covered in the same soft rubber, but underneath, one was made of hard plastic and the other of squishy sponge. The cylinders were attached to pressure transducers that recorded the frequency and strength of the babies' "squeeze" on the objects. When these objects were placed, one at a time, in the babies' hands, they spent more time squeezing the hard object. But when the objects were gently placed in their mouth, they much preferred the squishy one, squeezing it more than the hard one.[15] You can imagine how newborns' oral preference for soft things could be helpful for getting started with feeding.

Babies are sensitive to touch, and as parents, we know this intuitively. Holding, stroking, patting—these gentle touches can communicate so much care to a baby. Touch can even help lessen a newborn's reaction to what is normally a painful procedure. In a randomized controlled trial, newborns held snugly skin-to-skin with their moms during a routine heel stick procedure (to collect blood for newborn screening) cried 82 percent less than those swaddled in a blanket in a bassinet.[16] As parents, we get lots of time to try different ways of soothing our babies, and we can learn to use the power of touch to comfort them as they adapt to the world.

WHAT DOES A NEWBORN HEAR?

Newborns know their mothers' voices. Even at 38 weeks, still in utero, a fetus can differentiate its mother's voice from that of other women. Play a recording of mom reading a poem, and the fetus's heart rate increases by five beats per minute. Play the sound of a strange woman reading the same poem, and its heart rate *decreases* by four beats per minute.[17] At birth, babies also prefer the sound of their native language to a foreign one, as well as the sound of a familiar story—one that their mothers recited many times during pregnancy—to a new one.[18]

In one experiment, newborn babies were given headphones and pacifiers that worked like little remote controls. If the babies sucked faster on the pacifier, it turned on a recording of their own mother reading Dr. Seuss's *And To Think That I Saw It on Mulberry Street*. Slower sucking turned on a recording of another woman reading the same story. In this study, 8 of 10 babies preferentially used the pacifier to tune in to their own mother's voice.[19]

There's much less research on how fetuses and newborns respond to fathers' voices. However, a 2014 study found that fetuses in late pregnancy (about 38 weeks) had a similar increase in heart rate when listening to recordings of their mothers or fathers reading the story *Bambi*, indicating that either parent's voice can capture the attention of a fetus in utero. The study found that after birth, newborns preferred their mothers' voices over their fathers' voices, measured by how often the infants turned their heads toward each voice.[20] The person carrying the pregnancy has an obvious advantage here; they've spent nine long months in constant contact with the developing fetus, who eavesdropped on their every word. The voices of other parents are usually less prevalent, and more muffled, on the prenatal soundtrack. Regardless, babies will learn, with exposure, to recognize the voices of those who care for them after birth, including those who become parents through adoption or surrogacy. That fetuses are listening to the voices they hear in utero might inspire nonpregnant parents to talk, read, or sing to their partners' bellies, or provide recordings of their voices to a surrogate mother carrying the pregnancy.

Newborns prefer familiar sounds, and these sounds may also help them to feel less stressed. In one study, 5-day-old babies were subjected to a heel stick. During the procedure, one group heard the sound of a maternal heartbeat, as it sounds in utero. Another heard a Japanese drum at the same volume and rhythm as the heartbeat, but with a different frequency of sound. The third group heard no sound. After the heel stick, all the babies showed a rise in salivary cortisol, a marker of physiological stress, but the group that heard the maternal heartbeat had a much smaller rise in the stress hormone.[21] What is familiar is comforting. This isn't surprising, because we know it to be true for ourselves as well.

WHAT DOES A NEWBORN SEE?

Vision is the least developed of the senses at birth. Visual development requires maturation of different parts of the eye as well as integration with multiple parts of the brain, and this happens rapidly over the first year of life. At birth, visual acuity, or clearness of vision, is not very good.[22] This is why newborns pay more attention to high-contrast, black-and-white images; they simply can't see more subtle gradations in brightness.

Visual acuity is assessed in older children and adults with those familiar eye charts that have letters of decreasing size. In infants, it is measured using cards with black lines of varying thickness, called the Teller Acuity Test.[23] A baby is shown a gray card with black-and-white stripes on either the left or the right side of the card, and if she can distinguish the stripes, she'll preferentially gaze toward them. Studies show that newborns can see high-contrast lines as thin as one-sixteenth of an inch, giving them a visual acuity of about 20/400 at birth. (For many children, their vision won't mature to 20/20 or better until 3 to 5 years of age.) Newborns also can't fully distinguish most colors at birth, although color vision quickly improves in the baby's first year.[24]

Toy companies have caught on to newborns' attention to high-contrast images and thus market lots of newborn-specific toys with bold black-and-white patterns, but there's no evidence that you need to provide this extra visual stimulation for your baby. Your home has plenty of natural black and white patterns: the stripes of window blinds, the rotation of a ceiling fan, and the edge of a doorway.

Babies are even more interested in human faces, particularly when they come with interactions from caring adults. In a classic 1975 study, infants just a few minutes old were shown several simple black-and-white images.[25] One had the features of a human face, two were scrambled versions (eyes at the bottom, mouth at the top, for example), and a blank version had just the outline of the face. The images were moved in an arc across each baby's line

Normal visual development in infants

AGE	CHARACTERISTICS OF VISUAL DEVELOPMENT
Birth	• Innate preference for human face • Sensitive to bright lights; sees best in dim lighting • Can resolve and pays attention to high contrast black-and-white patterns • Will follow slow-moving, close objects or faces • Able to see most colors
2 months	• Holds eye contact and studies the features of your face • Watches people from a distance • Begins to study own hands (called "hand regard"), marking early visual-motor integration
3 months	• Shifts from auditory to visual dominance • Seeks your attention by making eye contact and moving limbs • Shows more interest in simple objects, though still prefers faces
4–6 months	• Loves seeing the faces of other babies and own mirror image • Shows recognition of familiar people on sight alone and smiles in response • Sees an object of interest and will reach for and grasp it, then bring it closer for inspection • Shows understanding that an object hidden from view still exists (object permanence)
6–12 months	• Understands that a two-dimensional picture can represent an object • Follows the direction of your gaze to see what you are seeing • Reads the expression on your face to look for positive or negative responses to a situation • Shows an understanding of connections between words and objects • Looks from an object to a parent to communicate wanting it • Shows a toy to a parent to share in the wonder of it

Source: P. Glass, "Development of the Visual System and Implications for Early Intervention," *Infants and Young Children* 15, no. 1 (2002): 1–10.

Note: Vision is the least mature sense at birth, but visual development occurs rapidly within the first year of life. Visual acuity, or clearness of vision (assessed in adults with eye charts of different-sized letters), is about 20/400 at birth and doesn't reach 20/20 until 3 to 5 years of age.

of sight. When they were shown the correct face image, the babies were more likely to turn their heads to follow it, compared with the scrambled or blank image. What is most extraordinary is that these infant research subjects preferred the image of a human face even though they hadn't seen a real one yet; all the people in the delivery room were decked out in facemasks, hair caps, and gowns. (It tells you something about standard practices in a 1970s delivery room that this experiment was conducted before the babies even met their mothers.) More recent studies have replicated the finding that newborns have an innate preference for the human face.[26] Your face will best hold your baby's attention if it's within about 10 inches of her face, and dim lighting will encourage your baby to open her eyes and look around.[27]

Newborns also prefer a face that is socially engaged. If you show newborns two photos of the same woman, one with eyes open and one with eyes shut, they much prefer the one with eyes open.[28] They will also choose a face with a direct gaze, available for eye contact, over one with eyes averted to the side.[29] And newborns quickly learn to identify their own mothers' faces; within hours of birth, they recognize and prefer the face of their mother to that of a stranger. However, a newborn's ability to recognize the right mother's face is not based on visual information alone; it also requires having heard her voice. In one experiment, mothers were asked not to talk to their newborns at all but to otherwise care for them as usual. (Can you imagine how unnatural this would feel?) Several hours after birth, these babies were shown photos of their mothers and a stranger, and they showed no preference for their mom's face.[30]

These studies underscore the importance of eye contact and talking with our infants from the first day of their lives. And when you think about it, none of this is surprising. After all, it's how we humans best get to know one another: face-to-face, in conversation. Why should babies be any different? They're watching, listening, and making neural connections between the pattern of our faces and our familiar voices, often known from the womb. If it feels awkward talking to your newborn, know that there's no need to wax poetic or impart wisdom to your infant. Just narrating what you're doing, like describing the steps of a diaper change or naming the parts of her body as you bathe them, is plenty.

WHAT DOES A NEWBORN BABY SMELL?

The importance of a newborn's sense of smell was demonstrated in an elegant study of 30 mothers and babies that was published in the *Lancet* in 1994.[31] After each baby was born, one of the mother's breasts was washed and dried using an odorless soap. The baby was then placed on the mother's chest, nose at midline and eyes at nipple level, and observed as she wiggled toward one or the other breast. All 30 of the babies found their chosen nipple on their own and made mouth contact with it, and just 5 of them required some help latching on. Which breast did the babies choose? Of the 30 babies, 22 chose the unwashed breast, indicating a preference for the breast that carried the mother's odors. The same test repeated at 3 to 4 days of age revealed the same preference, showing that the baby was still using scent to find the breast. However, the older babies had clearly honed their skills; it took them, on average, just two minutes of "crawling" to start nursing, whereas the newborns had needed an average of 50 minutes to begin to nurse.[32]

Newborn babies also like the smell of amniotic fluid, which they've been swimming in, tasting, and inhaling up until birth. In one study, the smell of amniotic fluid significantly decreased the amount of time newborns spent crying when separated from their mothers.[33] In another, when one of the mother's breasts was rubbed with amniotic fluid, most 2- to 5-day-old babies crawled toward that breast rather than the untreated one. However, at 5 to 10 days old, the babies chose the natural-smelling breast over the one treated with amniotic fluid.[34] Around this age, researchers have also found that breastfed babies preferentially choose the smell of their own mothers' breasts over a stranger's. They're even attracted to the smell of their mothers' armpits![35]

The odors and flavors in both amniotic fluid and breast milk are affected by the mother's diet. For example, when women ate garlic during pregnancy, their amniotic fluid (obtained by amniocentesis) was deemed garlicky by a panel of adult sniffers. The same was true of breast milk from garlic-eating mothers.[36] Babies might shift their smell preference from amniotic fluid to breast milk a few days after birth because they're homing in on the specific flavors present in breast milk, which are associated with the satisfaction of a full belly.

IT GOES BOTH WAYS: GETTING TO KNOW YOUR BABY

We've marveled at how babies relate to their world and begin to learn about their important people, but what about us? We're using our senses to learn about our new babies as well, and studies show that new parents are really good, right off the bat, at identifying their new babies. For example, one study conducted a few days after birth found that mothers with their eyes and nose covered were able to pick out their own babies solely by stroking the back of their hands.[37] When the mothers wore gloves, they were no longer able to identify their babies.

Before I became a parent, I thought that all newborns looked the same. But when I had my own babies, I realized that this isn't the case at all. Science supports my epiphany. In one study, both mothers and fathers, after being with their new babies for at least 10 minutes, could almost always pick their own newborn's face from a lineup of seven new-baby photos. Fathers were just as good as mothers in this study at identifying their babies, which was notable because the study was conducted in Israel in the 1980s, when fathers visited their new babies in the hospital only once per day. In the study, they hadn't seen their babies for an average of 16 hours before taking this test, whereas the mothers were much more involved in their babies' care and had spent more time with them.[38]

Sweet newborn baby smell draws us to our newborns as well. We don't know exactly why newborns smell so good. It could be amniotic fluid, the vernix coating their skin, or a combination of several chemical signals. Whatever it is, we like it. Researchers have used functional magnetic resonance imaging (fMRI) to measure brain activity in women while smelling the odor on a shirt worn by an unfamiliar 2-day-old infant. They found that the smell triggered activation of reward pathways mediated by dopamine in all of the women, but this activity was stronger among new mothers in several areas of the brain.[39] Such signaling may help moms be more attuned to their own newborn's particular smell. In an older study, when mothers were handed three onesies worn that day by newborns in the hospital nursery, 100 percent could pick out the shirt from their own baby.[40]

Just as parents quickly learn to recognize their babies by touch, sight, and smell, they're also good at identifying them by the sounds of their cries. A 2013 study published in *Nature Communications* found that parents can pick out the sound of their own babies' cries from a sampler of crying infant recordings with 90 percent accuracy, and mothers and fathers scored equally well on this parental cry perception test.[41] This result was different from that found in several earlier studies, which had concluded that mothers were better at recognizing their babies' cries and thus were assumed to somehow naturally and instinctually be more attuned to their babies' needs.[42] But the more recent study included an important variable in their analysis: how much time parents spent with their infants. The authors found that this was the most important variable in determining parents' accuracy in identifying their babies' cries. Not surprising; it takes time to get to know the idiosyncrasies of another person. With time and experience, you'll learn to distinguish your baby's different cries, with distinct pitches and patterns communicating specific messages: feed me, change me, rock me, help me sleep.

FROM BIOLOGY TO BOND

So far, the focus of this chapter has been biology: how our babies sense us and the world, how we sense them, and how these biological forces bring us together in the first days after birth. It is human attraction in its purest form. However, it's only the beginning. Building a real relationship with our babies is a much longer and more complex process, but observing and trying to understand your baby is the first step in building that relationship.

At first glance, newborns may seem to be capable of little more than eating, burping, crying, sleeping, and pooping, and indeed, they spend most of their time engaged in one of these activities. But at the same time, they are experiencing the world with intense sensitivity. That sensitivity allows them to learn at a rapid rate, but it can also be overwhelming, and newborns are easily overstimulated.

Knowing this is a reminder that we don't need to add stimulation to a newborn's world. Your quiet, familiar voice is enough sound. Your face, gazing at your baby, is enough to see. Filtered light through a window is enough light and color. Resting against your chest is enough touch. And even this may be too much sometimes. Babies sometimes turn their faces away from stimulation if it becomes too much, and that's a sign that they need a break from sensory input. If you don't get that message, they'll probably use their most effective means of communication—crying. All of this is normal, everyday stuff for a baby; what matters is how we respond.

You can use your knowledge of your baby's senses to soothe her and help her to regulate stress. For example, a randomized trial compared newborns' salivary cortisol as a measure of stress in response to two soothing methods. In one, the infants were given a gentle massage by a researcher trained in infant massage, but she didn't make eye contact with or talk to the baby. These babies had increased cortisol after the massage—they appeared to be *more* stressed. The second soothing method also included massage, but the researcher talked to the baby and interacted using eye contact throughout. She also adapted her touch to each infant's cues, moving on to massage a different part of the body if the baby seemed uncomfortable, for example. In these babies, salivary cortisol went down, indicating less stress.[43] Engaging your baby's senses in a gentle and responsive way can help her feel more comfortable in the world.

Observing infants is key to understanding their needs and re-sponding appropriately. Even everyday activities, like diaper chang-es, dressing, and bathing, can be stressful to a new baby, but you can mitigate this by showing sensitivity to your baby's signals.[44] One study, for example, scored maternal sensitivity and cooper-ation during a baby's bath. How well did the mother observe and respond to the baby's signals? Did she follow the baby's pace and attention in the bath, or did she constantly begin new interactions and activities? The baby's salivary cortisol was measured after get-ting out of the bath as an indication of how stressful the transition was. All the babies showed a rise in cortisol after the bath, but the ones whose mothers were more sensitive and cooperative during bath time recovered to normal cortisol levels more quickly.[45]

This sensitivity to your baby—reading her cues and responding appropriately—takes time and some trial and error to learn. And it depends a lot on the baby, too. Some babies are more reactive and need more help in regulating their physiological and emotional states than others. Regardless, sensitive observation and respon-siveness can help you and your baby get through the day with less stress and more connection.

When Cee was born in 2010, there was a lot of evangelism around "attachment parenting," a philosophy promoted by William and Martha Sears, a pediatrician and nurse whose books have sold millions of copies around the world. They tell us that in order to build strong attachment relationships with our babies, we should embrace several practices, such as baby-wearing, bed sharing, and breastfeeding. These practices can work beautifully for many fam-ilies, except when they don't. As we'll discuss later in the book, breastfeeding certainly has benefits, but for a variety of reasons, it doesn't work well in all families. Likewise, bed sharing may be lovely for some, but there are very real concerns about its safety, and many parents find they sleep better when the baby is in her own bed. As for baby-wearing, carrying my babies snuggled to my chest (or strapped on my back when they were older) was often both sweet and practical, but sometimes my back ached from the constant weight of carrying another human, or my shirt drenched with sweat under the heat of said human, and I was glad to have a stroller as another option. Still, the prescriptive practices of attachment parenting fueled the so-called "mommy wars" and led too many of us to spend far too much time worrying that we were failing our babies.[46]

There's actually little evidence that these parenting practices alone do much to promote bonding or build attachment, but there is abundant evidence that parental sensitivity does.[47] This is why I emphasize the importance of observation and responsiveness—they form the foundation of attachment. A secure attachment relationship means that your baby knows you can be relied on when she needs you, and in having this security she is empowered to explore on her own as she grows, knowing that she can always come back to you. You soothe your baby when she's upset; you feed her when she's hungry; and when she smiles at you, you smile back. This is how we listen to what babies are saying to us, in their own ways, and respond in the best ways we can to let them know that we care.

Babies are fascinating. They already know and can do so much when they come into our care, and they learn more every day from the world and from us. Just as much as it's a responsibility and a lot of work to care for them, it is a privilege to watch them grow. Sensitive observation, starting from the first day of life, rewards us with moments of marvel, a calmer baby, and a stronger relationship.

5

VACCINES AND YOUR CHILD

Making Science-Based Decisions

Soon after they were married, my paternal grandparents had three boys in quick succession. The first was my father, Richard, born in October of 1948. Next came Frankie, 18 months later, and then within the next year, Larry. Three boys in the span of three years—close in age and close friends.

In the black-and-white photographs from their childhood, it is Frankie's face that I study the closest. Frankie died when he was 6 years old, so I know him only through photographs. He is smiling in nearly every one.

As a kid, I never thought very much about Frankie. I figured that the death of a child wasn't unusual during the "olden days." My grandparents had seven children in all, and in my childish mind, it seemed like that might compensate somehow for the loss of Frankie. But then I became a mother myself, and when I think about losing one of my children, I feel like my heart might explode. I told my grandmother this as we sat down to talk about Frankie in 2014, and she nodded. "Each one is special," she said.[1]

My grandmother, Margaret Green, was just a few months shy of 90 years old when I interviewed her about Frankie. Her mind was still sharp and her hugs firm. She died a couple of years later, so I'm grateful that I had the opportunity to talk with her about Frankie,

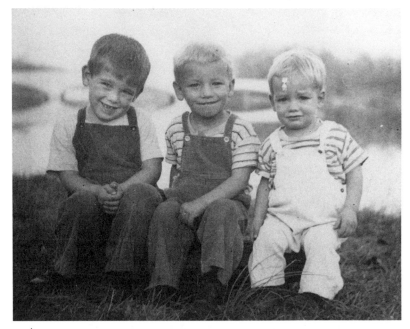

Three brothers (*from left to right*): Richard, Frankie, and Larry Green, circa 1953 or 1954, in Princeton, New Jersey. Frankie died in 1956, at age 6, of encephalitis caused by measles.

Source: Photo by Margaret Green, used with permission.

because she was the only person on earth who could tell me what he was like. My grandfather passed away almost 25 years ago, and my own father died a few years later. Margaret's small apartment was packed with shoeboxes full of photographs and old letters, but most of the memories of Frankie were carried close to her heart. So we sat and talked about him, a little boy who never grew up, the uncle I never met.

My grandmother remembered how Frankie adored his older brother, my father, and how one day they played hooky from school together, entertaining themselves in the town of Princeton, New Jersey. They must have been in first grade and kindergarten then, and according to my grandmother, they got in "mild trouble" for this mischief, but really she was grateful for her boys' spirit and close friendship. She remembered how desperately Frankie wanted a pair of toy six-shooter pistols the Christmas before he died, and how when she suggested that the right-shaped stick might work instead, he sweetly shook his head and said, "No, Mom, I don't think so." My grandparents gave Frankie his six-shooters that Christmas, and Margaret is thankful they did. And she remembers Frankie riding a merry-go-round for the first time, beaming at her with each turn: "I can still see his face, and that happy, happy smile."

Margaret also remembered when all three boys came down with measles in May of 1956. How lucky, the neighbors said, for the boys to get measles at the same time. In those days, measles was a rite of passage, a part of childhood. Nearly every child suffered through it at some point, but once they had, they would be immune for life. Parents often intentionally exposed their children at "measles parties" so that the whole playgroup would get the disease over with at once. It wasn't hard to infect a group of children quickly, intentionally or not. Measles is one of the most contagious pathogens on earth. Those infected can spread the virus for several days before and after the characteristic rash appears. With every cough or sneeze, the virus flies around in airborne droplets, where it can survive, suspended in air, for two hours.[2]

Having measles meant being stuck at home for a couple of weeks, at first with symptoms that seemed like little more than a common cold—cough and runny nose—but then progressing to a fever and often an eye infection. Several days later, measles clearly announced itself as an itchy rash that spread all over the body.[3] There was no doubt that this was uncomfortable, but "it was also a special time," my grandmother told me. The boys got ice cream and presents, and she read them lots of books. "And the three of them were together," she said.

After a week or so, the boys appeared to be getting better, their rashes subsiding. My grandfather had just been offered a job at Johns Hopkins, and he drove to Baltimore to look for a place for the family to live. Margaret continued nursing the boys back to health on her own.

She vividly remembers the night when Frankie's case of measles took a turn for the worse. "I settled all three boys down to bed. These were sick boys, but they were recuperating quickly, and they were all on their way to being completely well. I got Frankie settled and got him his glass of water and then went to bed myself. But as I was getting ready for bed, I heard this kind of funny noise and went in just to check one last time. He was draped halfway out of the bed, which was strange, and I rushed over to pick him up and get him settled and realized that he was unconscious."

Frankie never woke up. He suffered from one of the cruelest complications of measles: encephalitis, or inflammation of the brain. Sometimes it is a primary infection, occurring at the same time as the rash phase of the illness. The measles virus invades the brain and replicates there, directly damaging neurons and causing brain swelling and inflammation. Frankie probably died of a second type of measles encephalitis, which appears when the patient seems to be on the mend. In this case, the infection damages the myelin sheath that coats nerves and allows conduction of nervous signals. Both types of encephalitis are very serious, even with the best modern medical care. Those who survive often suffer permanent brain damage, hearing loss, and seizure disorders.[4]

As Margaret remembers it, Frankie was hospitalized, in a coma, for about a week before he died. Finally, after an urgent call from the hospital, she left the other children with a neighbor and hurried to see her boy. The pediatrician met her at the door to say that Frankie had already died. Then the doctor took Margaret to her own home and put her to bed in her guest room to let the news sink in before she went back to Richard and Larry and tried to explain where their brother had gone.

It's an unfathomable loss, and although it came as a shock to my grandparents and Frankie's brothers, his death, sadly, wasn't unusual. Frankie's was one of more than 600,000 reported cases of measles in the United States in 1956.[5] Actual numbers were probably much higher, thought to reach three to four million cases per year, since many went unreported. In the decades before the introduction of the measles vaccine, about 48,000 people were hospitalized with measles each year; 7,000 had seizures, 2,000 suffered permanent deafness or brain damage, and 500 died.[6] Every year. In 1956, Frankie was one of 530 lives lost to measles in the United States, most of them children.[7]

There are other, more common, complications of measles, like pneumonia in one out of every 20 infections and ear infections in one in 10. As Dr. C. Everett Koop, pediatric surgeon and former US Surgeon General, recalled, "Children would have measles . . . and they would develop an infection in their ear . . . Out of their ear would drip, for years, a foul-smelling gray-green pus, and it lasted until some of them were adults."[8]

Measles was a routine part of childhood, but that didn't make it any less scary. And had Frankie been born just a few years later, his death could have been prevented by the measles vaccine.

When my grandmother heard that some in my generation of parents worry about the safety of vaccines, she thought about Frankie. She also lived through polio outbreaks that crippled children and rubella outbreaks that caused thousands of miscarriages, stillbirths, and birth defects, and she had a hard time understanding why parents today hesitate to vaccinate their kids. And I think that we can't discuss the current vaccine controversies without first acknowledging the history of parenting under the dark cloud of deadly childhood diseases, just a couple of generations ago.

If my grandmother's pain over her lost child seems too much like ancient history, we need only look to 2020 for a stark reminder of the power and pain that can be wrought by a microscopic virus. As I write this in December of 2020, we are in the midst of the global COVID-19 pandemic, caused by a coronavirus previously unknown to humans. We've seen firsthand what happens when a pathogen against which we have no protection—not from natural immunity nor a vaccine—tears around the globe. COVID-19 has already infected more than 70 million and robbed more than 1.5 million people of their lives, and it shows no sign of loosening its grip on the world. It has derailed the education of children, thrown our families into chaos, ground economies to a halt, and deprived us of the basic human needs of socialization and a hug every so often. And while we have some tools for stemming the destructive tide of this pandemic, like wearing masks, staying physically distant from others, and testing and tracing infections, it is this week's approval of the first COVID-19 vaccine to be available in the United States, UK, and Canada that finally gives us a light at the end of the long pandemic tunnel. But we know it will take months to vaccinate enough people to bring this pandemic under control, and in the meantime, thousands are dying each day from this virus.[9] Today, I'm writing from a place of uncertainty and sadness, somber respect for infectious disease, and gratitude for the hard work of scientists to bring us a vaccine.

One of the few saving graces of COVID-19 is that it has largely spared children from serious infection.[10] That's unusual for infectious diseases, which are generally more dangerous for children. Such is certainly the case for measles, which is why we can be so grateful that we have a vaccine to prevent it.

DEVELOPMENT OF THE MEASLES VACCINE

Even as Frankie fought and lost his bout with measles, scientists were hard at work on a vaccine. Harvard professor John Enders headed an infectious disease laboratory at Children's Medical Center in Boston. Dr. Enders was a brilliant virologist, and he was also a generous humanitarian.[11] He never tried to patent his work, and he believed that vaccine development benefited from shared knowledge and collaboration with fellow scientists. In 1954, he and two colleagues were awarded the Nobel Prize in Physiology or Medicine for their work on growing poliovirus in cell culture, techniques that led to the development of the polio vaccine.[12] While this was a great accomplishment, Enders was actually more interested in measles. He considered it the more pressing problem since, worldwide, 8 million children died of measles each year.[13]

So Enders and his colleagues set out to collect samples of the measles virus from boys at a boarding school in Boston, where close living quarters meant frequent outbreaks. The scientists finally isolated a strain of measles swabbed from the throat of an 11-year-old boy named David Edmonston, and this same strain led to the measles vaccine.[14]

Scientists first worked on getting the isolated measles virus to grow in human cell cultures, but to make a safe vaccine, they needed to attenuate, or weaken, it. Since humans are the only natural host for the measles virus, they started growing their strain of measles in chick embryo cell cultures. In this environment, the virus had to change to survive, making it progressively weaker in humans. After three years of work, the attenuated Edmonston strain of measles was ready to test for its potential as a vaccine. It was first tested in monkeys, and then Enders and his research fellows tested it on themselves. They all showed a strong antibody response and had no adverse effects. Subsequent tests on children showed that they were completely protected in the next outbreak, although many developed a high fever and rash in response to the new vaccine.[15]

True to his nature, Enders shared the vaccine material with scientists around the country and encouraged them to work on refining the vaccine and getting it into production. Maurice Hilleman, who headed virological research at Merck Pharmaceuticals, was ultimately responsible for developing the measles vaccine in use today. When he started working with Enders's vaccine material, he considered it "toxic as hell," given the high incidence of side effects.[16] Hilleman felt pressured to get the vaccine out quickly, but he insisted on taking the time to make several modifications to reduce side effects and ensure the vaccine was safe. His version of the vaccine was first licensed for use in the United States in 1963, and a further attenuated version followed in 1968. In 1971, the measles vaccine was incorporated into the MMR combination shot, which also includes vaccines for mumps and rubella.[17]

The measles vaccine was remarkably successful. Two doses of MMR induce immunity to measles in 99 percent of people, and after release of the vaccine, the incidence of measles dropped dramatically.[18] By 2000, measles was considered by the World Health

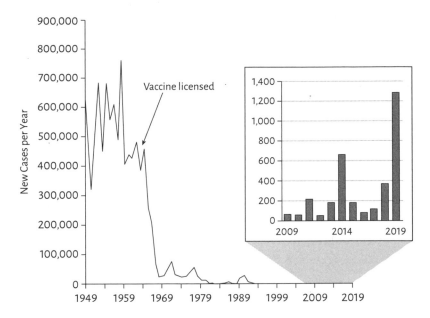

Measles cases reported in the United States between 1949 and 2019. The measles vaccine was first licensed in 1963.

Sources: Centers for Disease Control and Prevention (CDC), "MMWR Summary of Notifiable Diseases, United States, 1993," *Morbidity and Mortality Weekly Report* (*MMWR*) 42, no. 53 (1994): 1–73; National Center for Health Statistics, *Health, United States, 2018* (Hyattsville, MD: CDC, 2019); CDC, "Measles Cases and Outbreaks," last updated November 5, 2020, https://www.cdc.gov/measles/cases-outbreaks.html.

Organization to be eliminated from the United States, meaning that the disease no longer existed continuously in the country, though it was occasionally imported from other countries, causing isolated cases and small outbreaks.[19] Between 2000 and 2010, there were an average of 71 cases per year, almost always traced to international travel.[20] The virus would enter the United States with infected individuals, who were usually unvaccinated and unaware they were carrying the disease since the early symptoms can seem like a common cold. But with most of the population vaccinated, measles couldn't spread very far, and outbreaks were rare and easily contained.

In the past decade, however, we've witnessed a disturbing trend of larger and more frequent measles outbreaks around the United States. With more parents opting out of immunizing their kids, clusters of unvaccinated people have allowed the disease to spread. In 2011, there were 220 cases of measles in the United States, many imported by travelers from Europe, especially France, which was experiencing a large outbreak that year. In 2014, there were 667 cases, more than half concentrated in unvaccinated Amish communities in Ohio.[21] If parents in mainstream communities felt insulated from that outbreak, any illusion of protection was shattered by a 2015 outbreak thought to originate at Disneyland, the amusement park in southern California. That outbreak spread to seven US states, as well as Canada and Mexico, ultimately causing 147 confirmed cases of measles.[22]

And the measles outbreaks keep growing. There were 1,282 cases in the United States in 2019—the worst year for measles in this country since 1992—again centered in unvaccinated communities.[23] The situation is even worse in Europe, where large, sustained outbreaks caused the United Kingdom, Albania, Czechia, and Greece to lose their measles elimination status in 2018.[24]

The irony is that as some American and European parents are choosing not to vaccinate their kids, children in other parts of the world continue to suffer due to lack of vaccines. Worldwide, measles killed 142,300 people in 2018, most of them children under 5 years of age. That number was down from 535,600 in 2000 due to a concerted effort to get the MMR vaccine to more children, though progress has stalled and the number of cases has increased in the last few years. About 99 percent of measles deaths occur in Africa, the Middle East, and Southeast Asia, where the percentage of children receiving the first dose of measles vaccine lies between 74 percent and 89 percent, leaving too many vulnerable to infection to control the spread of the disease.[25]

Because of the highly effective vaccine, measles is entirely preventable, and it's theoretically possible that it could be eradicated from the earth, as smallpox was. But this requires that the vaccine is accessible to all children worldwide, and that their parents see its value and agree to vaccinate them.

HOW VACCINES HAVE CHANGED CHILDHOOD

Frankie died of measles, but my father and his brother fully recovered. During the course of their infections, their immune systems responded by developing immune cells that produced antibodies to the measles virus. These cells would stay around for the rest of their lives, ready to respond to another exposure to measles. Of course, this immunity came at a price, given the high incidence of complications of the disease, which my dad's family knew all too well.

The measles vaccine also induces immunity to the measles virus, but it does so in a much gentler way, without the risks that come with a full-blown infection. Vaccines contain components of the infectious pathogen, weakened in some way. Our immune systems still recognize the pathogen and produce antibodies to fight it, but it doesn't make us sick. A vaccine effectively educates our immune systems about the pathogen so that if we are exposed to the disease in the future, we're ready to respond. With a vaccine, we not only acquire immunity without getting sick, but we also get to control the amount of exposure to the pathogen by using the smallest dose possible, and we get to choose the timing of exposure, aiming to induce immunity as soon as a child's immune system can safely and effectively do so. This is why we give babies so many vaccines—because infections are usually most dangerous in the first years of life. If we waited until later in childhood to vaccinate our children, we would be leaving them unprotected from diseases during a very vulnerable time.

Measles is but one of at least 14 diseases that your child may be vaccinated against in the first two years of life.[26] As each vaccine was approved and recommended for children, there was a subsequent drop in the numbers of both cases and deaths, most reaching a 99 percent to 100 percent decrease compared with pre-vaccine levels.[27] For these diseases, the historical numbers of cases and deaths—each one representing someone's beloved child—are so large that they are incomprehensible to us today. Each year in the United States, the modern childhood vaccination schedule is thought to prevent nearly 20 million cases of disease and 42,000 deaths and to save $69 billion in direct medical costs and indirect costs to society due to missed work, lost productivity, and disability.[28]

Sometimes people who question the value of vaccines point out that prior to vaccines, the death toll from infectious diseases had already been dramatically reduced due to improved nutrition, sanitation, clean water, antibiotics, and advances in medical care. This is true. However, these advances still left an awful lot of people suffering through these diseases and their complications, and although modern medicine and public health measures may have improved the chances of survival, children like Frankie were still dying.

We also have examples of vaccines that have been introduced in just the past few decades, a time when there haven't been overwhelming advances in sanitation or nutrition. *Haemophilus influenzae* type b (Hib) used to be the leading cause of bacterial meningitis—when bacteria invade the fluid surrounding the brain and spinal cord—in children under 5, infecting 20,000 children and killing approximately 1,000 per year in the United States before the introduction of the vaccine in 1985. The vaccine has decreased the incidence of this terrifying disease by 99 percent.[29] A vaccine against pneumococcal bacteria, which can cause pneumonia, meningitis, and blood infections, decreased the incidence of these invasive bacterial infections by 91 percent after its introduction for infants in 2000.[30] Pneumococcal bacteria also cause ear infections, and the addition of this vaccine to the routine childhood schedule has helped to make ear infections far less common in young children. That's saving children from the discomfort of ear infections and their parents from the inconvenience and economic hardship of lost work, and it's reducing antibiotic prescriptions in children—an example of the preventative power of vaccines and their potential to reduce our dependence on these precious medicines in an era of growing resistance to antibiotics.[31]

Rotavirus can cause severe diarrhea and vomiting in babies and young children. It doesn't discriminate; regardless of income, hygiene, nutrition, or water source, it infects nearly every child in the world within the first years of life (although severity of symptoms varies). In developing countries, where children often don't have access to good medical care, rotavirus is thought to kill half a million children each year.[32] In the United States, modern medicine saves most babies from dying of rotavirus, but before the vaccine, rotavirus still caused more than 600,000 doctor and emergency room visits, 55,000 to 70,000 hospital admissions, and 20 to 60 deaths per year—a heavy burden.[33] By 2010, there was a 96 percent decrease in the number of hospitalizations for rotavirus infections in US children under 2 years of age.[34] Improvements in hygiene or nutrition didn't prevent these illnesses; the vaccine did.

The success of vaccines means that many previously common diseases are now rare, but even with less disease circulating in our communities, unvaccinated children remain vulnerable. This is why doctors are more concerned when they see a sick child who isn't vaccinated; they know they're more likely to have a disease like Hib or an invasive pneumococcal infection. As a result, doctors are likely to run more tests, like a blood culture, lumbar puncture, and chest X-ray, and to start antibiotic treatment before waiting for the results, because these diseases can become so dangerous so quickly. Likewise, an unvaccinated child is 60 times more likely to contract measles and up to 20 times more likely to catch pertussis (whooping cough) than a vaccinated child, and communities with more unvaccinated kids are more likely to see outbreaks of vaccine-preventable diseases.[35] In the rare case that a vaccinated child still gets measles or pertussis (because no vaccine works 100 percent of the time for every person), studies show the illness will be less severe, of shorter duration, and less likely to result in hospitalization.[36]

Would it be more natural to let children fight off these diseases on their own, without the protection of vaccines? Maybe, but that's an awfully cruel side of nature to entertain. It also isn't natural to fly around in airplanes, carrying diseases around the globe, or congregate in crowded spaces like commuter trains, indoor playgrounds, and movie theaters, and this unnatural behavior puts us at constant risk for outbreaks. Without vaccines, more healthy children like Frankie would be dying, and we would spend much more of our time and energy nursing sick kids, quarantining them to protect the more vulnerable, and worrying about whether they'd survive the latest bout of illness. We'd use more antibiotics, with increasing rates of resistance. We'd be nursing more sick kids in NICUs and PICUs, trying to keep them hydrated, nourished, and breathing, and billing insurance companies or taxpayers for each day in the hospital. This model of handling disease is far more costly in lives, suffering, and dollars (and far more profitable for pharmaceutical companies) than the model of preventive medicine.

With vaccines, our children are intentionally exposed to germs in a controlled, well-tested way, strengthening their immune systems without the risk of the "natural" illness. Without them, we would return to the days of countrywide outbreaks of childhood diseases, and encephalitis sneaking in to steal away a little boy just after bedtime. Maybe that's more natural, but it sure isn't better.

HOW VACCINES PROTECT COMMUNITIES

High rates of vaccination protect our communities from the spread of disease. If most of the people in a population are vaccinated, then the odds are low that a single infected individual will infect others and cause a large outbreak. This is called herd immunity, and it's vitally important to public health because it is how we protect people who can't be vaccinated, including infants too young to receive vaccines, people who are allergic to vaccine ingredients, and those who are immunocompromised.

For each vaccine-preventable disease, we can estimate a threshold for herd immunity, or the percentage of the population that must either have natural immunity or be vaccinated to protect it from an outbreak. This threshold depends on how quickly the disease can spread from one person to another, how well the vaccine works (a small percentage of people won't respond to it), and how unvaccinated people are distributed in the population. If there are pockets with a lot of unvaccinated individuals, the chances of an infection spreading are greater.[37] For most diseases, we need about 80 percent to 85 percent of the population to be vaccinated to minimize outbreaks and protect susceptible individuals. Measles and pertussis have higher thresholds for herd immunity, around 92 percent to 95 percent, because they spread so easily.[38] In the COVID-19 pandemic, we've seen firsthand what happens when there is no natural or vaccine-induced immunity to a virus; as it spread in 2020, there was no place on the planet where it couldn't find a vulnerable host to infect.

In 2008, a 7-year-old unvaccinated boy returned from a trip to Switzerland to his home in San Diego, his parents not realizing he was infected with measles. If this little boy had encountered only people who were immune to measles, as 99 percent of vaccinated folks are, then he might have been the only person affected. Instead, his unvaccinated brother and sister were immediately infected, and then, between the three of them, they went to school, dance class, their pediatrician's office, and finally the emergency room. Several unvaccinated classmates were infected, as were children in the waiting room of the doctor's office—three infants too young to be vaccinated and one 2-year-old whose parents had decided to delay the MMR shot. Other children infected in this outbreak went to swimming pools, grocery stores, indoor playgrounds, and the circus. In these everyday activities, hundreds of people were exposed. Twelve children were ultimately infected with measles, all of them unvaccinated, and one infant was hospitalized.[39]

The San Diego boy's immediate community included many families who had chosen not to vaccinate their children. Together, they had low herd immunity, and that's what allowed this outbreak to spread as much as it did. The larger San Diego community had good vaccine coverage, with 97 percent of children receiving the MMR shot. Between high vaccination rates and the 21-day quarantine of infected kids, this outbreak couldn't spread further.[40] The story was different in 1989–91 when the United States experienced large outbreaks of measles, resulting in 55,000 cases and 136 deaths, mostly in unvaccinated preschoolers. At that time, vaccination rates in preschool-aged children were between 60 percent and 70 percent, far below the threshold for herd immunity.[41]

Today, we see time and time again that the communities hardest hit by measles are those with low immunization rates, and therefore less protection from herd immunity. That was evident in the 2018 and 2019 outbreaks in New York State, which began with a handful of unvaccinated travelers who brought measles infections from Israel, itself in the midst of a large outbreak. Across New York State, 98 percent of children were vaccinated, so most communities in the state were untouched by the virus. But when the virus landed in tight-knit Orthodox Jewish communities, where only 77 percent of children were vaccinated for measles, it could take root and spread, ultimately infecting 1,114 people. Most of those infected were unvaccinated, and about 10 percent required hospitalization because of complications from the disease. Many were babies too young to receive the measles vaccine.[42] So long as measles is rampant around the world, all it takes is one international traveler returning to a community with clusters of unvaccinated people to begin another outbreak.[43]

We also get to see herd immunity at work when a new vaccine is introduced. For example, the varicella, or chickenpox, vaccine is given between 12 and 15 months of age. For the first few months of life, maternal antibodies that passed across the placenta during pregnancy provide some protection to the baby, but when that wears off, babies are susceptible to varicella until they can be vaccinated. After introduction of the varicella vaccine in 1996, the incidence of varicella in unvaccinated infants less than 12 months old decreased by 90 percent.[44] These babies were benefiting from indirect protection by the vaccine, probably because their older siblings and playmates were vaccinated, so there was less varicella virus circulating around them. Likewise, after the rotavirus vaccine was introduced, rates of rotavirus infection dropped in unvaccinated children and even in adults.[45] The vaccine was directly protecting babies, and the people around them were benefiting indirectly, through herd immunity.

These are just a couple of examples. Herd immunity is happening all the time, with nearly every vaccine, in our immediate families and communities.[46] Of course, herd immunity also protects children whose parents choose not to vaccinate them because of personal or philosophical beliefs. This is a good thing; nobody would wish a preventable disease on anyone, let alone innocent children. But it's also a dangerous gamble for these families, and a community can sustain only so many of these "free-riders" (that's the academic term) before it is susceptible to a serious outbreak, threatening not just those who are unvaccinated by choice (or rather, their parents' choice) but everyone who doesn't have immunity to the disease, including young babies and those unable to be vaccinated for medical reasons. In a paper on herd immunity, researchers aptly commented, "A single unvaccinated child in a community of vaccinated children holds a strategically opportunistic high ground, protected from risk of disease by herd immunity while avoiding risk of exceedingly rare adverse events associated with vaccination. Yet, when too many parents want their child to be that child, the entire community is affected."[47] Parents who choose not to vaccinate their children might point out how naturally healthy they are, but they forget that the health their children enjoy rests on the protection provided by herd immunity. Vaccinating your child means contributing to the collective health of your community and protecting those more vulnerable.

UNDERSTANDING VACCINE RISKS

Although the benefits of vaccines are tremendous, they do carry some risk. But then again, nothing we do is 100 percent safe. Every car ride is a risk of collision; every meal a possible choking emergency; and every trip to the playground a potential broken bone. But of course, we still drive our cars, eat food, and let our children play, because we know that the benefits of these choices far outweigh their risks. Likewise, when we vaccinate our children, we want to understand the risks, ensure that they're smaller than the benefits, and minimize them as much as possible.

The risks of side effects or reactions from vaccines are well understood. They're listed on the CDC website and on the information sheets given to parents with each vaccine their child receives. And for the vast majority of people, the benefits of vaccine protection are much greater than the risks.

Consider the MMR shot. We've been using MMR for nearly 60 years, which has given researchers plenty of time to collect data on its side effects. A 2012 Cochrane review summarized data from more than 60 high-quality studies, including 15 million children.[48] This and other studies show that the MMR vaccine can cause common but mild side effects, like fever in 1 in 7 children, and a short-term rash in 1 in 20. There are rarer side effects, such as febrile seizure in 1 in 3,000 to 4,000 MMR recipients and a temporary blood clotting disorder in 1 in 40,000.[49] Febrile seizures can occur any time a child has a fever, and they aren't thought to be dangerous—although they can be very scary to parents.[50] However, these side effects are miniscule compared with the risks of the diseases themselves: for measles, a 1 in 20 chance of pneumonia and 1 in 1,000 chance of encephalitis; for mumps, a 1 in 7 chance of meningitis and, in boys and men, a 1 in 2 chance of testicular inflammation, often leading to atrophy; and for rubella infection during the first 20 weeks of pregnancy, almost certain harm to the fetus, causing miscarriage or major birth defects.[51]

Most other vaccines have only mild side effects. Very rarely a child will have a severe allergic reaction to a vaccine component, but the chances of this are about one in a million,[52] and there is a similar risk of allergic reaction every time your baby tries a new food or medicine. Still, the risks and benefits of vaccines can seem so intangible that it can be daunting to try to tally them up on our own. A helpful resource is the National Academy of Medicine (previously called the Institute of Medicine, or IOM), a private, non-profit organization that works outside the government to bring together unbiased, interdisciplinary, volunteer experts to assess health concerns. Their reports—each hundreds of pages long—are available to the public online, and they've assessed a number of questions regarding vaccines, including concerns about ingredients in vaccines and links with autism, SIDS, and immune dysfunction. In 2013, an IOM committee, specifically selected to exclude anyone who had financial ties to the pharmaceutical industry or had previously served on a federal vaccine committee, assessed the safety of the entire childhood immunization schedule; it found no evidence that the current schedule isn't safe.[53]

What the IOM did was systematically review all the research on vaccines to reach a scientific consensus. This is vital, because among the thousands of scientific publications on vaccine safety, there are a few concerning reports, and these will often be cherry-picked by anti-vaccine activists to build a story about the dangers of vaccines. Sometimes they're preliminary studies, sometimes their methodology is shoddy, and sometimes they're simply misinterpreted. In their reviews, the IOM committees included these papers but put them in context with the rest of the research to arrive at a scientific consensus.

In the appendixes of this book, I address several specific vaccine safety questions and concerns, including why the hepatitis B vaccine is recommended at birth in the United States (appendix B), the worry that we give too many vaccines too soon (appendix C), and concerns about links with autism (appendix D), the risk of SIDS (appendix E), and aluminum in vaccines (appendix F).

VACCINE TESTING AND SAFETY MONITORING

What about when a new vaccine is introduced? How do we know that its benefits will outweigh the risks? Let's walk through this process by looking at the history of the rotavirus vaccine, the most recent addition to the childhood schedule.

Globally, rotavirus kills nearly 500,000 children each year, and developing a vaccine has been a research priority since the 1970s. That research started in labs at universities and research institutes, where scientists worked out the intricate details of how the virus worked and developed potential vaccine strains. By the 1990s, the leading vaccine candidate, called RotaShield, was being tested by the pharmaceutical company Wyeth.[54] Before the Food and Drug Administration allows a new vaccine to be tested in humans, it first needs to be shown to be safe and effective in animals. Then it is tested in three phases of human clinical trials, the third phase including thousands of people tracked for several years. Any new childhood vaccine must be tested in children along with the rest of the immunization schedule to ensure that it works and is safe not only on its own but also in the context of other vaccines. If the trials go well, the company submits its data to the FDA.[55]

If the FDA approves a vaccine, the CDC works with an external group of advisors, the Advisory Committee on Immunization Practices (ACIP), to determine whether it makes sense to give the vaccine in the United States, given the prevalence and seriousness of the disease, and at what age it should be given. ACIP reviews vaccine recommendations every year, not just looking at new vaccines but also monitoring any new data on established vaccines.[56]

In early 1999, ACIP recommended that RotaShield be added to the immunization schedule for babies.[57] At this point, clinical trials including more than 10,000 babies showed that the vaccine worked very well and had an excellent safety profile. However, Wyeth, the FDA, and ACIP noted that a few infants had developed an intestinal condition called intussusception soon after getting the vaccine. This is a serious but treatable problem in which one part of the intestine slides into another part, like sections of a telescope. In the clinical trials, the intussusception cases appeared to be coincidental, but everyone would be keeping an eye on this when the vaccine was introduced.

After a vaccine is introduced, one way that its safety is monitored is through the Vaccine Adverse Event Reporting System (VAERS). VAERS allows anyone—usually doctors or parents—to submit reports of any outcome that is suspected of being related to a vaccination. The CDC and FDA watch VAERS for patterns that seem unusual, recognizing that many reports aren't necessarily linked by causation but could be coincidences.[58]

Within a few months of the release of RotaShield, VAERS had received 12 reports of intussusception. The CDC immediately began an investigation, and it suspended use of RotaShield in July of 1999. By October, Wyeth had taken it off the market. After the dust settled, it was estimated that RotaShield caused intussusception in about 1 in 10,000 vaccinated babies.[59]

The example of RotaShield illustrates a couple of things. First, the clinical trials and the multiple agencies that review safety and efficacy data serve a vital role, but they aren't foolproof. A 1 in 10,000 risk won't show up in a clinical trial of 10,000 children, but at least we know that any risk not identified at that stage is very rare. Second, after RotaShield was approved, the problem of intussusception was rapidly detected through VAERS, and the CDC acted quickly to investigate it and stop distribution of the vaccine. The system worked.

This didn't solve the problem of rotavirus, however. Without a vaccine, rotavirus would continue hospitalizing tens of thousands of babies in the United States. RotaShield's demise also had a significant global impact. Once US officials said that it wasn't safe enough for American children, it didn't have much of a chance internationally, where it might have provided much greater benefit even with the risk of intussusception. "I'd love to use it, we have 100,000 deaths each year of this disease. But when I have the first case of intussusception I will be tarnished in the press for having accepted a vaccine that was rejected in the US," one senior Indian health official said.[60]

Two more rotavirus vaccines were developed after RotaShield. This time the clinical trials were much larger, including more than 60,000 infants, to be more certain about intussusception risks. The newer vaccines showed no increased risk of intussusception and were recommended by the CDC and WHO for use around the world. Still, everyone kept watching for intussusception, and again, vaccine safety monitoring systems were used to carefully track the outcomes from these new vaccines. The CDC runs a program called the Vaccine Safety Datalink (VSD), a network of managed health care systems that tracks data on nine million people.[61] Researchers used the VSD system, along with additional safety data from the FDA, and concluded in 2014 that both new vaccines appeared to cause intussusception at a rate of 1 to 5 in 100,000 infants, a lower rate than RotaShield.[62] But as more studies followed up on this question, they failed to find a link between intussusception and the rotavirus vaccine. A 2019 Cochrane review—a meta-analysis combining 55 studies that included more than 200,000 children—found no increased risk of serious side effects, including intussusception, associated with the rotavirus vaccines.[63]

That's a relief, for sure. But the story of the rotavirus vaccine demonstrates the rigor that goes into testing new vaccines and then continuously monitoring them to ensure that they're safe. Every vaccine is held to this high standard for both safety and efficacy to ensure that the benefits of administering it to children far outweigh the risks, as was finally clear in the case of the rotavirus vaccine.[64]

Everyone—you, me, and the CDC—wants to know whether a vaccine has a serious side effect, however rare. The sheer number of acronyms in this section is a testament to the multiple regulatory agencies and monitoring systems that do their best to ensure the safety of every vaccine. So much work, data collection, and safeguarding is happening beneath the surface, and history has shown that when problems arise, they are quickly addressed. If you're worried about adverse effects of vaccines, understand that our public health agencies are too. They know they can't afford a major vaccine safety crisis, and none of us can afford to go back to the pre-vaccine era.

WHY WE STRUGGLE WITH THE CHOICE TO VACCINATE

Janie Oyakawa, an occupational therapist, lives in Prosper, Texas, with her husband and their six children.[65] A traumatic childbirth experience seeded her distrust in modern medicine, and she found like-minded "crunchy" moms, especially online, who were also re-nouncing mainstream practices in favor of parenting more natu-rally. She stopped vaccinating her kids. Her sixth child didn't see a pediatrician until she was almost a year old. Janie wrote on her blog, "I was very proud of that fact. I wasn't necessarily 'anti-vax,' I was just . . . done."[66] And she was worried. She read several books and internet sources that left her feeling uneasy about vaccine in-gredients, a possible link with autism, and the sheer number of vaccines babies get these days.

Janie was not alone in her concerns. Although the vast majority of parents in the United States continue to fully vaccinate their children, most also report being at least a little worried about vac-cines.[67] Why do we parents struggle so much with this decision?

I posed that question to University of Oregon psychologist Paul Slovic, who has studied the science of how we make decisions for his entire career, spanning nearly six decades.[68] He and others have found that there are essentially two ways that we approach decisions: fast and slow.[69] Dr. Slovic explained that we rely on the fast system for most of the choices we make throughout our days. "We make most decisions intuitively, on the basis of gut feeling, influenced by thoughts of the outcome, stories we may have heard, images that flick through our minds in a fraction of a second that carry feeling," he said. "The fast system was adaptive for millions of years over the evolution of humans. It was the way we dealt with risk before we had science."

I asked Slovic about the choice to vaccinate my child. If I relied on my fast system, with all its evolutionary success, to tell me whether I should let a nurse stick a needle delivering some element of an infectious disease into my baby's soft thigh . . .

Slovic interrupted me: "You wouldn't do it."

But, he told me, "Over eons of time, the brain evolved to pro-cess information in another way—in an analytic, deliberate way, and to create scientific methods to enhance our knowledge." For decisions about vaccinating our children, we need to call on this slow system. This is the system that helps us to weigh evidence in a rational way and to understand things that we can't see or feel in the moment.

Without science and critical thinking, we are easily led astray by common cognitive biases. For example, we tend to perceive something that is natural as safer than something that is made by humans, even though nature is full of toxins and brutal tragedies. We don't like to take risks that may carry unknown side effects, even if very rare, but we'll willingly take greater risks when we believe we understand and can control the potential for harm. One of the riskiest choices that we make in our daily lives is to drive a car, but we feel comfortable with this risk because it is familiar, understandable, and, to some extent, controllable (or at least we like to think that it is).[70]

And then there are the stories. For example, in your search for information about vaccines, you might happen upon a story of a child who was vaccinated and began to show signs of autism soon after. Even if you rationally know that the story might be untrue and that correlation is not the same as causation, it still plants a seed of doubt. "Stories carry a very powerful emotional impact. The perception of risk resides in us as a feeling as much as it does as a result of some analysis of the evidence, but we need to be aware that this feeling can be very misleading," Dr. Slovic told me.[71]

On the internet, it is far easier to find stories of adverse reactions—true or not—than it is to find stories of uneventful vaccinations, which happen in the thousands every single day, or stories of children dying of vaccine-preventable diseases. This inflates our perception of the risks of vaccines while at the same time deflating our perception of the risk of the disease.

Of course, the stories that flickered through parents' minds a few generations ago were quite different. My grandmother's stories were of Frankie and the family friends who had suffered from polio. A generation later, my parents were part of the counterculture movement of the 1960s and 1970s. They questioned authority, distrusted the government, and sought to raise their children naturally. I was born at home and breastfed. My parents raised grass-fed beef cows, tended a huge vegetable garden, and made farm-fresh, homemade baby food using a hand-cranked grinder. But there was no question that we would be vaccinated. My mother doesn't recall so much as a discussion about it. My hunch is that the consequences of these diseases, including the measles that killed Frankie, were still fresh in my parents' minds. But now, the stories of suffering from vaccine-preventable diseases are trapped in history books and lost with our grandparents. Vaccines are victims of their own success. When they work, nothing happens. There's no story.

My parents also didn't have the internet. If they had, they might have made a different choice. There is just as much misinformation as accurate information on the web, and it can be difficult to distinguish between the two. If you're worried about vaccines, you can find confirmation for that concern online, even if it isn't backed by good science. And being human, we tend to judge information as more reliable if it is consistent with our preexisting beliefs rather than to seek out information that challenges our beliefs.[72] As parents, we have to hold a very high standard for quality of vaccine information.

Janie Oyakawa eventually reversed her decision on vaccines, but it took both an emotional connection and critical thinking for her to reassess her beliefs. She developed an online friendship with a tattooed, baby-wearing mama who tended backyard chickens, but then she discovered that her new friend was also a vaccine researcher at Johns Hopkins. That gave her an image—a story—of a proudly vaccinating parent that contradicted the others in her head. Then she attended a vaccine lecture by a chiropractor and saw how he cultivated fear in his audience. Janie wasn't fooled. "The latent science major" in her started finding holes in his argument, and she knew it was time to reassess her decision on vaccines.[73]

What Janie could finally appreciate was that science gave her the tools to cut through the emotions and stories and to evaluate the evidence for what it really is. Science uses rigorous methods to test vaccines and investigate concerns that arise. We ask researchers to invest years of advanced training in infectious diseases, immunol-

HOW TO FIND RELIABLE INFORMATION
ABOUT VACCINES

If you search for vaccine information, you will find a mix of reliable and unreliable sources. The internet is an equal-opportunity platform: anyone can put information there without backing it up with good science. Books aren't necessarily better. They're often not fact-checked, and anyone can self-publish or find a publisher that is more concerned with book sales than scientific accuracy. It's up to you to figure out whether you're looking at a reliable source or misinformation. Here are some tips for finding good information about vaccines.

Look for sources that . . .

- Are written by or include the perspective of experts with some credentials—such as an MD or PhD in a related field—and who are affiliated with a university or other respected institution.

- Cite peer-reviewed studies. Use PubMed or Google Scholar to check whether a study's findings are consistent with how the research was represented to you. Look for human studies; beware of the use of animal or cell culture studies to prove a point.

- Are current.

- Don't rely on anecdotes, no matter how compelling.

- Aren't selling products like supplements, e-books, or e-courses claiming to unlock the secrets to good health.

- Don't promote conspiracy theories or ideas completely different from the scientific consensus. (If so, ask yourself, If this source is correct, how many thousands of smart people must be wrong? How likely is this?)

And finally . . .

- Don't assume that a website with a neutral-sounding name offers unbiased information. For example, the National Vaccine Information Center (NVIC) is notorious for spreading anti-vaccine messages and inaccurate information.

- If you're not sure about a source, consider bringing the information you've found to your pediatrician. He or she can help you assess its accuracy.

RECOMMENDED READING ON VACCINES

I have only one chapter in this book to discuss vaccines, but there is so much more to learn. You can spend years trying to navigate around the Internet looking for reliable information on vaccines and decades reading the scientific literature. I've found it most helpful to sit down with a good book that explores the science, politics, and history of vaccines in detail. Here are some of my favorites:

- *Vaccines Did Not Cause Rachel's Autism: My Journey as a Vaccine Scientist, Pediatrician, and Autism Dad* by Peter J. Hotez (2018)
- *On Immunity: An Inoculation* by Eula Biss (2015)
- *The Panic Virus: A True Story of Medicine, Science, and Fear* by Seth Mnookin (2011)
- *Vaccines and Your Child: Separating Fact from Fiction* by Paul A. Offit and Charlotte A. Moser (2011)
- *Deadly Choices: How the Anti-Vaccine Movement Threatens Us All* by Paul A. Offit (2010)
- *Vaccine: The Controversial Story of Medicine's Greatest Lifesaver* by Arthur Allen (2008)

If you're looking for vaccine information on the internet, start with these sites:

- Centers for Disease Control and Prevention (CDC), Vaccines and Immunizations page, cdc.gov/vaccines
- The History of Vaccines, historyofvaccines.org
- The National Academies Press (search for vaccine topics of interest to access reports), nap.edu
- Institute for Vaccine Safety at Johns Hopkins Bloomberg School of Public Health, vaccinesafety.edu
- Vaccine Education Center of the Children's Hospital of Philadelphia, https://www.chop.edu/centers-programs/vaccine-education-center

ogy, and epidemiology, and even then, other scientists check their work and test it again. They do study after study to ensure vaccine safety and efficacy. When Janie focused on the science, she found very clear evidence that the benefits of vaccinating far outweigh the risks, and she felt confident getting her kids caught up on their vaccinations.

For me, choosing to vaccinate my children is about a few things. It's a tiny tribute to Frankie and his short life. It's an acknowledgement of what a privilege it is to be a parent in an era when we can protect our children and our communities from terrifying diseases. It's also because I know that, despite reading hundreds of scientific papers on vaccines, I'm not a vaccine expert. The experts in this field have devoted their lives to the science of disease prevention, and they're also parents who vaccinate their own children without hesitation. They go to work every day to improve the health of children, and I trust their knowledge on vaccines. I will not look to celebrities or conspiracy theorists for advice about the health of my children. Most of all, my choice to vaccinate is about critical thinking and evaluation of the scientific evidence. Among all of the topics I cover in this book, the choice to vaccinate on schedule is backed by the strongest, clearest, biggest pile of evidence. It's one of the best things you can do to protect the health of your child and others in your community.

6

SLEEP SAFELY, SLEEP SWEETLY
Safety at Night and the Bed Sharing Debate

Cee was 3 weeks old when I felt like I was being swallowed into a fog of cumulative sleep deprivation. My mother had returned to her own life several thousand miles away, and my husband was flying around the country for job interviews. I was facing newborn night duty alone, and between diaper changes and breastfeeding and soothing Cee back to sleep, I found myself piecing together my sleep in 30-minute increments.

During one endless night, after I'd nursed Cee in my bed in the wee hours, we fell asleep together. I woke to find sunlight streaming across the bed and my baby still sleeping sweetly next to me, her eyelids newborn translucent.

"Crap!" I thought. "We're cosleeping. I don't want to cosleep!"

But it happened again the next night and the night after that. When my husband returned home, he was relegated to sleeping on the couch, while Cee and I shared our bed.

With Cee in my bed, I felt more rested, and I no longer resented her frequent night awakenings. Sleeping next to her made it easier to breastfeed during the night, and she often went back to sleep without a fuss when she could feel my body close to hers.

Still, I was uneasy about sleeping with Cee. I worried that I might roll onto her or pull a blanket over her head during the long night, layered with consciousness and unconsciousness and the border-land between. With this at the back of my mind, I slept fitfully next to her, fretting about the position of her small body and mine. I often woke to feel my heart pounding like a jackhammer, and the only thing that would calm it was seeing the gentle rise and fall of Cee's chest as she breathed peacefully in her sleep.

I called my mom to ask her advice. Besides being my mother and a wise woman in general, she worked for a social service agency supporting mothers and babies, so she talked about babies' sleep as part of her job.

"Alice, the safest place for Cee to sleep is in her own bed," she said, her voice gentle and empathetic, but also firm.

She was right, I thought, and from then on, I put Cee back in her bassinet next to my bed after our nighttime feedings. I was more comfortable with this arrangement, and it turned out that Cee adjusted easily to sleeping on her own. Our flirtation with cosleeping was over, and my husband happily reclaimed his side of our bed.

Cosleeping wasn't a good fit for us, but many parents feel differently. A few months after Cee was born, my friend Esmee gave birth to a little boy named Miller. Miller slept in the crook of Esmee's arm on the night of his birth. Home from the hospital, he joined his parents in their bed, and two years later, they still couldn't imagine it any other way. Esmee believed that the safest place for her baby to sleep was right next to her, and she didn't care what her mother or anyone else had to say about the matter.[1]

Even now, as my two children sleep soundly in their own rooms and only rarely need me in the night, I am still fascinated with the debate around where babies should sleep. Peek into bedrooms around the world, and you'll find babies spending the night snuggled against their mamas, often breastfeeding on demand through the night. You'll also find babies sleeping in cribs in their own rooms, many going for long stretches without parental contact. Can we say which one is better? I dove into the research to answer this and other questions about sleep safety.

Before I go on, let me clarify the vocabulary around this topic. The term *cosleeping* means different things to different people. To avoid confusion, I will use the term *bed sharing* to specifically mean that the baby and at least one parent sleep in the same bed and *room sharing* to mean that they sleep in the same room but on a different surface.

INFANT SLEEP IN CULTURAL CONTEXT

We can't talk about infant sleep practices without first putting them into cultural context. After all, cribs are a relatively recent invention in the history of human parenting. Our evolutionary foremothers probably slept with their babies out of necessity, to keep them warm and safe. And in modern times, many mothers and babies around the world still sleep in close proximity—in the same bed, or at least the same room.

For example, a 1992 study in the journal *Developmental Psychology* reported that among Mayan families in rural Guatemala, it was normal for a mother to share her bed with her youngest child, breastfeeding as needed through the night.[2] After two or three years, a new baby might be born, and the toddler would move into a bed with the father or siblings. When researchers told these Mayan families that babies in the United States often sleep alone, they were horrified. "Most of the families regarded their sleeping arrangements as the only reasonable way for a baby and parents to sleep," the researchers wrote. In these families, nobody slept alone. Even a widowed grandmother or single auntie was likely to have a child in her bed.

On the other side of the world, in a more industrialized and technologically advanced society, it's traditional for Japanese babies to sleep with their mothers as well—if not in the same bed (usually a futon mat on the floor), then at least in the same room. The sleep habits of Japanese families reflect their priorities for relationships. Historically, Japanese culture has valued the mother-child bond, as opposed to the husband-wife bond, as the "most intimate family relationship." Fathers worked long hours and often preferred to sleep in a separate room away from the rest of the family in order to be rested for the workday.[3] Even as gender roles have become more egalitarian in Japan, with more mothers working outside the home and sharing the work of parenting with their partners, bed sharing and room sharing remain very common.[4] Shared sleep is the norm in many non-Western countries.

But in Western countries, the cultural norm over the past several generations has been for babies to sleep alone in a crib—at least that's the norm you see in mainstream parenting books and websites. The usual advice is for newborns to sleep in a bassinet in their parents' bedroom to make frequent night feedings easier, but then to move to a crib in their own bedroom as soon as possible. Western cultures tend to value a baby's ability to fall asleep independently and to sleep through the night on his own. In many families, if bed sharing occurs, it is not because parents *want* to sleep with their children but because they live in tight quarters, they've exhausted other options for coping with sleep problems, or they've conceded to their children's preference for staying close at night.[5]

But while solo sleep may appear to be the mainstream cultural norm, bed sharing remains common in Western countries. Recent estimates from Europe have put the rate of at least occasional bed sharing between about a quarter to half of infants. In Australia, bed sharing rates are documented as high as 40 percent to 80 percent. In the United States, a 2015 survey found that 61 percent of mothers say they bed-share at least some of the time, and 24 percent say they bed-share often or always.[6] In some families, it's also cultural; bed sharing is much more common among the Maori of New Zealand and Australian Aboriginal families, and in the United States, it's more common in African American, Hispanic, and Asian families. Some parents, like Esmee and her husband, are also choosing to bed-share as part of their parenting philosophy, believing it will build a closer bond with their baby. Others do it, not out of any kind of philosophical conviction, but just because they find that it works to get their family more sleep, and few things matter more during the early days and weeks of parenting.

123

When did parents start putting babies to sleep in cribs? There isn't a clear answer to this question, but scholars have identified several possible reasons for this shift.[7] For example, there are horrifying accounts, going back 500 years, of poor mothers in urban Europe confessing to priests that they intentionally smothered their babies in bed because they simply couldn't afford to feed another child. Lacking reliable birth control methods, this was the only way they could control their family size. The Church responded by campaigning against bed sharing, and some countries banned it. In the following centuries, there was an increased emphasis on the concept of "romantic love" and a greater desire for parental privacy. By the early twentieth century, Freud was also sounding the alarm that exposing infants to sex might cause lasting psychological harm, and having multiple bedrooms in a family home was seen as an indicator of status and wealth. Finally, there was the belief that infants who slept alone would develop greater independence and self-reliance, attributes highly valued in industrialized Western nations.

While these factors may have contributed to the Western cultural shift in infant sleep practices, they seem outdated to today's parents. There is no evidence, for example, to support the idea that babies that sleep alone become more independent and self-reliant adult members of society. To my mind, the one serious objection to bed sharing that remains is the concern that it isn't safe.

CONFLICTING SAFETY ADVICE

When my mom told me that Cee wasn't safe sleeping with me, she was only repeating the advice of the American Academy of Pediatrics.[8] This recommendation isn't an arbitrary judgment on what should go on in our bedrooms at night; it is based on many studies showing that bed sharing is associated with an increased risk of infant deaths from SIDS and other sleep-related infant deaths, such as those caused by suffocation.

Some researchers and parenting advice authors disagree with this recommendation. They say that bed sharing is the natural way for mothers and babies to sleep, that it facilitates bonding and breastfeeding, and that it can be done safely. For example, the website AskDrSears, written by Dr. Bill Sears and family, states that bed sharing is safer than putting your baby to sleep in a crib.[9] Notre Dame anthropologist James McKenna is a staunch advocate of bed sharing, and he's openly critical of those who discourage it. "The public wars being led by governmental agencies and by medical groups against bed sharing are nothing less than disrespectful and vitriolic of parents who choose to bed share safely," he wrote.[10]

Faced with this contradictory advice, you and I are left to make our own decisions on the long and lonely nights of caring for a baby. We all want to keep our babies safe, but we might also find the idea of sleeping next to them appealing and even necessary. We can't help but wonder, how good exactly are the data behind the recommendations against bed sharing?

Before I tackle this question, I want to warn you that this is not an easy topic to discuss. Whatever the reasons and risk factors for sudden infant deaths, each is a tragedy to the children and the families that survive them. It is my intent to understand these deaths so that we can do our best to prevent them, not to assign blame or to scare you into one or the other choice.

SUDDEN UNEXPECTED INFANT DEATHS AND THE SLEEP ENVIRONMENT

Sudden infant death syndrome, accidental suffocation or strangulation in bed, and sleep-related deaths with unknown cause are collectively known as sudden unexpected infant deaths (SUID, also called SUDI in Europe and Australia). Together, they are among the most common causes of death among babies between 1 month and 1 year of age in the United States and many other developed countries.[11] In 2010, SUID rates varied from a low of 0.19 deaths per 1,000 live births in the Netherlands; 0.45 to 0.50 in Australia, Canada, England, and Wales; 0.60 in Japan; 0.95 in the US; and 1.0 per 1,000 live births in New Zealand.[12] In the United States, there are huge racial and ethnic disparities in SUID rates, with American Indian, Alaska Native, and Black infants having a two- to fivefold risk of dying in their sleep compared with white, Hispanic, Asian, and Pacific Islander infants.[13] These disparities track with infant mortality and other metrics of maternal and infant health and are likely caused by a combination of factors, including social determinants of health and the chronic stress that accompanies exposure to systemic racism.[14]

SIDS is generally defined as an infant death that can't be explained after an autopsy, scene investigation, and review of medical records. This makes SIDS a "diagnosis of exclusion," meaning that it's defined not by what it is, but what it isn't. To make things more confusing, an autopsy alone can't usually provide evidence of suffocation, and while evidence at the scene of death may point to an obvious cause, this isn't always the case. Because there are usually no conscious witnesses at the time of death, how to classify these tragedies becomes a matter of interpretation. Medical examiners and coroners in different parts of the world and even different jurisdictions within the same country have varying practices and policies around infant deaths. Presented with the same medical evidence and scene of death, one coroner will call a case SIDS, another may call it suffocation, and another might simply call it "undetermined."[15] This inconsistency has made it difficult to research SUID and SIDS, identify causes, and track trends in its incidence.

Further complicating the issue, there's been a "diagnostic shift" over time in the classification of SUID cases. For example, in the United States, the incidence of SIDS has appeared to decline steadily since 1990, but the incidence of deaths classified as accidents or with unknown cause has increased, and the overall SUID rate has remained about the same since around 2000. The same shift has been seen in Australia, England, and Wales, and at least some of this change seems to be not in the actual causes of deaths but simply in how they are labeled.[16]

No matter how these deaths are classified, there's no question that there's too many of them, and progress in keeping babies safe while they sleep has been frustratingly slow. It's also clear that many of these deaths could be prevented, either by putting the babies down to sleep on their backs (more on that in a moment) or by ensuring that their sleep environments were safer.

Before we get into the bed sharing controversy, it's worth discussing some obviously unsafe sleep environments for babies. One of the most dangerous sleeping spaces is on a sofa or couch. Studies estimate that babies are about fifty- to seventyfold more likely to die while sleeping on a sofa than in a crib. In the United States, 13 percent of SUID deaths happen on a sofa, a large number considering that this isn't a typical place for babies to sleep. Most of the time, these deaths happen with an adult snuggled up with the baby.[17] You can imagine a scenario that begins so sweetly—maybe an accidental afternoon nap together or a parent nodding off during a middle-of-the-night feeding—but ends tragically.

Any type of soft bedding that could conceivably obstruct a baby's mouth or nose, like blankets, pillows, sheepskins, and bumper pads, also make a baby's sleep environment unsafe. Deaths classified as suffocation often have soft bedding involved, and while these deaths happen most often in bed sharing scenarios, they can also happen in cribs with soft bedding or bumper pads.[18] Bumper pads may be cute and make a crib look cozier, but they're unnecessary and can be deadly.[19] (There are "breathable" crib liners and bumpers on the market now, but there's no research to say whether they're safe, and in my view, it's just not worth the risk.)

Despite the many swings, bouncers, rockers, "lounger" pillows, and other inclined sleeper products marketed to parents, these also aren't safe sleep surfaces for babies. This includes car seats, which should absolutely be used to keep babies safe in vehicles, but not as a place to sleep (especially unsupervised) once you've arrived at your destination. A 2019 study reported that 348 infants died while sleeping in sitting devices between 2004 and 2014 in the United States.[20] Also in 2019, a Consumer Reports investigation linked at least 73 infant deaths to sleeping in the Fisher Price Rock 'n Play Sleeper and other inclined sleep products. Fisher Price recalled their product, and retailers like Amazon stopped carrying similar inclined sleepers.[21] However, these sleepers remain in circulation through hand-me-downs and yard sales, and similar sleepers are still sold. Then there are infant swings. I know the only reason we allow these bulky plastic and metal fixtures to take up half of our living rooms is because they seem to help some babies sleep, but they almost always have inclined seats.

The bottom line is that any sleep surface that puts the baby at an incline may carry an increased risk of asphyxia, such as if the baby's head turns into the soft sides of the sleeper or downward in a way that could obstruct the airway.[22] While deaths in these devices are relatively rare, it's just best to avoid them and help your baby learn to sleep well on a flat surface. At least you can take some solace in the money you'll save and the landfill-bound plastic you'll avoid by just not buying these products in the first place. It's also a common belief that sleeping at an incline may be helpful for babies with reflux, but a small study found the opposite—babies placed in a car seat after feeding spit up *more* than those laid flat on their backs.[23]

The safest, and simplest, sleep environment for a baby is a crib (or a cot, depending on your part of the world) or bassinet with a firm mattress and a fitted sheet. In a US study published in 2012, only 13 percent of infants that died in their sleep of suffocation were sleeping in a crib or bassinet.[24] Fifty-two percent were in an adult bed, 19 percent were on a couch or chair, and most were sleeping with an adult at the time of death. Those numbers make solo sleep in a crib look relatively safe compared with sharing sleep on a surface not designed for babies.

An adult bed has many more potentially hazardous factors in play: bedding, pillows, headboard, not to mention a parent or two and maybe another child. Major causes of accidental infant deaths during sleep include an adult rolling onto the baby, soft bedding or pillows blocking the baby's airway, and the baby becoming entrapped, such as between a mattress and the headboard or wall.[25] Whether a bed sharing environment can ever be as safe as solo sleep in a crib is controversial, but taking some care to eliminate obvious risks can go a long way toward making it safer. The safest bed sharing environment is probably a firm mattress on the floor, with no bed frame, and little or nothing in the way of blankets and pillows that might cover a baby's head. Any sleep partners should be unimpaired by drugs or alcohol and should not be particularly heavy sleepers. Nonparent adults, children, and pets are less likely to be aware of the baby during the night and should not bed-share.[26]

UNDERSTANDING SIDS

Eliminating hazards from your baby's sleep environment can clearly reduce the chances of suffocation or entrapment during sleep, and it can also reduce the chances of SIDS. But why SIDS happens is still a mystery, though researchers are working hard to understand it. Most babies will wake up if they're struggling to breathe, but babies that die of SIDS don't. Researchers have found several differences in SIDS victims that might have contributed to their deaths. For example, some studies have found that babies who die of SIDS have alterations in brain stem serotonin, which could affect their ability to arouse from sleep.[27] Others have found signs of immature neurons, increased cell death, abnormal heart rhythms, greater inflammation, and even microbiome differences in SIDS babies.[28] So far, these differences are only measured after death, but if they can help untangle the cause (or causes) of SIDS, that science may one day give us the tools to identify and protect babies more vulnerable to SIDS early on.

In the meantime, the working model explaining SIDS is the Triple Risk Model, which states that for SIDS to occur, three types of risk converge:[29]

1. *Critical period of development*: By definition, SIDS occurs in babies less than 12 months of age, but most deaths happen between 2 and 4 months, and 90 percent occur before 6 months of age, a period of rapid maturation of cardiorespiratory control and sleep-wake cycles.

2. *Vulnerable infant*: Some babies are born with greater vulnerability to SIDS because of intrinsic risks like being born prematurely or low birth weight, being exposed to tobacco smoke in utero, or having genetic defects such as the brain stem abnormalities mentioned above.

3. *Exogenous stressor*: This could be due to the baby sleeping prone (on his tummy) or on his side, a soft sleep surface or bedding, head covering or overheating, or exposure to environmental tobacco smoke. Bed sharing is thought to increase the risk of exogenous stress.

The first component of the Triple Risk Model—the critical period of development—is unavoidable; all infants must pass through the developmental phase when the risk of SIDS is highest. For the second—infant vulnerability—there are some factors that we can control, such as not smoking during pregnancy and seeking prenatal care, but other aspects that are out of our hands and unknown to us, such as an underlying brain stem abnormality. It is the third component of the Triple Risk Model—exogenous stressors—that is contingent on the decisions we make around caring for our babies, so that is where we tend to focus our SIDS prevention efforts. Based on the Triple Risk Model, a baby could have an underlying brain stem abnormality, but if he always sleeps in a safe environment, he will probably remain safe from SIDS. As parents, understanding and minimizing these exogenous stressors can go a long way toward reducing our babies' risk of SIDS.

Case-control studies are used to identify risk factors for SIDS. In a case-control study, researchers monitor SIDS deaths as they occur. When an infant dies of SIDS, several infants that were born around the same time in the same population are recruited as controls. Parents and caregivers of both the case infants (those who died of SIDS) and the control infants are interviewed. Were the babies exposed to smoking during pregnancy or after birth? Were they sleeping on their backs or tummies? Where were they sleeping when they died? Were they sleeping alone or with another person? Did their parents drink or use drugs? These factors are tallied up for the case and control infants, and then statistical analyses determine differences between the two groups. The results are presented as odds ratios, which give the odds of SIDS occurring in babies with the factor of interest. The higher the odds ratio, the greater the risk associated with that particular factor.

Case-control studies have some serious limitations, though. Most importantly, they can show which factors are *associated* with SIDS deaths, but they can't establish *causation*. In addition, they rely on parents' memory and honesty for information. For example, in their interviews with researchers, parents might decide to omit the fact that they had a couple of drinks or more before bed. Or they just might not remember what exactly happened on the night in question. On the other hand, parents of the babies who died of SIDS may be more likely to remember details, because the horror of finding your baby dead might intensify memories around the event. (This difference in remembering is called recall bias.) In other words, case-control data are only as reliable as parents are honest and accurate.

A randomized controlled trial would give us a more accurate picture of the role of a factor like bed sharing in SIDS, but it would be unethical and nearly impossible to do. We can't randomize babies by sleep habits. That would mean instructing some parents to bed-share and some to put their babies in cribs, and as you can imagine, it is unlikely that parents would follow those instructions, given differences in parenting styles and infant temperament. Another barrier to this kind of study is that it would have to be huge. Since only about 1 in 2,000 infants die of SIDS, we'd need to study hundreds of thousands of families to detect a difference in SIDS rates between bed-sharing and crib-sleeping infants. This leaves us with case-control studies. Imperfect as they are, they are considered the best tool we have for studying population-wide risk factors associated with SIDS.

A BRIEF HISTORY OF SIDS RESEARCH
AND ADVICE

In the 1970s and 1980s, SIDS rates were at an all-time high in Western countries, and researchers turned to case-control studies to try to figure out why. One risk factor that popped up over and over was sleeping prone, or tummy down. Babies that died of SIDS were much more likely to have been placed to sleep on their tummies or to have rolled there from the side position than the surviving controls. In the early 1990s, Back-to-Sleep campaigns urged parents to put their babies down for sleep on their backs, and within a couple of years, SIDS rates had plummeted.[30]

This bit of SIDS history illustrates "modern" parenting advice gone wrong. In 1955, Dr. Benjamin Spock recommended in his book *Baby and Child Care* that babies be placed to sleep on their backs. This was customary in most of the world at the time and probably throughout human history, because parents feared their babies would suffocate on their tummies. However, in his 1956 edition, Spock changed his tune and told parents to put their babies to sleep in the prone position, citing concerns that a baby sleeping on his back might choke on his own vomit.[31]

Tragically, nothing about Spock's advice was evidence-based. There weren't any good studies to support his ideas. But prone sleep seemed to work great, since babies sleep longer and deeper on their tummies,[32] and Spock's advice was quickly adopted by parents. Unfortunately, we now know that prone sleep decreases that critical ability to arouse from sleep, putting babies at greater risk for SIDS.[33]

Dr. Spock couldn't have known how harmful his advice would be, and he wasn't alone in recommending prone sleep. However, he had such a huge audience that he does bear some responsibility for this mistake. His book was printed in 42 languages and sold 50 million copies.[34] By 1970, there were two case-control studies pointing to prone sleep as a risk factor for SIDS, but Spock continued to recommend tummy sleeping until 1978. A 2005 study estimated that at least 60,000 infant deaths could have been prevented had the Back-to-Sleep campaign started in 1974.[35] The campaign didn't begin until the early 1990s, so it took some time for the science to make its way into parenting advice books like Spock's and public health advice, and that cost babies' lives.

I include the story of Dr. Spock and prone sleep for two reasons: to illustrate the utility of case-control studies and as a cautionary tale. The case-control studies—with all their flaws—are what alerted researchers to the dangers of prone sleep. And it's a cautionary story in that Spock gave the advice that seemed logical to him, with tragic results. It's a reminder that we can't always trust the narrative that makes the most sense to us or that we'd like to believe is true. Instead, we should use a wide lens and an open mind to look at all the science available before drawing conclusions.

BED SHARING AND SIDS

The success of the Back-to-Sleep campaign encouraged researchers to look for other factors that might be putting babies at risk for SIDS. Since the 1980s, epidemiologists have investigated thousands of SIDS deaths in case-control studies, trying to understand why some babies die of SIDS while others do not.

Overwhelmingly, these studies find that babies that die of SIDS are more likely to have been bed sharing than the surviving (control) babies. But they also show that, in most cases, there are one or more other factors in the bed sharing environment that increase the risk. In other words, it's hard to tell if it is bed sharing per se that is dangerous, or if it is the circumstances in which we bed-share—factors that we could change to minimize the risk of SIDS.

There are two recent meta-analyses that combine data from multiple case-control studies to examine the risk of bed sharing in various circumstances. Both were published by research teams led by medical statisticians from England, one by the late Bob Carpenter of the London School of Hygiene and Tropical Medicine and the other by Peter Blair of the University of Bristol. Carpenter's study was published in 2013 and combined results from 19 studies from the UK, Europe, Australia, and New Zealand, including a total of

1,472 SIDS cases and 4,679 controls.[36] Blair's study was published a year later and pooled two UK studies for a total of 400 SIDS cases and 1,386 controls.[37] Though Blair's study was smaller, it included more complete data on parental alcohol use. Bigger is usually better when comparing two studies, but that generalization doesn't necessarily hold here.

The two meta-analyses are in clear agreement that bed sharing in combination with tobacco exposure or a parent impaired by alcohol increases the risk of SIDS. Blair's study, for example, estimated that a baby who bed-shares with an adult smoker has a fourfold increased risk of dying of SIDS, and sleeping next to an adult who's had more than two drinks increases the risk a full eighteenfold. Likewise, bed sharing on a sofa or in a soft chair also increases the risk of SIDS by eighteenfold. If there are multiple risk factors, such as sleeping on a couch with a smoker, the risk multiplies. These risks were even greater for infants less than 3 months old.[38]

But what if you're a nonsmoking, sober, breastfeeding mother, sleeping with your baby in a bed that's carefully arranged to be free of excess bedding and pillows? These were the conditions in which I considered bed sharing with Cee, but unfortunately, it's this scenario where the most controversy and least clarity lie. Carpenter's study concluded that even without the risks associated with smoking and drinking, a breastfed baby less than 3 months old who bed-shares has a fivefold increased risk of SIDS compared to one who sleeps in their own bed. After 3 months of age, however, bed sharing without those additional hazards doesn't increase risk, according to Carpenter's study. Carpenter and his colleagues concluded, "Our findings suggest that professionals and the literature should take a more definite stand against bed sharing, especially for babies under three months."[39]

Blair's study, on the other hand, concluded that bed sharing in the absence of other known hazards (smoking, drinking, sofa-sharing) does not increase the risk of SIDS, even for infants less than 3 months old. "An important implication of our findings is that to give blanket advice to all parents never to bed-share with their infant does not reflect the evidence," Blair and colleagues concluded, arguing that it's more important to educate parents about the specific conditions in which bed sharing is particularly risky.[40]

So, two well-respected groups of researchers conducted studies attempting to answer the same question and arrived at different answers. If you really wanted to believe that bed sharing was inherently safe or unsafe, you could select the study that supports your preferred narrative and wave it around as evidence supporting your view. Advocates on both sides of this debate can sometimes be seen cherry-picking the data in this way.

My preference is to simply acknowledge that there's still uncertainty on this question. Researchers are trying to figure it out, but given the limitations of case-control studies and the inherent difficulty of studying a rare event in a complex world, we may never know the answer for sure. But in the meantime, while researchers debate this question and argue about the best advice to give to parents, we're left wondering whom to believe, and ultimately, might distrust one side or the other or, worse, distrust science in general. And we still need to get some sleep.

Science can't always give us a clear answer, but in this case, it still gives us a great deal of information. What we can say is that bed sharing, even in the absence of other hazards, *may* increase the risk of SIDS in young infants. However, SIDS is very rare with careful bed sharing. Carpenter's study estimates that a baby whose parents have followed all the "rules" (breastfeeding, room sharing but not bed sharing; no smoking or alcohol) has a one in 12,500 chance of dying of SIDS. For the same baby, bed sharing increases the risk to one in 4,348.[41]

You might look at that roughly threefold increase in risk and decide that given the unthinkably catastrophic nature of SIDS, it's just not worth it to bed-share, especially in the first three to four months of life, when babies are most vulnerable to SIDS. That's the view of the AAP, as well as pediatric and public health professionals in Canada, who advise parents that bed sharing should be avoided.[42] But this risk analysis becomes more complex if you find that bed sharing also comes with some benefits. For example, some parents find that their baby struggles to sleep without body contact, and every repeated attempt to set the baby down into a bassinet or crib is met with wails and a wakeful baby. In this case, the risk of being up with a sleepless baby night after night and suffering the effects of chronic, severe sleep deprivation (think postpartum depression, car accidents, falling asleep in exhaustion with the baby on a couch, etc.) might easily outweigh the relatively small risk of bed sharing in an otherwise ideal situation. The choice to bed-share isn't risk-free (nothing in life is), but it's possible that it could sometimes be the less risky choice.

The risk of falling asleep while holding your baby on a couch or soft chair is very real and serious. Blair and colleagues noted that in some cases of infant deaths on sofas included in their study, the parents told investigators that they were holding the baby on the sofa specifically to avoid bed sharing.[43] Sadly, their babies might still be alive today if they'd laid down on a firm mattress with the baby instead of a couch. In their 2016 policy statement on SIDS prevention, the AAP acknowledged this risk. If you're feeding your baby during the night and you think there's a chance that you'll doze off, consider the safety of the environment around you. You'll be safer and more comfortable if you feed in a bed that you've set up with safety in mind, just in case, than trying to prop yourself up on a couch and hoping for the best.[44]

Unlike the US and Canadian advice against bed sharing, the UK and Australia have taken a more nuanced approach toward educating parents about SIDS prevention.[45] Acknowledging that bed sharing is common, despite decades of advice against it, they emphasize the situations in which bed sharing is particularly risky (e.g., with a smoker or someone who has been drinking). They also discuss sleep options in a nonjudgmental way, which allows for more open conversations about how to reduce risks. One concern with the North American approach is that "banning" bed sharing comes across as being out of touch with the reality of parenting and could also get in the way of honest conversations between health professionals and families about how to make the bed sharing environment safer.

Toward that end, it might be helpful to consider some possible explanations for the risks of bed sharing with young babies. A few studies have looked closely, using infrared cameras and physiological monitors, at the behavior of sober, breastfeeding mothers sleeping with their babies in their own homes. They have found that it was common for bed-sharing babies to end up with their faces covered by blankets during the night and, as a consequence, to have brief periods of low oxygen and high carbon dioxide—conditions that are thought to precede SIDS deaths.[46]

For example, among 40 bed-sharing infants observed for two consecutive nights, 22 of them had a total of 102 incidents of head covering by blankets, with most cases caused by a parent's movement, and some babies slept like this for hours. In contrast, there was only one incident of head covering in a matched group of 40 babies who slept in cribs.[47] Another study found that of 20 infants observed for one night of bed sharing, 7 of them had a parent's limb resting on them for part of the night.[48] All of these incidents occurred on nights when parents knew they were being video recorded, so they may have been more careful than usual.

Clearly, bed sharing introduces more variability into the environment and increases the chances that a baby's breathing might be challenged by a change in oxygen availability during the night. In these sleep studies, all the babies were able to respond to these small respiratory challenges by increasing their breathing and heart rates or by moving or crying to wake a parent. It is probably the intrinsically vulnerable infants—like those exposed to cigarette smoke, born prematurely, or having an unrecognized brain stem abnormality (unrepresented in these small studies)—who might fail to arouse and correct the problem.

Since we can't usually know in advance which babies are vulnerable due to something like a genetic defect, it seems prudent to arrange a baby's sleep environment to prevent head covering as much as possible. Putting your baby to sleep in a crib without blan-

THE SCIENCE OF MOM

kets is the surest way to do that. Another option is to use a sidecar cosleeper that attaches to the side of your bed and provides your baby with a separate sleep surface, away from your blankets and limbs. If your baby bed-shares with you, eliminate or at least minimize blankets and arrange them in such a way that they are never close to him. Wearable sleep sacks are a genius invention; they keep the baby warm without risking face covering. Whatever your interpretation of the science and wherever your baby ultimately sleeps, I think everyone agrees that making the sleep environment as safe as possible should be a priority.

SAFE SLEEP RECOMMENDATIONS

- Always put your baby down for sleep on his back and on a firm and flat mattress.

- Breastfeeding and giving your baby a pacifier for sleep (even if it falls out after a few minutes) are associated with a reduced risk of SIDS.

- The safest place for your baby to sleep is in a crib or bassinet in your room. Room sharing is recommended for at least the first six months of life, and the AAP recommends this arrangement for the first year.

- Avoid sleeping with your baby on a couch or chair, or feeding in this position if you think you might fall asleep, because this dramatically increases the risk of SIDS and suffocation.

- Babies who are born prematurely or exposed to cigarette smoke (before or after birth) have a greater risk of SIDS, especially if bed sharing. Bed sharing with adults who are impaired by alcohol, drugs, or medications is also associated with a much higher risk of SIDS.

- Some, but not all, studies have found that bed sharing during the first 3 to 4 months of life is associated with an increased risk of SIDS, even in the absence of other hazards. Wherever your baby sleeps, know that SIDS risk is greatest during this time, so use extra care.

- Safety considerations for cribs and bassinets: Ensure your baby's bed meets current safety standards. Do not put bumper pads, bedding, pillows, stuffed animals, or toys in the crib. A tightly fitted sheet is all that is needed. Avoid putting your baby for sleep in an inclined device such as a car seat (except when traveling), swing, or stroller (except when strolling).

- Safety considerations for the bed sharing environment: Minimize the use of pillows and blankets, and keep them well away from the baby. Ensure that there's no space where the baby could become entrapped between the mattress and wall or bedframe. Avoid using side rails, since they can create a space for entrapment. Never leave a baby to sleep alone in an adult bed, and avoid bed sharing with other children, nonparent adults, and pets.

- Keep your baby warm using pajamas and a sleep sack rather than loose bedding. Don't overbundle him; dress him just enough to stay warm. The head is an important area for heat dissipation, so avoid using a hat for sleep. Ideal room temperature is thought to be 61° to 68°F, or 16° to 20°C.

Sources: H. Ball and P. S. Blair, "Health Professionals' Guide to 'Caring for Your Baby at Night,'" UNICEF UK, 2017, www.unicef.org.uk/babyfriendly/baby-friendly-resources/sleep-and-night-time-resources/caring-for-your-baby-at-night; American Academy of Pediatrics (AAP) Task Force on Sudden Infant Death Syndrome, "SIDS and Other Sleep-Related Infant Deaths: Updated 2016 Recommendations for a Safe Infant Sleeping Environment," *Pediatrics* 138, no. 5 (2016): e20162938.

THE CASE FOR KEEPING YOUR BABY CLOSE AT NIGHT

In the 1980s, British pediatrician D. P. Davies was working in Hong Kong, where he was surprised to find that SIDS was virtually absent from childhood mortality statistics. Davies surveyed forensic pathologists and pediatricians at the major hospitals in Hong Kong, and all agreed that SIDS was very uncommon. For a closer look, they tracked babies that died of SIDS during 12 months in 1986–87, finding a total of 21 deaths, approximately one-fifth the rate in the United States at that time.[49] What were these Hong Kong families doing right, or more to the point, what were American families doing wrong?

Life wasn't all rosy for a baby in Hong Kong in the 1980s. Breast-feeding was rare, living conditions were extremely crowded, and rates of respiratory infection were high. However, smoking and prone sleep were uncommon, and most babies were born into supportive extended families. Davies speculated, "I wonder whether there might be some benefit to such high-density living. Babies are left alone much less. Sleep patterns might be different, effecting subtle modulations to physiological responses concerned with ventilatory control. The question 'When can I put baby into his own room?' is virtually never raised. Might closer overall contact with the sleeping baby somehow lessen the risks of sudden death?"[50]

Similar observations have been made in other cultures. A survey of nearly 5,000 families in 17 countries found that bed sharing and room sharing were common in many, but not all, countries with low SIDS rates.[51] Close sleeping arrangements are also common in Asian immigrant communities in the United Kingdom and among Pacific Islanders in New Zealand. These groups have low rates of SIDS, particularly compared with their neighbors of European descent.[52]

From these cross-cultural data, we can only speculate as to the role of close sleeping in SIDS rates. It may be other things about the way babies are raised, like prone sleep or lack of smoking, that explain these observations. On the other hand, if bed sharing were truly a major independent risk factor for SIDS, we would expect to find higher SIDS rates in countries where bed sharing is common.

But just because bed sharing occurs often in cultures with low rates of SIDS, it does not mean that bed sharing as practiced currently in Western cultures is safe. Perhaps if we mimicked the sleep practices of cultures with low SIDS rates, this would be a good starting place for safe bed sharing. I asked Dr. Rachel Moon, lead author of the AAP's statement on safe sleep, if she could imagine a safe bed sharing environment. "A pallet on the floor," she responded.[53] At first I laughed a little. "I'm serious," she said sternly. "In other countries, where they sleep with their babies and quite safely, that's what they do. In Japan, the futons are not like the futons they sell in the US. Here in the US, they're kind of foamy and cushiony, and in Japan, they're flat, and they're hard as rock. And that's what they sleep on." This may sound extreme, but if we believe bed sharing to be safe because it is found to be safe in other cultures, then we should be prepared to adopt as much of those sleep environments as possible. (Having now been to Japan, I can confirm the accuracy of Moon's description of traditional futons, although I did notice that it's common to sleep under a thick duvet on cold nights. It's also worth noting that autopsies are not routinely performed on infants that die of SUID in Japan, so they use the SIDS diagnosis less often and designate many cases as "sudden death, cause unknown."[54] A recent analysis found that the overall rate of SUID in Japan was lower than in the United States and New Zealand, but higher than Australia, Canada, England and Wales, Germany, and the Netherlands.[55])

Beyond the cross-cultural data, there's more evidence that sleeping close together might protect babies. The same European case-control studies that showed bed sharing was a risk factor for young infants also showed that putting a baby to sleep alone in another room, separate from his parents, roughly doubles the risk of SIDS. In one study, the authors estimated that 36 percent of SIDS deaths could have been prevented if babies had slept in the same room as their parents. In fact, sleeping in a separate room turned out to be a more important risk factor than bed sharing, which accounted for 16 percent of deaths. Add just those two risks together—sleeping too far and sleeping too close—and more than half of SIDS deaths could be prevented, according to the authors' estimates.[56] Other studies have found similar results.[57]

Nobody knows why room sharing might be protective, but researchers speculate that it allows some sensory exchange between caregiver and baby. Perhaps babies are more likely to wake, or sleep more lightly, and parents are more likely to check on them. Importantly, studies find that sharing a room with other children doesn't protect babies from SIDS. The presence of an adult devoted to caring for the baby seems to be a critical component of the protection of sleeping close.

In the United States, the AAP recommends room sharing (without bed sharing) ideally for the first year of life, but at least the first 6 months.[58] Similarly, Australia recommends room sharing for the first 6 to 12 months, and Canada, the United Kingdom, New Zealand, and the Netherlands suggest room sharing for the first 6 months.[59] The room sharing recommendation is somewhat controversial, however, because just as many parents find it hard to keep the baby out of their bed, others find they want the opposite: space from the baby at night. That's because babies can be loud sleepers, and many families find that everyone sleeps better when the baby is in a separate room. I'll address how room sharing affects parental and infant sleep in the next chapter, but if you're struggling with the room sharing recommendation, remember that most SIDS deaths happen between 2 and 4 months of age, and 90 percent occur by 6 months, so if there's a protective effect of room sharing, it's likely most important in those first 6 months.[60]

THE PHYSIOLOGY OF SLEEPING CLOSE

Anthropologist James McKenna is one of the most vocal advocates of the benefits of bed sharing. He began his career studying the social behavior of monkeys and apes, but when his son was born in 1978, he turned his attention to understanding the sleep of human infants and their mothers.[61]

In the 1980s, McKenna began detailed sleep physiology studies of breastfeeding mothers and babies at the University of California, Irvine. Until McKenna's work, Western scientists had observed infant sleep patterns only in the context of solitary sleep. As an anthropologist, McKenna recognized that this was not the way mothers and babies had evolved, and nor was it the norm around the world. And as a father, McKenna was probably aware that it was not uncommon for American parents to bring their babies into bed with them.

142

In McKenna's studies, both the mothers and their babies were outfitted with a series of electrodes, belts, and thermocouples to take physiological measurements while they slept, including heart and respiration rates, brain activity, eye movements, muscle tone, and body temperature. Throughout the night, they were also video recorded by infrared cameras. McKenna and his colleagues recruited new moms, including some who routinely bed-shared at home and others who routinely slept separately. Each dyad spent three consecutive nights at the sleep lab, the first to allow the participants to adapt to the lab conditions, and the second and third to test, in random order, the effects of sleeping both together and apart.

McKenna and colleagues found that when infants slept next to their mothers, they spent a little less total time in deep sleep than they did when they slept alone in a crib. They also had more short arousals from deep sleep but fewer arousals during active, or REM, sleep. Like their infants, bed-sharing moms also woke more often, usually in response to their babies, but these arousals were short and didn't reduce their total sleep time. Bed-sharing dyads also breastfed more during the night.[62]

McKenna contends that human infants evolved to sleep with their breastfeeding mothers and believes that these observed physiological differences are adaptive and beneficial. He thinks that the more frequent arousals observed in bed-sharing babies may protect against SIDS, preventing babies from sleeping too deeply for too long and giving them practice in regulating their breathing during the night.[63]

McKenna's research and ideas flipped the conventional Western thinking about infant sleep on its head, and many parents embraced his ideas. Breastfeeding moms had been sleeping with their babies all along, though perhaps quietly, and now there was science to tell them that maybe what *felt* right also *was* right for babies. Undoubtedly, many sleep and SIDS researchers felt challenged. Sleep researchers had been working on the assumption that when babies slept through the night, that was a good thing, and here was a guy telling them that frequent wakings were healthy for babies.

Meanwhile, SIDS researchers were finding an association between bed sharing and SIDS, and McKenna was directly challenging their assumptions about that relationship.

What McKenna has taught us is that we can't really understand infant sleep if we only study infants sleeping in cribs. But there is still so much that we don't know. SIDS does seem to be related to a failure of babies to arouse from sleep, and it makes sense that if bed-sharing babies spend less time sleeping deeply and arouse more frequently, this might protect them. It makes sense that if an attuned mom is waking and briefly checking on her baby frequently during the night, this could decrease the chances that the baby will die in his sleep. But we don't know if any of this is true. And unfortunately, the numbers still tell a different story.

Although sleeping in the same room—close, but not on the same surface—has repeatedly been shown to be protective, among the many case-control studies of SIDS, only one has so far found bed sharing to be protective (and only in babies older than 3 months, in a very small sample size).[64] It's possible that there are some elements of bed sharing that are truly protective, like lighter sleep and more opportunities to check on the baby. And it may be that other elements of bed sharing, like the risk of the baby's face being covered with bedding, are hazardous.

If our foremothers slept with their babies from the dawn of our species, they probably also experienced both benefits and risks from the practice. Of course, the benefits of bed sharing in a cold cave would have far outweighed the risks, but for us, the risk-benefit calculation is a bit different. Bed sharing advocates often say that human babies were "designed" to sleep with their mothers. But babies weren't designed; they evolved. If they evolved to be sleeping with their mothers, then this was probably an adaptive practice within the circumstances of their lives. It doesn't mean that it was or is a risk-free practice or that it is necessarily the best way for our babies to sleep in modern times. Babies didn't evolve sleeping in cribs, but most of our current data indicate that a crib next to the parents' bed is the safest place for babies to sleep.

McKenna's hypothesis is a fascinating one, and it's such an attractive idea, calling to mind the picture of a peaceful mother and baby sleeping together, hearts beating in synchrony. But it is still just a hypothesis, one we should study further, while keeping it in context with the data we have and the realities of life in the twenty-first century.

DOES YOUR BABY NEED A BREATHING MONITOR?

Before Cee was born in 2010, we bought a $20 baby monitor so that we could hang laundry or toss a tennis ball for the dog in the backyard while she napped. The sound quality was a little staticky, but it did the job. But by the time Max was born in 2014, I found myself accosted with ads for a whole new class of baby monitors, which promised to track my baby's heart rate and breathing while he slept. With brand names like Owlet, Angelcare, and Snuza and price tags as high as $400, these monitors market peace of mind for parents who worry about SIDS (which, of course, is all of us). Price tag aside, I could see how this could be reassuring—to be able to glance at my phone and know my baby is still breathing. But here's the thing: there's little research on these monitors and no evidence that they can prevent SIDS. For this reason, the AAP doesn't recommend them as a strategy to reduce the risk of SIDS. These monitors are not tested or regulated as medical devices, and some pediatricians and researchers say that's a problem if they give inaccurate readings that either give parents a false sense of security or scare them with false alarms, which could lead to unnecessary anxiety and trips to the hospital for healthy babies. A 2018 study tested two of these commercial monitors against a hospital-grade monitor. One (Baby Vida, now unavailable) performed very poorly, often reporting normal oxygen levels when the baby was quite low in oxygen. The other (Owlet) performed much better but was sometimes inconsistent. If you do choose to use one of these monitors, know that it isn't a substitute for safe sleep practices, and talk with your child's doctor about how you should react if an alarm goes off.

Source: C. P. Bonafide et al., "Accuracy of Pulse Oximetry-Based Home Baby Monitors," *JAMA* 320, no. 7 (2018): 717–19.

BED SHARING AND BREASTFEEDING

One of the most commonly cited benefits of bed sharing is that it facilitates breastfeeding. Human milk is rapidly digested, so breastfed infants need to feed frequently.[65] This is especially important during the first few months, and the need for regular refills continues through the night as well as during the day.

In general, moms who bed-share are more likely to breastfeed for longer durations.[66] A UK study found that babies who bed-shared throughout the first year had five times the odds of still breastfeeding at 12 months compared with those who slept alone.[67] In the United States, mothers who bed-shared were 2.5 times more likely to be exclusively breastfeeding compared with those who room-shared without bed sharing.[68]

These studies show a strong correlation between breastfeeding and bed sharing, though they can't show that bed sharing directly *causes* more breastfeeding. It's likely that the two practices mutually reinforce each other, and in many cases, they're both part of a larger philosophy about caring for a baby. Bed sharing can make breastfeeding easier, and the more frequent feedings necessary for breastfed babies may make bed sharing a more attractive choice. Regardless, there's no question that if you're breastfeeding a baby every couple of hours, keeping that baby right next to you is easier than getting out of bed to walk across the room or down the hall. Just lift your shirt, pull baby in closer, and voila—you're feeding. Many mothers find they barely need to wake up for this maneuver.

Video studies have also shown that breastfeeding mothers have a specific and consistent way of bed sharing with their babies. They usually sleep side-lying, knees drawn up and body curled in a C-shape, arm tucked around the baby. Bed sharing, breastfed babies rarely sleep in the dangerous prone position but rather on their backs or sides, at the level of the mother's breast and well-below her pillow. This position keeps the baby in a convenient position for initiating feeding, and it also may protect him from the hazards of the bed, such as the pillow, headboard, and edge of the mattress.[69]

Once I got the hang of it, I found breastfeeding relaxing, and even in the middle of the day, I often found myself dozing off within a minute of latching on my baby. It's worth reiterating, especially for breastfeeding mothers, that the most dangerous place to fall asleep with your baby is on the couch or a plush chair. In a US survey of more than 6,000 moms, most of them breastfeeding, 55 percent said they fed their babies at night on a chair or sofa. Of these, 44 percent said they sometimes fell asleep while feeding.[70] As we've already discussed, if you think you may fall asleep while feeding, then it's best to feed in bed, cuddling your baby in that C-shape position, just in case you fall asleep. Studies show that when you bring your baby into your bed for feeding and comfort and then return him to his own bed for sleep, there's no added SIDS risk.[71] If you do fall asleep, your baby will be in a safer environment than on a couch, and you can return him to his bed as soon as you awaken.

Breastfeeding for at least two months, whether exclusive or mixed with some formula-feeding, also reduces a baby's risk of SIDS by about half; continuing for at least 6 months further reduces the risk.[72] This may be because breastfed babies arouse more easily from sleep than those fed formula, or perhaps it's because breastfed infants tend to have fewer respiratory infections, which can increase SIDS risk.[73] This is a factor to add to your personal risk-benefit analysis for bed sharing; if bed sharing means you're more likely to continue breastfeeding, then the protection of breastfeeding may help offset the risk of bed sharing.

RECONCILING THE DEBATE IN THE REAL WORLD

When I began the research for this chapter, I hoped that, with enough reading and thought, I could eventually arrive at a clear understanding of where babies should sleep. As is probably obvious by now, I haven't found the One Right Answer to this question.

In my quest for answers, however, I spent some time talking with Dr. Rachel Moon, the chairperson of the AAP's Task Force on SIDS and the lead author of their policy statement recommending against bed sharing. As a practicing pediatrician and mother of two children, both of whom were exclusively breastfed as infants, Dr. Moon is well aware of the challenges of infant sleep. Still, she sees the question of bed sharing as a fairly simple one: in her view, it just isn't safe. "Nine times out of ten, it [bed sharing] will be okay," she told me. "But I come from a different perspective because I spend my life talking to people where things haven't gone okay . . . If you've seen one of those cases, you just don't want to take the chance. Why take the chance?"[74] Moon carries with her the weight of grieving families. She knows as well as anyone that the data aren't perfect, but in her mind, bed sharing just isn't worth the risk. The worst-case scenario is just too grave.

A bed sharing advocate like James McKenna, on the other hand, spends his time working with families for whom sleeping with their babies is a valued practice. Both Moon and McKenna have the best of intentions in the way they approach this topic, but both have unavoidable emotional biases. The difference is that McKenna is telling us what many of us want to hear: that it is natural to keep our babies close and that they're safe there. Moon's message is far less romantic and reassuring. From a public relations standpoint, I think that Moon has the more challenging job.

The truth is that no study design can fully describe something as complicated as how a mother and baby sleep. Scientists and parents can argue about the safety of bed sharing all they want, but we may never know who is right. And to be honest, I'm not sure it really matters. If it were only about safety, I believe that most parents would take the AAP's advice to heart and avoid bed sharing, just as most have adopted the Back-to-Sleep recommendation. But bed sharing is a more complex behavior. Parents have been sleeping with their babies forever, and there are cultural, biological, and physiological reasons why we may be drawn to hold our babies close at night. Parents will continue to bed-share, with or without the approval of the AAP.

Since I can't provide you with a single recommendation on this complex topic, I'll leave you with this advice: whatever route you choose, do your best to make it safe. Science can never quantify all the risks and benefits of bed sharing or, for that matter, any parenting practice. It can give us some clues at the population level, but you have to factor in how you and your baby feel about the matter as well.

POSTSCRIPT: REFLECTIONS THROUGH
A SEVEN-YEAR LENS

As I wrote in this chapter, except for a brief flirtation with bed sharing in early infancy, Cee slept in her own bed. That worked well for us, and it didn't stop us from breastfeeding for two years. By the time Max was born, I'd researched and written this book, and frankly, reading study after study about SIDS made me more terrified to bed-share.

And yet, I have to be honest and tell you that biology and fatigue took over, and I did bed-share with him. Maybe it was because the mechanics of breastfeeding were easier the second time around, or I was more tired with two kids, but I just could not stay awake while I fed him at night. As part of my strategy to stay awake, I would sit straight up in my rocking chair, denying myself a blanket on my lap so that I would always be just a little chilly. I tried listening to podcasts or audiobooks, but still, I fell asleep every time. The only thing that worked to keep me awake—sometimes—was Facebook: that addictive infinite timeline keeping my finger scrolling, scrolling, and the light from the screen artificially stimulating my brain. But even then, I'd still sometimes wake an hour later, finding myself slumped in the chair with my phone slipping out of my hand, and frantically check to be sure Max was still in my arms and still breathing.

Trying to follow every safe sleep rule meant I was inadvertently breaking one of the most important ones and endangering my baby, not to mention increasing my anxiety levels. I hadn't intended to bed-share with Max, but I finally admitted that he would be safer if I fed him in my bed, arranged with safety in mind. I gave myself one firm pillow and a small, lightweight blanket, and I slept in a sweatshirt so that I could keep the blanket at waist level. I made sure Max always started each night in his own bed, and he usually slept his longest stretch there. When he woke to feed, I brought him into my bed, doing my best to remember (but often forgetting) to set a quiet, 10-minute alarm on my phone as a reminder to return him to his own bed. And sometimes, I fell asleep with him next to me in my bed, then moved him back to his bed as soon as I woke again. As Max grew, his feedings became fewer and quicker, and it was easier for me to stay awake and return him to his bed. For a couple of months, though, I had to compromise and choose the path that would best minimize our risks.

7

IN SEARCH OF A GOOD NIGHT'S SLEEP

(*Or Something Like It*)

I have a vivid memory of a conversation with my mother in a dark hallway during Cee's first week of life. It was some wretched hour in the middle of the night, during which Cee was feeding every 60 to 90 minutes. Each time she woke, the labor-intensive routine of breastfeeding (when we were both still getting the hang of it) and helping her settle back to sleep left little time for either of us to sleep between feedings. My husband would groggily get up to change Cee's diaper if I elbowed him hard enough, but otherwise he was remarkably good at sleeping through most of this. To be fair, he was already back at work, caring for sick children in the hospital, and needed the sleep. But that reality didn't change my growing sense of fatigue and despair that I would never feel well rested or clear-minded again.

My mom was staying with us to help for a few weeks, and she must have woken with Cee's cries that night. She peeked into my bedroom. "Is everything going okay, Alice?" she asked.

I felt the back of my throat tighten and surprise tears well up in my eyes. In fact, everything was not going okay. I was exhausted, my nipples were sore, and I felt that surely it wasn't supposed to be this hard. Weren't newborns supposed to sleep all the time? Was there something wrong with my baby? Or with me? Or my milk?

As we talked in the hallway, my mom responded in what I now know was the most perfect way she could have answered my concerns. She didn't offer a solution or even reassurance that it would get better anytime soon. She simply said, "This is completely normal. This is how newborns sleep and feed."

Somehow, knowing that Cee's sleep was normal made it bearable. Of course, right around the time I started to understand newborn sleep, her sleep patterns changed. I had so much to learn, and this was just the beginning. Between two kids born four years apart, we would spend nearly a decade of our lives strategizing how to get enough sleep for everyone in our family, and it's still sometimes a struggle. But, by far, the first year was the most challenging.

Having a baby changes everything about sleep, and nothing can quite prepare us for this. I coped with our sleep struggles by learning as much as I could about the science of infant sleep. I found a wealth of fascinating research that helped me to understand what normal infant sleep looks like, how it changes as they grow, and how parenting shapes babies' sleep development. I put that knowledge into action to help my family find a good night's sleep, and I hope this chapter can help you do the same.

WHY SLEEP MATTERS

I can't overstate the importance of sleep to parents. It's one of our most basic physiological needs, and becoming a parent doesn't make us magically immune to the effects of sleep deprivation. If anything, sleep becomes even more vital to our well-being, as we recalibrate our lives to the demands of parenting. It's as if we're sailing our little boats into an unfamiliar harbor filled with surprisingly choppy waters and hidden obstacles: the loneliness and monotony of caring for an infant, hormonal changes, new tensions with our partners, financial strain, and fragile mental health. These are challenging waters to navigate, but it's so much more doable when we've had a decent night of sleep.

When we haven't had enough sleep, our brains don't function as well. We're more likely to struggle with regulating our emotions, with learning, and with remembering things.[1] Sleep deprivation renders us more susceptible to illness, more prone to weight gain, and more likely to get into a car accident.[2] It makes it harder to muster the energy to exercise or put a decent meal on the table. And for new parents especially, sleep deprivation is associated with more marital strain and a greater risk of depression for both mothers and fathers.[3] The effects of cumulative sleep deprivation build and build.

I've learned to prioritize sleep for the whole family, because I know that without it, our physical and mental health is endangered. Our little boat is much more likely to end up snagged on a rock or overtaken by the metaphorical sea monster that swallows my patience and makes me snap with rage when we're late getting out the door in the morning and my toddler refuses to put his shoes on.

I'm a better person and a better parent when I've had enough sleep, a truth that extends from the first light of the morning to the last moments of the day, when I know I can be more calm and consistent at bedtime if I'm not already exhausted. This is supported by research, too. A 2019 study published in the *Journal of Family Psychology* found that mothers who go to bed later and get less and more variable amounts of sleep are less sensitive and emotionally available to their 6-month-olds at bedtime. This, in turn, could be expected to affect how well the baby sleeps; other studies have shown that sensitive parenting at bedtime leads to better infant sleep.[4]

All of this is to say that it's worth making sleep a priority at every stage of your child's development. One of the unique challenges of caring for a newborn is that your sleep is broken by frequent night waking. Research has shown that when people get eight hours of sleep that's fragmented by being awoken four times during the night, their cognition and mood are impaired just as much as if they'd only gotten four hours of sleep.[5] Especially during the newborn stage, organizing your night in shifts so that you can get at least a four-hour stretch of uninterrupted sleep can make a huge difference. This might mean expressing milk and going to sleep at 8:00 p.m. so your partner can do the first feeding. Or it might mean asking a visiting relative if they'll wake up at 5:00 a.m. to take a shift with the baby, which was the invaluable gift my mother gave to me in the first couple weeks of both of my babies' lives.

The biology of breastfeeding and a lack of family leave for non-lactating partners often conspire to make the work of nighttime caregiving fall disproportionately to the breastfeeding parent, and this inequity can become a habit that persists even after the baby has weaned. This is too bad, because research shows that when fathers are more involved in infant care (both day and night), babies and their mothers get better sleep, with fewer night wakings.[6] This is a win for everyone: mothers are better rested, babies' sleep is more consolidated, and both parents have time to bond with the baby.

LOOKING OUT FOR YOUR MENTAL HEALTH

Pregnancy and having a baby represent a time of vulnerability for mental health. After all, whether it's your first or fourth, a new baby represents a major life change. It changes your physical body and hormone levels, and it temporarily throws a wrench into the routines that normally support wellness, like getting enough sleep, eating well, being physically active, and finding fulfillment in work and hobbies. In the weeks after your baby is born, it's very common to experience feelings of worry, sadness, and fatigue. If these symptoms are mild and subside within a couple of weeks, you can chalk them up to normal "baby blues." However, if your symptoms last beyond two weeks, you could be suffering from postpartum depression or another mood disorder, and you should seek help from your health care provider.

Common symptoms of postpartum depression include persistent sadness, anxiety, and irritability; trouble sleeping (even when your baby is sleeping); difficulty bonding with your baby; and constant worries about being able to properly care for your baby. Depression can begin before, during, or after pregnancy, and altogether, affects about 1 in 10 women in the 12 months after having a baby. Its cause is multifactorial, and it's not your fault. It's caused in part by hormonal changes and is more common in women with a history of past depression, those experiencing additional life stress (e.g., marital, financial, emigration), those without good social support, and those with family members who have experienced postpartum depression. Though less common, fathers can have postpartum depression, too.

Postpartum depression is an illness, affecting your health and your ability to enjoy life. It's also associated with more trouble with breastfeeding and bonding with your baby, and with impaired cognitive, language, and behavioral development in children. Depression is not something to ignore or try to tough out on your own. If you're struggling, please seek professional help and know that postpartum depression is very treatable through counseling, medications, or a combination of the two.

Asking for more support from your partner, family members, and friends can also make all the difference; they can prepare meals, take on other household chores, care for the baby while you sleep or get out for a walk, or just give you more company and conversation. Caring for a baby was never meant to be a solitary task, and building your child's village of caring adults early on will nurture your child and buffer you from the stress and strain of constant parenting.

Postpartum psychosis is a rare and severe mental illness that can affect women after giving birth. It's a medical emergency characterized by delusions, hallucinations, paranoia, and confusion. If you or your partner is experiencing these symptoms, get help right away. And regardless of other symptoms, if you ever have thoughts of harming yourself or your baby, please go to an emergency room, dial 911, or call the National Suicide Prevention Lifeline at 1–800-273-TALK.

Sources: A. Viguera, "Postpartum Unipolar Major Depression: Epidemiology, Clinical Features, Assessment, and Diagnosis," *UpToDate*, last updated October 13, 2020, https://www.uptodate.com/contents/postpartum-unipolar-major-depression-epidemiology-clinical-features-assessment-and-diagnosis; National Institute of Mental Health, "Perinatal Depression," accessed December 29, 2020, https://www.nimh.nih.gov/health/publications/perinatal-depression/index.shtml.

SLEEP IN EARLY INFANCY:
WHAT IS NORMAL?

Newborn babies sleep as much as 16 to 18 hours of the day, but they don't always sleep when we hope they will.[7] Instead, they sleep just about as much during the day as they do at night. Their sleep is also fragmented into short cycles, and they often wake up hungry.

Breastfed babies feed especially frequently. Human milk is more easily digested than formula, so breastfed babies need their small tummies refilled often, both night and day.[8] Frequent nursing also helps to establish milk supply. In one study, breastfeeding mothers were encouraged to feed their babies frequently during the first weeks of life, and at 15 days old, their babies were drinking more milk and had gained more weight than babies fed on a three- to four-hour schedule.[9] And because only the baby can tell when she's hungry and when she's full, all newborns, whether breastfed or formula-fed, should be fed on demand, day and night.

Newborns cycle between active (rapid eye movement, or REM) sleep and quiet (non-REM) sleep, their sleep split about equally between the two types. They usually fall asleep in active sleep, when you'll see their eyes moving beneath closed lids, animated expressions crossing their faces, and twitches and movements in their limbs. They also wake easily from active sleep, so if your baby falls asleep in your arms, trying to set her down immediately during this stage might be the end of the nap or the beginning of another bedtime routine.[10]

After about 20 to 25 minutes of active sleep, newborns shift into quiet sleep. Their breathing becomes slow and rhythmic, and their bodies are still. In this deeper sleep, you can usually transfer a baby from your arms without waking her. She'll be in this phase for about another 20 to 25 minutes, after which she may continue to another active-quiet sleep cycle. However, making the transition from one cycle to the next is tricky for newborn babies. They'll often wake at this time and either be truly awake or need help getting back to sleep to begin another cycle.[11]

156

Thankfully, sleep patterns mature rapidly in the first few months of life. By the second month, babies get better at transitioning from one cycle to the next without waking, and they often have a long sleep bout during the first part of the night. They'll begin to start their sleep in quiet sleep and spend more time there. Active sleep will decrease and shift toward the early morning hours, which may mean your baby is more restless during the second part of the night.[12] As their stomachs grow, they can go longer between feeds, allowing their sleep to consolidate into longer periods.[13]

During these first few months, babies gradually start sleeping more during the night and less during the day. They're adapting to the outside world, where nights are dark and quiet and days are bright and busy. These light and dark signals help babies develop a circadian rhythm, synchronizing them with the 24-hour day-night cycle. When daytime light hits the circadian control center of the brain, it coordinates wakefulness throughout the body, including an increase in body temperature and cortisol and suppression of the sleep hormone, melatonin. When nighttime brings darkness, melatonin is released, allowing the body to rest and sleep.[14]

In the 1990s, psychologist Kate McGraw was working in the Sleep Study Unit of the University of Texas Southwestern Medical Center. She was so interested in the development of infant circadian rhythms that she enlisted her own newborn as a study subject. She and her husband observed their son, Tyler, day in and day out for the first six months of his life. They took his temperature hourly and collected his saliva weekly to measure his melatonin production. They exposed him only to natural sunlight, using no artificial lighting during the night, and they kept their whole family on a predictable schedule of sleeping and eating. Tyler, on the other hand, was breastfed whenever he was hungry and slept when he was tired. McGraw watched as baby Tyler began to show signs of a circadian rhythm, and she and her colleagues reported their findings in a paper published in 1999 in the journal *Sleep*.[15]

Just one week after his birth, Tyler's body temperature was dropping to its lowest point during the night, just as happens in adults. A week or so later, he was sleeping more at night and being more wakeful during the day. Consistent wake periods of 90 to 120 minutes emerged in the morning and before bedtime in the evening; these were peak play times for Tyler. By day 45, he showed a strong melatonin rhythm—high during the night and low during the day. By the end of his second month, he was basically sleeping from sundown to sunrise, with a few brief awakenings during the night for feedings.[16]

This study was fascinating because of its detail, but Tyler was just one infant among many. Other studies, though, have shown similar timing for the emergence of a circadian rhythm, although the careful control of Tyler's natural and social environment may have helped him find his rhythm a bit earlier than average. There's also a lot of inherent variation among babies, but most are sleeping much more during the night than during the day by the time they are 2 or 3 months old.[17]

HELPING YOUR BABY LEARN NIGHT FROM DAY

During your baby's first few weeks, sleep feels very disorganized. Some naps will be long and some short. Your baby may be sleepy during the day and wakeful at night. Your goal during this time is to help her rest when she's tired and to feed her when she's hungry. It's a simple but exhausting job. The good news is that as you show your baby the natural signals of night and day, she'll quickly begin to develop a circadian rhythm and sleep patterns that are more sustainable.

At night, keep the lights as dim as possible and the environment quiet and relaxed, even if you're feeding frequently. Breastfed babies also have the benefit of melatonin in nighttime breast milk, which drops to undetectable levels during the day. Since it can take babies a month or two to develop their own melatonin rhythm, milk melatonin can help bridge this gap to promote nighttime sleep.[18]

During the day, let your baby be part of the activity of the house. Even as she sleeps, keep her in a light room. One study found that among 6- to 12-week-old babies, those who were exposed to more light between noon and 4:00 p.m. slept better at night.[19] After the first few months, most babies nap better in a quiet and dark place. You will want to respect that, but by then your baby should—hopefully—have the day and night straightened out.

Giving your baby these natural signals of light and activity allows her to develop a circadian rhythm that matches your own. Illustrating the importance of environmental and social cues, one study found that both preemie and full-term babies develop strong day-night rhythms within 9 to 10 weeks of coming home from the hospital, despite the relative neurological immaturity of the preemies.[20] One baby in this study still hadn't developed a circadian rhythm at 5 months of age and was just as wakeful during the night as during the day. It turned out that when this night owl woke during the night, he was fed in a bright room; he was getting confusing signals about day and night.

Despite all the studies on infant sleep, little work has been done on wakefulness. But from a practical standpoint, an awareness of how long your baby can handle being awake is important to timing good sleep. Baby Tyler, whose sleep and wake cycles were tracked by his scientist mom, showed distinct periods of 90 to 120 minutes of wakefulness in the morning and in the late afternoon by the time he was 1 month old.[21] As wakeful periods emerge in your baby, those times of day will be best for playing and interacting. And as the wakeful period winds down, keeping an eye on the clock and your baby's signs of tiredness will allow you to prepare her for sleep before she becomes overtired. The amount of time that your baby can comfortably be awake will increase as she grows; one study found that, on average, the longest period of wakefulness was about 2 hours at 3 months of age and 3.5 hours at 6 months.[22]

It's also never too early to develop a soothing bedtime routine, a consistent sequence of calming rituals that you use each night and before naps to get your baby ready for sleep. A small 2016 study looked specifically at the effects of a 15-minute nightly massage with lotion in the first month of life. By the end of the first month, the babies receiving the massage *and their mothers* were both going to sleep faster, waking less during the night (two times instead of three), and getting about an hour more sleep each night.[23] Notably, the study was sponsored by Johnson and Johnson, a company that sells baby lotion, and this could have biased the findings. Still, a massage can be a sweet way to wind down and connect with your baby, and any brand of lotion would do. If massage isn't your thing, any routine that you and your baby both enjoy will likely help, so long as it's soothing and predictable, with the same sequence each night.[24] A randomized controlled trial showed that a routine of bath, massage, and snuggles helped older infants and toddlers to fall asleep faster, sleep more during the night (an average of 36 more minutes!), and wake in a better mood in the morning.[25] Not surprisingly, their mothers felt better, too, reporting less fatigue, anger, depression, tension, and confusion. (The study only looked at mothers' mood and not their partners.)

Reading to both my babies was always my favorite part of the bedtime routine, and my kids and I now agree that it remains one of our favorite times of the day. From Max's very first days through his toddler years, I always said the same thing as I put him in his crib to sleep: "It's going to feel so good to rest." That became a sort of mantra to remind us both that sleep was a *good* thing, not something to resist. And we still sing "Twinkle, Twinkle, Little Star" to our kids before we say goodnight. Cee, now 10 years old, says she wonders if she's getting too old for a lullaby, but she still asks for it every night.

SLEEP IN THE FIRST YEAR: WHAT IS NORMAL?

Once your baby can tell her nights from her days, sleep should get a lot easier. The most rapid sleep consolidation happens within the first several months of life, and by 3 to 4 months, many babies are sleeping for nice 8- to 10-hour chunks without waking their parents.[26] However, the fact that many babies do this doesn't mean that your baby will or even should. When it comes to infant sleep, there is a wide range of normal.

SUPPORTING HEALTHY NEWBORN SLEEP

- Help your baby learn the rhythm of days and nights. Let your home be bright, with normal activity, during the day. At night, keep it dark and quiet, with lights and screens very dim or off.

- Understand newborn sleep cycles. When your baby is in active sleep, she may wake easily, and she may be noisy. Don't assume that every grunt and sigh represents a wakeful, hungry baby. Before intervening, watch to see whether she's just moving in her sleep, waking briefly, or is asking for your help.

- Observe your baby to learn how long she can be awake before she gets tired. Help her get comfortable for sleep before she's over-tired.

- Develop a simple, soothing bedtime routine.

- Use a phone app (or pen and paper) to keep a log of your baby's sleeping and feeding so that you can see patterns emerge and have a little predictability for your days and nights.

When I polled my blog readers about when their babies began sleeping for eight-hour stretches, the responses ranged from as early as 5 weeks to well into the toddler years. It's not a scientific sample, but it gives you an idea of how pointless it is to worry about what is normal. If your baby sleeps that long at 2 months, she's normal; lots of babies catch on early. But then again, if she doesn't sleep through the night until 2 years, she's normal, too. Although there are things you can do to help your baby sleep through the night sooner, as we'll discuss later in this chapter, there's also a lot of inherent variability from child to child. Between 6 months and 4 years of age, genetics explain about half of the differences in sleep patterns from one child to the next.[27]

It is also completely normal for a baby to be sleeping through the night for some time and then to start waking again in later infancy, just when you think you have your sleep back.[28] These sleep set-backs can occur because of teething, illness, developmental leaps like learning to crawl (and wanting to practice during the night), and separation anxiety, among other things. Max stopped napping entirely for a couple of weeks when he was around 6 months and discovered that he could get from one end of the room (or crib) to the other by rolling. A 2015 study documented that babies start waking more during the night when they learn to crawl, a phenomenon that many parents, including me, have also observed. The researchers estimated that it could take as long as three months for the babies to return to their previous sleep trajectories after mastering this new motor skill.[29] Many babies are still waking their parents at least once each night at 12 months.[30] In fact, half of toddlers (12 to 35 months) and one-third of preschoolers (3- to 5-year-olds) in the United States wake their parents at least once on a typical night.[31]

Breastfed babies usually take longer to sleep through the night, a factor that has not always been considered in studies of "normal" infant sleep patterns. When anthropologist Helen Ball surveyed British mothers about their babies' sleep habits, she found that two out of three babies were no longer waking their parents for a feed by 3 months of age.[32] However, 96 percent of these dreamers were formula-fed, and sleeping through the night at this age was rare for a breastfed baby. Among the babies still waking at 3 months old, about half were formula-fed and half were breastfed. Formula feeding may help with sleep consolidation, but it isn't a golden ticket by any means.

One helpful tip that emerges from sleep research is that an earlier bedtime correlates with more nighttime sleep. This was shown in a 2016 study in which caregivers of 841 babies and toddlers logged their children's sleep on a phone app.[33] Pooling all that data, the researchers found that morning wake time was consistently between 6:30 and 8:00 a.m. for most children. Bedtime was more variable; most 5-month-olds fell asleep anytime between 6:00 and 10:00 p.m., and the earlier the bedtime, the more sleep they logged. This is absolutely consistent with my experience: babies and toddlers don't sleep in. After a late night, their internal clock somehow wakes them at their usual time in the morning, even if they desperately need more sleep and will be cranky until their first nap. If you want your baby to sleep more at night, aim for an earlier bedtime. Bedtime is also usually easier if you start it before your baby is exhausted. I don't have studies to back this up, but my experience is that an over-tired baby has a harder time going to sleep and, ironically, is more likely to wake during the night.

Compared with nighttime sleep, there's less research on babies' napping patterns, but a 2012 meta-analysis provides a helpful summary of available studies, and the phone app study reported similar findings.[34] Most babies take three to four naps per day in the first few months, decreasing to two naps—one in the morning and one in the afternoon—by around 8 to 10 months. By 18 months, most have dropped to just one afternoon nap. Of course, there's a lot of variability in the exact timing of these trajectories, but this gives you an idea of what to expect. If you notice that your baby is having a harder time falling asleep at naptime or nighttime, it may be time to experiment with dropping a nap.

SLEEPING TOGETHER OR APART: HOW BED SHARING AND ROOM SHARING AFFECT SLEEP

The AAP recommends room sharing without bed sharing—baby sleeping in the same room as the parents but in a separate bed—for the first year of life as the safest sleep arrangement, with the lowest risk of SIDS or suffocation. This plan works well for some parents, but some want the baby out of their room sooner because they find it hard to sleep with a noisy baby so close. Others want the opposite—to sleep *closer* to the baby, in the same bed. Bed sharing often isn't the original plan, but some parents discover that physical closeness at night makes it easier to monitor, feed, and soothe the baby, and the carefully decorated nursery ends up abandoned for many months.[35] Ultimately, where your baby sleeps is a personal choice, one that should include an evaluation of safety concerns (discussed in chapter 6), sleep quality of the baby and parents, and family dynamics.

Most studies show that bed-sharing babies and their mothers tend to wake more often than solo sleepers. However, it's not clear whether these arousals result in less nighttime sleep; some studies find less sleep with bed sharing, some find more, and some find no difference.[36] Despite a more fragmented night of sleep, night wakings can be less disruptive with bed sharing, especially for breast-feeding mothers, and many families choose to bed share because it helps them get enough sleep. In breastfeeding moms and babies, sleep cycles can become synchronized so that the baby's waking can feel less jarring, and some moms find that they can doze restfully while their babies nurse, accepting this as normal and expected.[37] Others don't adapt well to frequent wakings and find serving milk all night to be exhausting. Just as many parents swear that bed sharing is the key to sleep, many others choose not to bed-share because they say it interferes with good sleep.[38]

The link between bed sharing, breastfeeding, and night waking was nicely demonstrated in a 1986 study published by Harvard child psychologist Marjorie Elias and colleagues.[39] Though small and dated, this study makes for fascinating reading for those of us interested in how parenting practices affect babies' sleep. Elias and her colleagues studied 32 breastfeeding moms in suburban Boston. Half of the mothers were recruited from the local La Leche League (LLL) breastfeeding group and the other half were considered the "standard care" group. Although both groups were overwhelmingly white, middle-class, and well educated, their parenting practices were quite different. Standard care moms nursed their babies about five to seven times per day during the first year, and most weaned between 7 and 20 months. LLL moms breastfed about 11 times per day during the first year, and all but one were still breastfeeding at 24 months. About 25 percent of the standard care moms bed-shared for at least part of the night during the first year, while bed sharing was as high as 88 percent in the LLL group. In other words, the LLL moms were practicing a more intensive style of parenting, emphasizing frequent breastfeeding and physical closeness.

164

These different parenting philosophies and practices were reflected in the babies' sleep patterns. Compared with the LLL babies, the standard care babies had longer sleep bouts during the night and, beginning at 10 months, had more total sleep per 24-hour period. The researchers tried to tease apart the effects of breastfeeding and bed sharing on sleep patterns, but they found that both were important. When they looked at the longest sleep period (without waking a parent) of 2-year-olds, they found that those who both breastfed and bed-shared slept for an average of 4.8 hours at a time; those who breastfed but slept alone slept for about 6.9 hours; and those who were weaned and slept in their own beds slept for 9.5 hours.[40] Based on this study, if your breastfed and bed-sharing baby is waking frequently, it probably isn't because she's incapable of sleeping through the night but because the cozy bed with her favorite person and favorite food isn't exactly encouraging it.

That bed sharing is associated with less sleep is not a Western phenomenon; it's observed around the world. A cross-cultural survey of almost 30,000 parents of infants and toddlers found that bed sharing or room sharing was much more common in families living in Asian countries, who also reported more night wakings and less sleep compared with the "predominantly Caucasian" sample made up of families from Australia, Canada, New Zealand, the UK, and the United States.[41] Even among one of the few remaining hunter-gatherer societies on earth—the Hadza of Tanzania—a recent study found that with more people (mothers, fathers, children) sleeping together in the same bed, the adults got less and more fragmented sleep.[42] The Hadza people said this situation wasn't a problem for them, and it may not be a problem to you, either. But if you're struggling with sleep deprivation, the consistent link between sharing a sleep space and more fragmented sleep highlights a potential solution.

Even sleeping in the same room as your baby can put a damper on your ability to get a good night's sleep, a fact that's received more attention given the advice to room share for at least the first 6 months for prevention of SIDS. A 2017 study surveyed parents of 6,236 in-

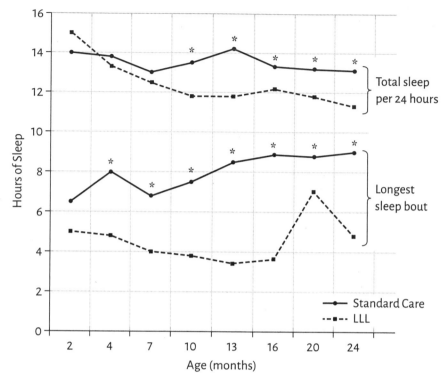

Impact of parenting style on developing sleep patterns. The La Leche League (LLL) babies were breastfed more frequently and for a longer duration in childhood, and most were bed-sharing. The standard care babies were breastfed less frequently, weaned earlier, and less likely to bed-share. Across infancy, LLL babies had shorter sleep bouts, and in late infancy, shorter total sleep per day. Asterisks indicate statistically significant differences between groups at a time point ($P < 0.05$).

Source: M. F. Elias et al., "Sleep/Wake Patterns of Breast-Fed Infants in the First 2 Years of Life," Pediatrics 77, no. 3 (1986): 322–29

fants aged 6 to 12 months in the United States and 3,798 infants in an international sample from Australia, Brazil, Canada, Great Britain, and New Zealand. In both the US and international samples, parents reported that babies who slept in a separate room went to sleep more quickly, slept for longer stretches at night, woke less, and got more overall sleep.[43] Another study, published in 2017, tracked the sleep of 230 Pennsylvania infants at 4, 9, 12, and 30 months.[44]

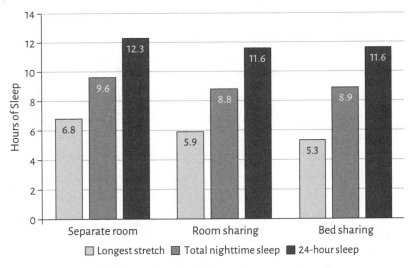

Parent reports of infant sleep in different locations, based on survey responses from parents of 6,236 infants aged 6 to 12 months in the United States. Infants who slept in a separate room had a longer stretch of nighttime sleep and more total nighttime and 24-hour sleep.

Source: J. A. Mindell et al., "Sleep Location and Parent-Perceived Sleep Outcomes in Older Infants," *Sleep Medicine* 39 (November 2017): 1–7.

It found that infants moved to their own room by 4 months got a similar total amount of sleep, but their longest stretch was 46 minutes longer than the room sharers, indicating better sleep consolidation. By 9 months, infants who slept in a separate room were sleeping for longer stretches and getting more sleep overall, and the effect was strongest for those who had moved to their own room by 4 months. Even at 30 months, the infants who had moved to their own room by 9 months were sleeping 45 minutes more than those who had room shared at that age. That suggests that when infants sleep more independently from a younger age, they're able to develop more consolidated and longer sleep.

However, it's important to recognize that these studies can only show associations, not causation. Both studies also found that babies who slept in a separate room had earlier bedtimes and more consistent bedtime routines, and they were more likely to fall asleep on their own (i.e., not rocked or fed to sleep).[45] All these practices have been shown to help babies sleep better, and they also might be harder to implement with the baby in your room. It's possible that it's not where the baby sleeps that's important so much as how and when the baby falls to sleep. It's also true that many parents don't have a separate room for the baby; if you live in a tiny city apartment or in a room of a family member's home, sharing a room may be your only choice.

Other studies have asked mothers and babies to wear small wristwatch-like actigraphs, similar to a Fitbit, or have taken video recordings to objectively assess sleep patterns; these methods are considered by researchers to be more accurate than simply surveying parents with questionnaires. Interestingly, these studies have shown that babies can sleep just as well room sharing as in a separate room. However, they very clearly show that their mothers don't—their sleep is more disrupted, with shorter sleep stretches and more frequent wakings. In a 2018 study from Israel, room sharing mothers also reported more separation anxiety and less help from their babies' fathers.[46] Likewise, in a 2016 US study, room sharing mothers reported more marital and coparenting distress, and on video recordings of their bedtime interactions with their babies, they were also less sensitive or more irritable with their babies at bedtime.[47]

Again, these studies only show correlations. We can't assume that room sharing causes these issues, but it's worth considering the possibility. Many factors affect how we arrange our baby's sleep, and where the baby sleeps can in turn affect parents. If you're feeling trapped by your baby's sleep arrangement, if it's affecting your ability to get a good night's sleep, if you think it might be causing stress in your marriage, if you're finding it hard to be a sensitive and responsive parent night after night, then it may be worth considering a separate sleep space for your baby—if that's possible in your living situation.

What about for the baby? Is one or the other pattern—the frequent feeding and waking associated with bed sharing (and to some extent room sharing) or the more consolidated sleep found in babies that sleep alone—better for babies? Beyond the observational evidence that room sharing may protect babies from SIDS (discussed in the previous chapter), we really don't have much evidence either way. When breastfed, solo-sleeping babies have more consolidated sleep, they tend to make up for fewer night feedings by indulging in a big morning feed, and there's no apparent difference in their growth rates.[48] Although bed sharing is often promoted as a way to build a stronger attachment relationship, what little research we have on this idea shows that this isn't necessarily the case.[49] Wherever your baby sleeps, what seems to be most important to attachment and good sleep is emotional availability—being sensitive to your baby's cues and responding appropriately.[50] In this sense, the best sleeping arrangement is probably the one that feels right for you and works well for your baby.

In many families, bed sharing works well in infancy but loses its sweetness as the baby approaches toddlerhood. I talked about this with a local pediatrician, who told me that she valued bed sharing with her babies herself. Her children were born while she was in medical school and residency, and they slept in her bed to make up for their time apart during the day and to help maintain her milk supply. But, she told me, she sees moms in her clinic every week who are breastfeeding and bed sharing with 12- to 18-month-olds and are just exhausted. "These babies wake frequently, especially in the second half of their sleep," she said. "They are used to nursing to sleep, and they need that every time they wake during the night."[51] Some parents ride out this period, knowing that their children will eventually outgrow it. Others "night wean," continuing to bed-share but explaining to their toddlers that the milk bar is closed for the night. Still others decide it is time for their baby to have her own bed, and the frequent wakings often resolve on their own.

NIGHT WAKING AND SELF-SOOTHING

In the late 1960s, a young psychiatrist named Thomas Anders was studying infant sleep patterns in the newborn nursery at Montefiore Hospital in New York City. Another researcher was working

169

under the same mentor, only she was studying the development of sleep in kittens. As Anders told me, a romance developed between the two, and they were married. Their first child, Michael, was born in 1972.[52]

In his research on the sleep of newborn babies, Anders had been using a technique called polysomnography, a set of physiological measurements that required attaching an array of harmless electrodes to a baby's body. In those days, newborn babies spent their nights in the hospital nursery, and most moms agreed to let Anders conduct these studies as their babies slept. However, he had a hard time getting moms to bring their babies back into the sleep lab for longitudinal studies, to see how the infants' sleep developed over the first months of life. Parenting is hard enough in those early days, and the last thing those moms wanted to do was bring their little babies into a hospital sleep lab and put them to bed with a bunch of electrodes. Even for the sake of science.

So when his first child was born, Anders thought: "Here's the perfect subject for a longitudinal study." But, he told me, "When it came time to put the electrodes on him and do the polygraphic recordings, both my wife and I sort of looked at each other." They knew that the recordings wouldn't hurt their baby. But the electrodes had to be attached with a type of glue, which would get stuck in his hair, and the whole thing was probably irritating to a baby. Anders and his wife couldn't quite bring themselves to make their son a guinea pig in this way.[53]

What I love about this story is that the experience of becoming a parent pushed Anders to find a new and better way to answer his research questions. He ditched polysomnography and instead began using what was then a brand-new technology: time-lapse video. He could skip all the electrodes and glue and wires. All that was needed was a video camera mounted above the baby's crib at home. Watching these videos of babies sleeping, Anders could easily differentiate active sleep from quiet sleep.[54] At the time, he was interested in how sleep architecture changed with age, thinking that this might be a window into how a baby's brain was developing.

As he watched these videotapes, tracking cycles of active sleep, quiet sleep, active sleep, quiet sleep, and so on, Anders noticed something totally new and unexpected. He noticed that every single baby woke up at least a few times during the night, even the ones who had appeared to be "sleeping through the night."[55] Before this discovery, sleep researchers assumed that babies who slept through the night really did just that—slept the entire time. Instead, Anders found that all babies woke up at some point during the night. Their longest sleep bouts lengthened during the first year, but it was unusual for any baby to sleep for more than six hours at a time.[56] As Anders described it, "It is normal, it is physiologic, and it is expected that babies even at a year wake. I would think that these brief awakenings are necessary for the nervous system."[57]

All the babies in Anders's studies woke during the night, but what differed was how they responded to an awakening. Some babies cried when they woke, and Anders labeled these babies "signalers." Others woke, looked around, perhaps finding their thumb to suck, and then went back to sleep. Anders called these babies, the ones who didn't alert their parents to their awakenings, "self-soothers."[58] Now, this discovery may not sound so groundbreaking to you. You might have already read about self-soothing in one of the baby sleep books on your nightstand, or witnessed it yourself on your baby's video monitor—now a common piece of technology in baby bedrooms. But at the time, it was a really important finding. Anders had essentially defined, in an objective way, what generations of parents meant when they said their baby was a "good sleeper": a baby that woke in the night but was able to go back to sleep on her own. And with this discovery, Anders and others could begin to identify factors that were different between self-soothers and signalers.

WHAT MAKES A SELF-SOOTHER?

Overwhelmingly, and across cultures, babies that self-soothe usually have one thing in common: they are put in their beds at night while they are awake.[59] They aren't fed or rocked or bounced to

171

sleep. Instead, they manage the transition from wakefulness to sleep on their own at the beginning of the night, and having this skill, they're able to do the same thing in the middle of the night as well. It's as if they wake up, look around, and think, "Oh yeah, here I am in my crib still. Nothing interesting going on here. Yawn . . . Guess I'll go back to sleep." Signaling babies, on the other hand, are often actively soothed to sleep at bedtime and then gently set down in their cribs. When these babies wake up, they cry. Perhaps they are thinking, "Wait a second! Last thing I knew, I was nuzzled against my mama, drinking my favorite drink, listening to her sing my favorite song. Now I'm lying here alone in this crib. Mama? Mama! Bring back the milk and the warmth and the sweet melody!" In other words, the baby who falls asleep with help at the beginning of the night is likely to call out for help in the middle of the night. (As with everything in parenting, there are certainly individual exceptions to this rule, but in studies that look at this question in a group of babies, this pattern almost always emerges.)

Anders explained to me that "falling asleep is a learned phenomenon" and that, according to his data, most self-soothing babies learn to fall asleep on their own by about 4 to 5 months of age. And because self-soothing is a learned skill, it takes a little practice.

Your baby gets to practice self-soothing to sleep when you start putting her down in her bed while she's still awake. This may mean ending her feeding session before she falls asleep completely or even waking her up a bit as you put her to bed. It might mean avoiding previous "active" soothing methods, including rocking, bouncing, and walking to sleep. The goal is to let your baby try falling asleep on her own. Anders told me that at this stage, if the baby protests being put down to fall asleep, "You can quietly, soothingly, sit by the baby and talk to the baby, pat the baby . . . You can help the baby to not be so upset and fall asleep."[60] This might be the beginning of a gradual learning process, and you can offer your support without jumping in to take over for the baby.

One study from Anders's lab showed that at 12 months of age, babies were more likely to be self-soothers if their parents waited just a few minutes before responding to their night wakings when they were 3 months of age.[61] These parents weren't neglecting their babies; average wait time during this study was just three minutes. Maybe that was just long enough to give the babies a chance to try soothing themselves, maybe sucking a thumb or fingers, finding a pacifier, and so on. And most babies do make some attempts to self-soothe after waking during the night, even if for just a few seconds and regardless of whether or not they end up crying for help.[62] Many of the babies in Anders's studies who were usually signalers had occasional awakenings during which they quietly soothed themselves back to sleep without waking their parents. Most babies have some ability to self-soothe, and this can develop further over time with some brief opportunities to practice.

A more recent study of 120 London families, published in 2017, found that parents who waited at least one minute before feeding their baby after a night waking had infants who were sleeping much longer stretches and having fewer feeds at night (but making up for it with longer feedings during the day) compared with those who fed their babies within one minute of waking. At 3 months old, 89 percent of the babies who consistently had to wait to eat (1.5 minutes, on average) were sleeping at least five-hour stretches at night compared with just 42 percent of the babies whose parents fed them in less than a minute. These authors speculated that "an interval before feeding may increase wakefulness and feeding vigour, resulting in greater intake and physiological adjustments which extend sleep length and the interval before the next feed. The existing findings do not support the long-standing assumption that breast milk constituents require 3-month-old infants to wake frequently at night."[63]

A little wait time also recognizes that when babies are in active sleep, they can be incredibly noisy and active. They might grunt, whimper, cry (briefly), twitch, flail their limbs around, and even open their eyes, all without truly waking. A parent who comes running at every little peep might end up waking a sleeping baby, and if that happens enough times, waking can become a habit. With this in mind, if your baby wakes you during the night, you might take a few minutes to pause and listen before reacting. If she's fussing quietly, she may not really need your help. But if she sounds distressed, then there's not much point in letting her get more worked up.

A few randomized controlled studies have tested parent education programs that teach strategies to help infants learn to self-soothe, including putting the baby down awake and waiting a moment before responding after an apparent night waking.[64] When parents received this advice, their babies slept longer and woke their parents less often during the night by the time they were a few months old. Because these were prospective and randomized

TIPS FOR SUPPORTING SELF-SOOTHING

- Develop a soothing, consistent bedtime that you begin before your baby gets too tired, at about the same time each night.

- Feed your baby early in the bedtime routine, and then follow with a quiet activity or two like reading, massage, or singing. (It's difficult, if not impossible, to avoid feeding to sleep when your baby is very young. Enjoy those sweet milk-drunk moments. After a few months, you'll find you can separate feeding and sleeping.)

- Put your baby in bed sleepy but awake.

- Let your baby fall asleep in the same conditions where she'll spend the night: ideally, a cool, quiet, dark room. Using a white noise machine can be helpful as a signal that it's time to sleep and to muffle ambient noise, but keep it on all night or she might fuss upon waking to a completely silent room.

- When your baby wakes during the night, wait a minute or two before responding, especially if she's just making quiet noises.

- If you feed your baby during the night or respond to another need, do so quickly and quietly and then return her to bed sleepy but awake.

- If possible, having the nonbreastfeeding parent be the first responder to nighttime crying can help you figure out if your baby needs to be fed or just offered a bit a comfort.

studies, they clearly showed that parents can shape their babies' sleep patterns and that giving brief opportunities to self-soothe from a young age can lead to more restful sleep.

WHEN SELF-SOOTHING IS NOT THE GOAL

This is a good time to point out that much of what I'm saying here about desirable sleep for a baby, while rooted in the scientific literature, is still decidedly biased toward Western cultural beliefs and my own experiences. When Cee dropped her last middle-of-the-night feeding and started "sleeping" (or more accurately, self-soothing) through the night at around 8 months of age, I both celebrated the full night of sleep for myself and felt proud for her. To me, this was a developmental milestone that represented her growing autonomy and ability to self-regulate. There was also a part of me that mourned the loss of our quiet time together in the night, just as I mourned the passing of nearly every baby stage.

But not everyone shares my perception of self-soothing as a milestone or has the expectation that self-soothing is something with which babies should be concerned. For example, on the topic of how to respond to night wakings, attachment parenting advocates Bill and Martha Sears write, "If you get to your baby quickly before he completely wakes up, you may be able to settle him back to sleep with a quick laying on of hands, a cozy cuddle, or a warm nurse. If you parent your baby through this vulnerable period for night waking, you can often prevent him from waking up completely."[65] Based on what we know about self-soothing, this strategy might actually wake a sleeping baby or teach her to look for you upon waking rather than try to self-soothe. But lots of parents around the world approach nighttime parenting in this way, and their children will eventually self-soothe and sleep through the night, even if a few years down the line.

Understanding self-soothing also helps explain why breastfeeding and bed sharing may be associated with more night wakings. Several studies have shown that it is probably not breastfeeding per se that causes more wakings but rather breastfeeding to sleep, at least in older babies.[66] That's consistent with this same idea that if the baby falls asleep with the active involvement of a caregiver, she'll ask for the same kind of involvement after a normal night waking. Likewise, if a bed-sharing baby falls asleep snuggled against her mama, she will seek those same conditions upon waking in the night. And with bed sharing, it is much harder to wait a minute or two before reaching out to pat the baby or offering a breast. This means that the baby can grow accustomed to constant outside comfort and help with transitioning from one sleep cycle to the next.

If that help is always there and it doesn't interrupt the parents' sleep much, this system can work very well. This was demonstrated in a study comparing the sleep practices and problems of American and Japanese families.[67] In the Japanese families, most babies not only bed-shared but also fell asleep and remained in body contact with their mothers throughout the night. The mothers in these families reported few problems with bedtime struggles or night wakings. Some of the American families bed-shared too, but they were much more likely to report problems with it. One striking difference between the two cultures was that the American bed-sharing children were more likely to fall asleep outside the bed (e.g., rocked to sleep, pushed in a stroller, etc.). Since these falling-to-sleep conditions wouldn't be matched in the middle of the night, this might have caused more sleep disturbances, whereas the Japanese children could fall asleep knowing that they'd find things just as they left them if they woke in the night. If you're bed sharing, you might consider how you can match the going-to-sleep expectations with the middle-of-the-night expectations.

YOUR SLEEP PHILOSOPHY SHAPES YOUR CHILD'S SLEEP

In a 2009 study, Israeli researchers asked pregnant women to describe their philosophies about infant sleep, presenting them with 14 vignettes of baby sleep situations and asking them how they would respond.[68] For example: "Kevin is an 8-month-old boy. He is described as a very active and alert child . . . During the night, Kevin wakes up a number of times and has difficulty falling asleep." The women completed the questionnaire again several times during their babies' first year. None of the moms were extreme in their answers, but when the results were tallied, the researchers found that some moms put more emphasis on encouraging independent sleep and others were more likely to interpret night waking as infant distress and emphasize active parental soothing. They all turned out to be good, responsive moms; some were just more intense in their responsiveness than others.

The women who, while pregnant, expressed a sleep philosophy that assumed a waking baby was a distressed baby who needed parental assistance ended up being more involved in soothing their babies to sleep, and their babies woke more during the night at 6 months of age.[69] In a follow-up study, there were similar correlations between the mothers' sleep philosophies at 12 months and their children's sleep when they were 4-year-olds.[70] What this study shows is that your sleep philosophy helps to shape your child's sleep. If you believe your baby can self-soothe, and you let her try it, chances are good that she will self-soothe. If you think your child needs your help to sleep, then chances are that she will.

The authors of this study are quick to point out, "It would be wrong to conclude from these findings that parents should abstain from approaching their infants at night in order to facilitate good sleep patterns. Undoubtedly during the first months of life, infants need their parents for comfort and regulation, while gradually these functions shift from the caregiver to the infant. In the course of the infant's development, most parents sensitively balance between their infants' need for proximity and their need to develop separateness and autonomy. However, some parents find it difficult to keep this balance and adopt an unbalanced approach of either overinvolvement or avoidance."[71]

My personal philosophy is that, as a parent, it's my job to find that balance of when my child is ready to try something on her own and when she needs help. I believe that babies are born with the desire and ability to learn and grow, and we should respect that, even as we wish we could freeze in time these moments of sweet baby bliss. Overnight video studies show that some babies are capable of self-soothing even as young as a few weeks of age.[72] Babies are extraordinary, aren't they? We'll know what they are capable of only if we are willing to step back and give them a chance to try something on their own before we jump in to help.

Think of other developmental milestones, like learning to sit up. If, every time we saw our babies working at getting upright, grunting with effort, furrowed brow, we jumped in and propped them up, how would they learn? I think of nighttime parenting strategies as a continuum of responsiveness, and we parents must try to find our own sweet spot, where our babies know that they are loved and supported but also have a chance to grow and develop their own sense of autonomy. But all of that said, I'd much rather err on the side of being a bit too responsive. And, this is just my philosophy. It's what I'm comfortable with, and it is how I make sense of the daunting task of parenting a child day and night. Your philosophy might be different.

Whatever your philosophy, it's important to remember that every baby is different. We may be able to help shape our babies' sleep, but we can't control it. Some babies just naturally have a more difficult time soothing themselves, falling asleep, and staying asleep. That some children take longer to sleep through the night independently is in part a reflection of their inborn tendencies as well as how they are raised.[73]

WHAT ABOUT SLEEP TRAINING?

When Cee was a baby, I didn't know most of what I've written in this chapter. I didn't know that learning to self-soothe could be a gradual process and that it could start early in life. We followed the advice of many mainstream parenting books: do whatever works to soothe your baby for about the first three to four months; then, if your baby is having trouble sleeping, consider sleep training. Sleep training (also called controlled crying or controlled comforting depending on your part of the world) means asking your baby to fall asleep more independently and almost always involves some crying as she gets used to the change.

In the newborn stage, what worked to soothe Cee was bouncing on an exercise ball. Within a few weeks, we were bouncing Cee to sleep for nearly every single sleep, including the middle of the night, and she was requiring longer and longer stints of bouncing to get settled into a deep sleep. At 3 months of age, she had little ability to self-soothe—it's something she never had a chance to try—and my aching back was telling me that we had picked an unsustainable soothing method. I started trying to rock her to sleep, but she just screamed at me. She wanted to be bounced, and she didn't know how to settle without it. I knew that she had to learn to sleep in another way.

At this point, I finally had to admit that my presence wasn't helping Cee in her struggle to fall asleep. She needed a little space to learn to sleep on her own. And so we tried sleep training. For us, that meant putting Cee down in her crib after our usual bedtime routine, saying goodnight, and leaving the room. We returned at intervals of a few minutes to give her a little reassurance. She cried, but no more than she had while falling asleep in my arms in the rocking chair. And by the third night, she was fussing for just a few minutes before falling asleep.

Over the course of a few days, Cee went from being a baby who struggled to fall asleep, despite all our active soothing, to one who went to sleep easily on her own and woke only once in the night to nurse. (She continued to have one nighttime feeding until she dropped it on her own, around 8 months.) She went from having fragmented nighttime sleep of about 8 hours to sleeping 12 hours a night. We would often wake to the sound of her babbling contentedly in her crib after a good night's sleep, whereas before, our mornings had begun abruptly with the sound of her crying. I was finally getting some sleep, too, and I no longer had that horrible feeling of resentment that sometimes crept into my heart when I was bouncing Cee at 2:00 a.m., my back and neck aching in exhaustion. I was well rested and able to be a responsive, sensitive parent, day and night.

This was our story. In hindsight, I wish that Cee's path toward self-soothing had been more gradual and supported, beginning during the first months of life. (This was the approach we took with Max, and his sleep steadily became more independent and consolidated as he grew, without any major intervention on our parts.)[74] But I know that sleep-training Cee helped her, and us, to get the sleep that we needed, and it made our nights together more peaceful and sweet. Like every baby, Cee went through later periods of night waking when she was teething and learning to walk. If she woke and cried in the night, we comforted her. But by and large, her ability to self-soothe gave our family the gift of good sleep, and for that I am thankful.

Some people strongly oppose the idea of letting babies cry as they learn to fall asleep on their own. Since sleep-training Cee and writing about it openly, I have been told that it was cruel abandonment and that it may have damaged her brain or our relationship. Those comments made me feel horrible and defensive, but they also compelled me to find all the research I could on sleep training. I wanted to know, truthfully, how effective it is and whether it might be harmful to babies. Here's a quick summary of what I learned.

1. *Sleep training works.* There is an array of "methods," some gradual and some more abrupt. They all involve letting your baby work on self-soothing so that she can eventually fall asleep without your help, and they all are effective. A 2014 review summarized 12 trials of sleep training, including a total of 1,742 children aged birth to 5 years, and several more have been conducted since. Together, they find that sleep training leads to reduced bedtime struggles, fewer night wakings, longer sleep for both baby and parents, better maternal mental health, and even improved baby temperament and mood.[75]

2. *But, sleep training doesn't work for every baby.* Dr. Jodi Mindell, associate director of the Sleep Center at Children's Hospital of Philadelphia and one of the authors of the 2014 review just mentioned, has published more than 50 peer-reviewed studies on infant sleep. When I asked her if sleep training works for every baby, she replied, "Of course there will be babies who do not respond. Just like with anything—most do well, some receive no benefit, and a few will do poorly."[76] You are more qualified than anyone else to venture a guess at whether sleep training will work for your baby and to know when to throw in the towel if it doesn't seem to be working. And even a baby who knows how to self-soothe will probably go through periods of night waking again. For most families, sleep training improves sleep, but it isn't a magic bullet. And if your baby doesn't respond well to sleep training, it's a good idea to talk with your pediatrician to consider if there could be a medical reason for the sleep issues.

3. *There is no evidence that sleep training will hurt your child.* Those who think sleep training is harmful will cite scientific studies to back their assertions.[77] But if you read those studies, you'll find that they aren't about sleep training; they're about babies who were subjected to chronic neglect or abuse or were raised in orphanages, lacking strong attachment figures. Or they're about nonhuman primates or rodents separated from their mothers for extended periods of time. These are examples of chronic, toxic stress.[78] They're deeply saddening, but they don't tell us much about sleep training in the context of a loving family. When researchers in Australia actually evaluated children who were sleep-trained as infants, they found no difference in the stress levels, behavior, or relationship with their parents at 2 and 6 years old.[79] Another recent Australian study, while small, found no difference in babies' cortisol levels (an indicator of stress) one week and one month after sleep training, as well as no dif-

ference in mother-infant attachment a year later.[80] Anyone who claims that sleep training will cause long-term harm is not representing the science accurately, and they're ignoring the fact that chronic sleep deprivation could be harming you and your baby. You will make up for a few nights of tears with all the positive parenting interactions that come with a well-rested family.

4. *Sleep training is an imperfect solution.* Really. As much as I know it helped our family, it's still hard. It's a big change, and it is probably causes at least some temporary stress to babies.[81] It's stressful to parents as well, particularly if half of your friends are telling you that it is a Big Mistake that only Bad Parents make. I like to think that setting your baby up with good sleep habits from the start can help the transition to independent sleep be more gradual and gentle. When that doesn't work, sleep training is one solution, but it isn't the only solution. You might find that just working on a calmer and more consistent bedtime routine can help. Sharing more nighttime parenting with your partner, if possible, can also work wonders. Each family is different in what works for them.

5. *You don't have to abandon your baby in a dark room.* And you don't have to follow any rules or sign on to a specific method. You can follow your heart for setting gentle boundaries for sleep. It can be a gradual and supportive process—whatever works best for you and your baby. What's most important is that you're consistent in your approach, and that you and your partner are on the same page so that you support each other.

As you work through sleep struggles with your baby, try to remain open-minded, to observe and respect your baby's needs and abilities, and to work within your own zone of comfort and your parenting philosophy. Tom Anders gave me this wise warning: "I think that parental culture, belief systems, and values are really important ingredients to take into consideration. Good sleep is promoted by a calming, secure, comforting environment, and if parents are trying to impose some kind of a behavioral technique that isn't consonant with their own belief system, I don't think that's very helpful."[82]

SLEEP TRAINING AND OTHER BIG CHANGES

- First, lay the groundwork. Your baby should have plenty of time to be active during the day, and the evening should be calm and predictable, leading to a bedtime routine that gets you to lights out before your baby is overtired. If you haven't already, experiment with at least brief opportunities to self-soothe at bedtime and during the night. You may find that just focusing on these steps can improve sleep and you won't need a big sleep training intervention.

- Before starting sleep training, talk with your child's pediatrician. He or she has likely counseled countless other parents through sleep issues and can give you an idea of developmentally appropriate expectations for your infant's feeding and sleep needs.

- Find a strategy that works for you. Make a plan with your partner so that you're both comfortable and confident in your strategy and can support each other. The goal is to help your child move toward more independent sleep, usually falling asleep on her own without your active soothing. How you get there is up to you. It can be relatively quick, with only brief checks after lights out. Or it can be very gradual—perhaps starting with sitting right next to your baby's crib as she falls asleep and then gradually moving your chair farther away (although this strategy takes longer and is often more difficult to implement). Consider your child's temperament and your tolerance for her protests. There's not a magic formula; it's different for every family.

- Prepare your child for the change. Explain that she'll be learning to go to sleep in a different way. Tell her that you know that she can do it and you'll support her as she learns. Even a baby, who may not understand the meaning of your words, might understand from your tone that a change is coming. And verbalizing your plan can help you stick to it.

- Be consistent. Once you decide on a strategy, be ready to follow through. Know that it will be hard, but you've thought carefully about this, and you know that your family needs a change. Being confident and consistent will help your baby feel more secure in this change and allow her to adapt more quickly.

- Find support. Lean on your partner, talk to a friend who has been through this process, or join a supportive online forum. Find support from parents who understand your philosophy, so they can help you troubleshoot the process without judgment.

Whatever you do, do it mindfully, lovingly, and respectfully. And then, please, don't feel guilty about your choice. If you feel judged by others, remember that they don't live in your house at night, and they don't care for your child. You do, and you are capable of doing the right thing for your baby. You and your family need sleep. And if you find that whatever you're doing isn't working for you, don't be afraid to change course. There is no overwhelming evidence that any one choice in nighttime parenting is superior to another. The one thing we know is that if your choice is working for you, it is superior for your family.

RECOMMENDED READING

I've read just about every baby sleep book out there. These are my favorites. Each author has a different style and some differences in approach, so I encourage you to check them all out and see which ones resonate most with you. (Thank you, public libraries! But of course, if you can, buying books is a great way to support your favorite writers!)

- *It's Never Too Late to Sleep Train: The Low-Stress Way to High-Quality Sleep for Babies, Kids and Parents* (2019) by Craig Canapari, MD, drcraigcanapari.com

- *Precious Little Sleep: The Complete Baby Sleep Guide for Modern Parents* (2017) by Alexis Dubief, preciouslittlesleep.com

- *The Happy Sleeper: The Science-Backed Guide to Helping Your Baby Get a Good Night's Sleep—Newborn to School Age* (2014) by Heather Turgeon and Julie Wright

8

MILK AND MOTHERHOOD

Breast Milk, Formula, and Feeding in the Real World

When it came to breastfeeding, Cee was a natural. Within a couple of minutes of her birth, she started moving her cheek against my breast, rooting for milk. I cradled her clumsily, trying to remember the holds I'd practiced with a baby doll in my breastfeeding class a month before, but then a nurse came to my rescue, confidently arranging a pillow under my arms and guiding my hands into place around Cee's body. Cee did all the rest. She latched on and started nursing like it was what she was born to do. It was good that her instincts were so strong, because I'm not sure mine had kicked in yet.

I was determined to get everything right about motherhood—naïve, I know—and feeding was no exception. I always planned to breastfeed, and between the two of us, Cee and I figured it out pretty quickly. After the first couple of weeks of nipple soreness and constant nursing, we settled into pleasant feeding routines. I loved this time with her, and it was empowering to know that my body could nourish her so completely. Breastfeeding was a big part of my identity as a new mother. It was also a source of pride; I relished the approval from my pediatrician, family, and friends, and I enjoyed the supportive glances from strangers. (I know many mothers experience an overt lack of support when they breastfeed in public, so I consider myself lucky that I never did.) Because my experience was so positive, it was easy for me to be a little judgmental of those who didn't breastfeed, given the long list of purported benefits for both mother and baby.

Three years later, my brother and sister-in-law, Jordan and Cheryl Green, welcomed their own baby girl, Amy Bell. Cheryl planned to breastfeed and, like me, was surrounded by support, from Jordan, her grandmother, and her friends, among them lots of other mothers experienced with breastfeeding. But beginning at the hospital, Cheryl's plans quickly unraveled. Amy Bell struggled to latch on correctly, and although she appeared to be feeding, her weight was dropping rapidly. Within her first few of days of life, she lost 12 percent of her birth weight, and a lactation consultant urged Cheryl and Jordan to supplement with formula. For the next three weeks, Cheryl kept up an exhausting and labor-intensive cycle of attempting to breastfeed, pumping, and supplementing with formula. Everyone told her to keep trying, that it took time and practice. But still, Amy Bell didn't latch on, and very little milk came through the pump.[1]

Cheryl was scheduled to return to work at four weeks postpartum, and she didn't know how she would keep up these efforts on the job. Reluctantly, she and Jordan began exclusively feeding formula to Amy Bell. Months later, as Amy Bell neared her first birthday, Cheryl told me she still felt a little guilty about not breastfeeding for longer, and she wondered if she had missed out on a special bond with her daughter. But, she told me, it was also helpful to be able to share feeding responsibilities with Jordan as they both learned the routines of new parenthood.

For Jordan's part, he had been very attached to the idea of Cheryl breastfeeding their child. He grew up around breastfeeding, and he saw it as the normative and natural way for babies to be fed. But Jordan told me that after their experience, he appreciates that feeding, like all of parenting, is a "balance between ideals and practical realities." Thinking of his daughter's infancy, Jordan said,

"Now that I've watched her grow into an active, alert, engaged, and advanced baby, I feel confident that her needs are being met."[2]

Jordan was only bragging a little when he said that Amy Bell was advanced. As a baby, she seemed to hit nearly every milestone a little ahead of schedule, and she was hardly ever sick.[3] She picked up everything—letters, numbers, colors—quickly, and she started reading when she was just 3 years old, long before Cee. She and Cee are both beloved in our family, and nobody would ever think to wonder whether they'd been fed differently as babies.

Comparing my and Cheryl's breastfeeding stories, however, there is an impulse to call one a success and one a failure. That haunted me as I started working on this chapter. Cheryl's experience was riddled with challenges that I didn't face, and she tried harder than I ever had to. Her story of struggling to make enough milk is perhaps just as common as my happy story of breastfeeding for two years. And by any reasonable measure, Amy Bell and Cee are both big successes; they're happy, healthy, and well-nourished children, and both of our families found our own ways of adjusting to new parenthood.

But for new parents, it can be hard to find that perspective. Beginning in pregnancy (and often before), we all hear the same message: good mothers breastfeed—it's one of the most important gifts you can give your baby. This message translates into tremendous pressure, and we're quick to judge ourselves and each other if breastfeeding doesn't work out. This is unfortunate, because feeding our babies is one of the most important ways we care for them, no matter the source of the milk.

Breastfeeding and its role in modern parenting is in part a story about science: how science has paved the way for acceptable substitutes for breast milk while at the same time revealing its intricacies, which no substitute is likely to replicate. But it's also about how science is translated to real life and into public health messages intended to alter women's behavior. And what happens if breastfeeding, which should be the most natural way to feed babies, just doesn't work?

A SHORT HISTORY OF THE SCIENCE
OF INFANT FEEDING

The capacity to make milk to feed our young is part of what makes us mammals, and as humans, we evolved to produce a milk uniquely suited to meeting the nutritional and immunological needs of human babies. Breastfeeding is the biological norm, and it is how the majority of young infants have been fed throughout most of the history of our species.

There have always been substitutes for breastfeeding, though, and following their history is a fascinating way to follow the science of milk. For a long time, there was no science to guide infant feeding strategies; mothers and other caregivers just pieced together what they could. If a mother didn't make enough milk, had to work away from home, or died in childbirth, or if a baby had an oral handicap that impeded nursing, then other options were needed. Sometimes this meant another lactating woman, maybe a family member or friend, helped nurse the baby. Other times, it meant that a wet nurse was hired. In a particularly dark chapter of our history, enslaved women were forced to nurse their masters' babies. Records of wet nurses go back at least as far as the third or fourth century BC.[4]

But the cost of a wet nurse was out of reach for many families, and since wet nurses were being paid or forced to feed another woman's baby, their own babies were often denied enough milk. If human milk wasn't available, other substitutes were needed. Poor families and orphanages looked to milk from other species to feed hungry infants. Almost as soon as cows and other dairy animals were domesticated, their milk was used for infants. Orphanages kept herds of lactating goats or donkeys and often fed infants by placing them directly on the animals' teats to nurse. Infant feeding vessels have also been found in children's graves throughout the Roman Empire, dating back to 4000 BC.[5]

By the 1400s, soon after the invention of the printing press, printed books offered advice and recipes for homemade supple-

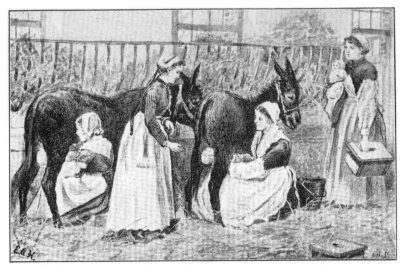

Foundling babies at the Hospice des Enfants Malades in Paris nurse directly from donkeys kept at the institution for this purpose.

Source: S. H. Sadler, *Infant Feeding by Artificial Means: A Scientific and Practical Treatise on the Dietetics of Infancy* (London: Scientific Press, 1896).

ments called pap or panada. These usually contained a cooked combination of several ingredients, including cow's or goat's milk, bread crumbs, flour, meat broth, honey, egg, and sometimes even wine or beer.[6] These concoctions could be used as the primary food for a baby or as a supplement to breast milk. Cross-cultural historical records indicate that two-thirds of preindustrialized societies introduced some solid foods to babies before 6 months of age, sometimes as early as a few weeks of life.[7]

Throughout most of history, it was probably self-evident that substitutes were inferior to breast milk and often resulted in illness. Ironically, this situation became especially dire in the eighteenth and nineteenth centuries, when it was a common belief that boiling cow's milk made it less nutritious. Raw milk was usually swimming in bacteria by the time it traveled, unrefrigerated, from farm to baby. During this time, babies fed breast milk substitutes suffered and died disproportionately from diarrhea, particularly during the summer months. In the seventeenth century, nearly all bottle-fed infants in New York City orphanages died.[8]

The history of breast milk substitutes is a reminder that they've always been needed, but only in very recent human history has science allowed for a safe alternative. In the late 1800s, Louis Pasteur's work showed that bacteria caused disease and that the pathogens could be killed with pasteurization. Water chlorination and modern sewage systems meant clean water for feeding and for washing bottles and nipples. By the early 1900s, the availability of kitchen iceboxes and canned evaporated milk meant that relatively safe formulas could be made at home.[9]

At the same time, the study of nutrition was exploding. Scientists were beginning to understand that not all milks are alike. Cow's milk has more protein and less sugar (i.e., lactose) than human milk, so scientists and pediatricians began recommending recipes meant to be a closer match. A common recipe that could be made at home called for one 13-ounce can of evaporated cow's milk, 19 ounces of water, and 1 ounce of Karo corn syrup. Scurvy and rickets were common problems, but by the 1920s, supplementation with fruit or vegetable juice and cod liver oil decreased the incidence of these vitamin deficiency diseases.[10]

As science revealed more and more about nutrition, homemade formula recipes grew more complex. Food companies stepped in to offer commercial products, relieving hospitals, institutions, and parents of having to make their own and creating a huge, profitable market. By the 1950s, commercial formulas had grown in popularity and had largely replaced homemade recipes. These products were, for the most part, nutritionally adequate, microbiologically safe, and consistent. For the first time in human history, babies could be exclusively fed a commercial breast milk substitute without a noticeable risk to their health. Most parents and pediatricians assumed that formula was just as good as, if not better (being more "scientific") than, breast milk. Mothers increasingly turned to doctors for infant care advice, and doctors recommended that they breastfeed their infants on a schedule, typically every four hours—too infrequent to establish a full milk supply for many mothers. If this breastfeeding schedule didn't seem to satisfy the baby, then supplementation with formula was needed, doctors usually advised.[11]

Other societal changes made formula feeding the preferred choice for the modern women of the era. By the mid-1900s, most women were giving birth in hospitals, where they were separated from their babies soon after birth and allowed only brief, scheduled visits for feeding, making it difficult to establish breastfeeding.[12] But women were also looking to break free of their endless and monotonous duties as full-time mothers and housewives. Particularly during World War II, formula allowed women to fill important jobs in the workforce, and after the war, they didn't want to give up their new careers. Breastfeeding went from necessary to optional to out of style. By 1970, it had reached an all-time low; just one in four infants were breastfed past 1 week of age at the time.[13]

But around the same time, women began fighting for more freedom from medical authority in childbirth and child-rearing, and a renewed appreciation for breastfeeding was part of this movement. Scientists, meanwhile, were taking a closer look at breast milk and finding that it was much more than just a collection of nutrients. While formulas based on cow's milk or soy can be made to contain similar quantities of protein, fat, and carbohydrate, these nutrients are of better quality and more easily digested in breast milk than in formula, in part because breast milk contains enzymes that aid in digestion.[14] The fatty acids found in breast milk are packaged within a unique triple-layer membrane that's embedded with molecules like cholesterol, sphingolipids, and proteins, many of which have been shown to play roles in brain development and support immunity.[15] Most infant formulas simply use vegetable oils as a source of lipids, which certainly provides fatty acids but lack the impressive packaging of milk fat. Breast milk is also packed with hormones, growth factors, and stem cells, as well as immunoglobulins to ward off pathogens.[16]

CHOOSING A FORMULA

A basic, iron-fortified, cow's milk–based formula works well for most babies. Soy-based formulas may be recommended in a few circumstances, such as for infants with lactose intolerance, a milk allergy, or a rare disease called galactosemia. And hydrolyzed formulas may be used for some infants with allergies or certain GI issues. Any of these formulas are safe and will meet infants' nutrient needs, as required by international standards and those set by the US Food and Drug Administration.

Formula companies work hard to differentiate their products in a competitive and profitable marketplace, often adding novel ingredients such as probiotics, prebiotics, and specific fats and proteins and advertising them as "immune-boosting" or "brain-building." These "structure/function" claims are intentionally vague and generally aren't backed by much evidence that the products they're touting are any better than the less expensive options on the shelf. Research on these new ingredients is promising, but at this time, evidence that they're beneficial is still limited.

The internet is full of recipes for homemade formula, which can *feel* like a healthier option compared with a commercial product containing an overwhelming list of ingredients, some unrecognizable. However, these homemade recipes are not formulated by infant nutrition professionals, and they leave too much room for error in nutrient levels and food safety. The same goes for using whole cow's milk, goat's milk, almond or other plant-based "milks," or stretching formula by adding extra water. These practices can cause nutrient deficiencies and strain the baby's kidney and liver function. Stick with breast milk or a commercial infant formula, prepared according to the package instructions.

Sources: S. A. Abrams, "Is Homemade Baby Formula Safe?," HealthyChildren.org, last updated February 25, 2019, https://www.healthychildren.org/English/ages-stages/baby/formula-feeding/Pages/Is-Homemade-Baby-Formula-Safe.aspx; A. Callahan, "The Quest for Better Baby Formula," *Knowable Magazine*, October 15, 2019, https://knowablemagazine.org/article/health-disease/2019/better-baby-formula.

We also now know that breast milk is a living substance, containing a diverse community of microbes that contribute to the infant's developing microbiome. In addition, human milk contains a rich collection of oligosaccharides, a family of as many as 200 different complex sugar molecules. Oligosaccharides are the third most abundant component in human milk, only exceeded in quantity by lactose and fat, but human infants don't have the enzymatic capabilities to digest them, a fact that puzzled scientists for decades. Why would the mammary gland expend the energy to make molecules that the baby couldn't use? It turns out that the oligosaccharides in human milk aren't there to feed the baby at all, but rather to nourish the healthy bacteria developing in the baby's gut. Some bacteria, such as the *Bifidobacteria* species, are especially well equipped to break down oligosaccharides, and these same bacteria produce short-chain fatty acids that nourish the infant's gut cells. They also outcompete less desirable bacteria, and the oligosaccharides act as decoys to bind pathogens in the infant's gut.[17]

Add to this fantastic complexity of breast milk the fact that it's dynamic; it changes in composition from the start to the end of a single feeding, from day to night (reflecting changing hormone levels and encouraging babies to sleep more at night and be more wakeful in the day) and over the weeks and months of lactation, in accordance with the changing needs of the infant.[18]

I read these studies about breast milk with a feeling of awe. We can now appreciate that breast milk evolved to include these complex components—the synthesis of which represents an expensive investment on the part of the mother—because they're good for babies. Although formula companies try to incorporate the latest in breast milk science into their products (and then market them as superior to their competitors' formulas), they'll never be able to fully replicate the individualized intricacies of a mother's milk, made for her baby. Health organizations now recommend exclusive breastfeeding for about the first six months of a baby's life, followed by introduction of solid foods and continued breastfeeding through the first or second birthday. But even if formula is not the same as breast milk, is it good enough to nourish our infants and support their healthy development? These are important questions for parents making decisions about feeding or grappling with its challenges (of which there are many), and they've been an active area of scientific research for the last few decades. This science, however, is difficult to do and even harder to interpret in a meaningful way.

HOW DO WE STUDY BREASTFEEDING?

One of the hypothesized benefits of breastfeeding is that it supports optimal brain development, whereas formula does not. It's easy to make that claim, and it's certainly conceivable given the many bioactive molecules found in human milk but not formula, but how do you test it? The best way would be with a randomized controlled trial (RCT)—the only study design that can provide evidence that one factor (breastfeeding) causes a specific outcome (higher intelligence scores). We would randomly assign one group of brand-new infants to be breastfed and another group to be formula-fed, and then we'd test the babies as they grew in order to compare their cognitive development. But this is a problematic study design for obvious reasons. Breastfeeding is much more than a medical intervention. It's a behavior that requires coordinated effort between mother and baby, and it is helped or hindered by a range of biological, cultural, and economic realities. Women's choices about feeding their babies are complex, and any researcher hoping to randomly dictate how a baby should be fed is bound to be disappointed. An RCT would also be unethical, because decades of research indicate that breastfeeding confers a range of health benefits. Conducting a true randomized trial of breastfeeding is pretty much impossible.

However, one group of researchers used some creativity to design an RCT of breastfeeding in a roundabout way. The study, called the Promotion of Breastfeeding Intervention Trial (PROBIT), was led by Michael Kramer of McGill University and conducted in the Republic of Belarus in the 1990s.[19] In the study, 31 maternity hospi-

195

tals and linked pediatric clinics in the Republic of Belarus were randomly assigned either to begin promoting and supporting breastfeeding using the WHO/UNICEF Baby-Friendly Hospital model (the intervention group) or to continue with their usual practices, which weren't particularly helpful for breastfeeding (the control group). This made PROBIT a randomized controlled trial without directly telling women how to feed their babies. PROBIT included more than 17,000 babies born in 1996–97, and follow-up studies have so far reported on the children's health into adolescence.

Although all women in the PROBIT study began breastfeeding after the birth of their babies, the intervention led to big increases in breastfeeding duration and exclusivity. For example, 43 percent of the intervention moms were exclusively breastfeeding at three months, compared with only 6 percent of the control moms. Because the trial was randomized, the intervention and control families were otherwise very similar, allowing PROBIT to look at infant feeding outcomes on a large, public health scale. It's a valuable study, so I'll mention the results several times as we parse the benefits of breastfeeding in this chapter. However, PROBIT did have some limitations. For one, it didn't include any babies who were never breastfed. For another, the intervention group also included many babies who received some formula, and the control group included babies who received breast milk, so some small effects of breastfeeding may not have been significant in the PROBIT data set because of the crossover between groups.

Beyond PROBIT, breastfeeding research is based primarily on observational studies. To investigate the question of cognitive development, for example, researchers can compare test scores in children who were breastfed and those who were formula-fed. But this kind of information, on its own, isn't really useful, because children who were breastfed and formula-fed in infancy may be different in lots of other ways besides the type of milk they drank as babies.

This is one of the major challenges to breastfeeding research. For example, a 2006 study of childhood intelligence and breastfeeding found that mothers who breastfed in the United States also had higher IQ and more education and provided a more stimulating and supportive home environment than those who formula-fed their babies.[20] Breastfeeding moms were also more likely to be white and older and less likely to be poor or to smoke. These differences demonstrate that in a country like the US, with such huge socioeconomic and racial disparities, breastfeeding is often a privilege. Children who are breastfed are more likely to be born into families in which mothers can afford to stay at home or work in the types of jobs that provide paid maternity leave, on-site child care, and the flexibility to pump breast milk during the workday. These disparities are all confounding factors that mean we can't draw a simple causal line from breastfeeding to health or intelligence in children. In the study just described, the breastfed children scored 4 to 5 percent higher on intelligence tests, but was that because of the breast milk or because they were born into more privileged families with so many other advantages?

Observational studies deal with confounding factors by including them in their statistical analysis, in effect trying to mathematically level the playing field. The 2006 study did an excellent job of this, and when the researchers accounted for all those confounding factors, it turned out that the breastfed kids scored just about 0.5 percent higher than the formula-fed kids, but this difference was no longer significant. (That is, the effect was so small and variable that, statistically, it wasn't different from zero.)[21] This is just an example; other studies of cognitive development and breastfeeding do find a bit more of a convincing benefit, which I discuss later.

Even the best observational studies can fall short, since breastfeeding is so strongly stratified by social class, and it's impossible to measure and account for every confounding factor. And yet, most of what we think we know about the benefits of breastfeeding is based on observational data. Many of these studies, particularly the older ones, do a poor job of controlling for confounding factors, so we always have to interpret their findings with caution and a healthy dose of skepticism.[22] In my review of the literature for this chapter, I've focused on the PROBIT study and observational studies that made a solid attempt at adjusting for relevant confounding factors.

BENEFITS OF BREASTFEEDING: THINGS WE FEEL PRETTY SURE ABOUT

There is good evidence that breastfeeding protects babies from gastrointestinal (GI) infections causing symptoms like vomiting or diarrhea. The PROBIT study reported that by 12 months of age, 9.1 percent of the babies in the intervention group (which had more breastfeeding) had experienced a gastrointestinal infection compared with 13.2 percent of babies in the control group.[23] Observational studies have also consistently found an association between breastfeeding and a lower incidence of gastrointestinal infections, with exclusively breastfed babies having the lowest chances of a GI bug.[24] For example, a 2019 study of 6,861 babies in the United States and the United Kingdom found that those who were breastfed for at least 3 to 6 months had approximately 40 percent fewer GI infections compared with those with no breastfeeding, and exclusively breastfed infants had 55 percent fewer infections.[25] This protection is especially important in developing countries, where lack of clean water and access to medical care means more babies get sick and fewer receive the medical attention they need, but it is relevant in developed countries as well. Wherever you're raising your baby, fewer instances of diarrhea and dehydration is a welcome benefit.

The PROBIT study did not find a reduction in respiratory or ear infections, such as those causing runny nose, cough, or fever, in the group with more breastfeeding. However, a protective effect of breastfeeding against these types of illnesses has been observed in many observational studies. So, it's less clear that this is a real benefit and not a result of confounding. So many factors contribute to babies' exposure and vulnerability to these infections, including whether they're in day care, vaccinated, or exposed to tobacco smoke, or whether they have older siblings who bring germs home to the rest of the family. However, observational studies that do a solid job of adjusting for confounders consistently find that breast-fed infants are less likely to come down with respiratory and ear infections, with greater protection for infants who are exclusively breastfed.[26] Most studies have found that the benefit of fewer gastrointestinal and respiratory infections is limited to the period of breastfeeding, with protection waning once the baby is weaned from breast milk.[27]

One reason that we feel confident about breastfeeding's role in reducing infections is that there's a clear biological mechanism for this benefit. Breast milk contains a host of molecules with immunological properties, including immunoglobulins from the mother, allowing her to pass on her immunity (gained from vaccination or in response to pathogens in their shared environment) to her baby. Some research suggests that a sick baby can even send signals via its saliva into the mother's breast, which in turn produces milk that's enriched in immune factors to help the infant fight off illness.[28] Human milk oligosaccharides, in addition to serving as prebiotics to feed healthy microbes in a baby's gut, also bind pathogenic ones to deter them from settling there.[29] Various other components attack bacterial and viral pathogens, inhibit bacterial growth, modulate inflammation, and stimulate the infant's developing immune system.[30]

The act of breastfeeding might also protect babies from ear infections. Breastfeeding requires the baby to create strong pressure in a rhythmic suck, swallow, breathe pattern, and this is thought to keep the Eustachian tubes in the inner ears aerated. Bottle feeding (whether breast milk or formula) creates less pressure, which can result in the pooling of milk in the Eustachian tubes and middle ear. Bottle feeding in a semiupright position can help prevent milk pooling and might reduce the risk of ear infections in bottle-fed babies.[31]

Gastrointestinal, respiratory, and ear infections are common and usually minor. They're pretty much inevitable, especially if your baby is in day care or you have an older child exposed to the many pathogens circulating at school. However, these infections can sometimes be serious, and ear infections in particular are the most common cause of antibiotic prescriptions in childhood.[32] This is a major public health concern, as the more antibiotics we use, the more we give antibiotic-resistant microbes a chance to grow and spread, causing more infections that are harder to treat as our drugs become less effective.[33] At a population level, supporting more families with breastfeeding is one strategy that can reduce our use of antibiotics. And though antibiotic treatment of these infections is often necessary, antibiotics do cause side effects like diarrhea, rashes, and allergic reactions, and they also indiscriminately kill a child's healthy gut microbes.[34] So, if breastfeeding can reduce the number of infants who experience the discomfort of illness *and* reduce our use of antibiotics, that's a significant benefit.

We also have some evidence that breastfeeding protects babies from SIDS, a rare but devastating outcome covered in detail in chapter 6. A 2017 meta-analysis of eight studies found that breastfeeding for at least 2 to 4 months reduced the odds of SIDS by about 40 percent, with additional reductions in risk with longer breastfeeding duration; breastfeeding for at least 6 months reduced the odds of SIDS by about 60 percent. This analysis found that exclusive breastfeeding did not further reduce the risk. In other words, formula supplementation of breastfed infants did not seem to increase the risk of SIDS.[35]

There is also good evidence that feeding preterm or low birth weight infants with human milk rather than formula is associated with a significant decrease in the incidence of necrotizing enterocolitis (NEC), a life-threatening condition in which the intestinal tissue dies.[36]

WHAT WE'RE NOT SO SURE ABOUT: LONG-TERM BENEFITS OF BREASTFEEDING

In 2014, Ohio State University sociologists Cynthia Colen and David Ramey published a study with the provocative title "Is Breast Truly Best?" It was a well-designed study including more than 8,000 children and looking at long-term outcomes, including body mass index (BMI), obesity, asthma, parental attachment, hy-peractivity, and a range of cognitive tests. When Colen and Ramey analyzed their data across families, incorporating statistical adjust-ment for confounding factors—including socioeconomic status, maternal education, prenatal care, and preterm birth, among oth-ers—they found that breastfeeding appeared to be beneficial for all of the outcomes tested except asthma (for which breastfeeding seemed to increase risk). However, they then limited their anal-ysis to a group of nearly 1,800 siblings who were fed differently as babies, some breastfed and some formula-fed, and everything changed about their results: breastfeeding seemed to have no im-pact on any of the measured outcomes. In other words, when they looked only at children who were raised in the same home, by the same parents, and with the same socioeconomic conditions, wheth-er they were breastfed or formula-fed mattered little to how they turned out later in childhood.[37] The sibling cohort study design is powerful because it significantly decreases the problem of the usual confounding factors. However, even this intrafamily design has limitations, as the reasons why a mother might breastfeed one child but not another could introduce new confounding factors.[38]

The release of Colen and Ramey's study caused a big stir. Me-dia outlets trumpeted the news: "Breastfeeding benefits have been drastically overstated"[39] and "Breast milk is no better for a baby than bottled milk."[40] Formula-feeding parents embraced the reas-surance that their kids would be just fine. Breastfeeding advocates picked apart the methods of the study with a rigor rarely applied to studies finding benefits of breastfeeding and worried that these new findings might derail breastfeeding promotion efforts.[41] The frenzy over this one study shows just how personal science can feel when it relates to our own parenting practices or to a cause in which we are invested.

Colen and Ramey's study was a big deal because it contradict-ed public health messages that have told us, over and over, that breastfed children have a life-long advantage over formula-fed chil-dren. The AAP's policy statement on breastfeeding, written by the organization's Section on Breastfeeding, lists improved cognitive development and prevention of obesity and asthma as long-term benefits of breastfeeding.[42] Michelle Obama's Let's Move! initiative, an inspiring effort at supporting healthier kids in the United States, listed breastfeeding as one of the first steps to preventing childhood obesity.[43]

But for those who had followed previous research on the long-term effects of breastfeeding, Colen and Ramey's findings weren't at all surprising. Outcomes like obesity, intelligence, and asthma are measured years after a baby ingested any breast milk, and a lot of other factors affect them in the meantime. Previous studies have found conflicting results for all these outcomes. Almost everyone seemed to miss the point that this was just one study among many to evaluate the long-term effects of breastfeeding, and it didn't detract from the well-established short-term benefits that we've already discussed.

Let's look at some of those other studies. In the PROBIT study, researchers looked at the two groups of children, the intervention group having higher levels of breastfeeding than the control group, at 6.5 years of age and found no difference in BMI, obesity, blood pressure, asthma, behavioral difficulties, or rates of dental cavities.[44] And again, at 11 years of age, there was no difference in BMI, obesity, or risk factors for heart or metabolic disease.[45] However, at age 6.5, the children in the intervention group had slightly higher verbal IQ scores, and their teachers gave them better ratings in reading and writing. At age 16, they also had a small edge in verbal function and memory compared with the control group.[46]

In short, PROBIT found, just as Colen and Ramey's study did, that the benefits of breastfeeding were mostly limited to infancy. The one exception was for cognitive development, a conclusion consistently supported by longitudinal cohort studies. A 2015 meta-analysis of 17 studies found that breastfeeding was associated with an increase in 3.4 IQ points. However, when they looked just at the nine studies that also measured and adjusted for maternal IQ, the benefit dropped to 2.6 IQ points.[47] Another study found that breastfed babies in both Britain and Brazil had a small but significant increase in IQ. Looking at both of these countries helped to reduce the effects of confounding factors, because breastfeeding is associated with higher education and socioeconomic status in Britain but is equally common across all social classes in Brazil.[48] Although Colen and Ramey, as well as another sibling cohort study, found no effect of breastfeeding on IQ, a third sibling study did find a significant effect.[49]

This question of breastfeeding and intelligence is an apt illustration of the value of looking at different types of studies, or "triangulating evidence."[50] No study design is perfect; all have limitations and biases, but they're not the same ones. If you look at several types of studies, all seeking to answer the same question, and they point to the same answer, you can feel more confident that you're on the right track. In this case, the RCT trial and observational data (including both longitudinal cohort studies and those comparing different populations) point to a small benefit of breastfeeding for intelligence. The fact that the sibling studies don't universally support this conclusion decreases our level of certainty, but this may be because of the unique limitations of that study design.

If breastfeeding does increase intelligence, it could be due to nutrients like docosahexaenoic acid (DHA), a long-chain polyunsaturated fatty acid that is necessary for brain and vision development and present in breast milk but wasn't added to infant formulas until the early 2000s.[51] More recent research has focused on human milk's unique fat globule structures, which contain components like choline, cholesterol, and sphingomyelin that are essential to brain development.[52] It could also be that hormonal differences in breastfeeding moms, such as increased oxytocin and prolactin, might help them be more relaxed and focused on their babies, and the greater amount of contact between mom and baby during breastfeeding might lead to more social stimulation that could enhance cognitive development.[53]

What about obesity risk in breastfed and formula-fed children? The evidence for this is also conflicting. The PROBIT study found no effect of the breastfeeding intervention on later obesity or risk factors for heart disease and diabetes, such as blood pressure and blood sugar levels.[54] Five sibling cohort studies, including the one by Colen and Ramey, found no effect of breastfeeding on obesity later in childhood, but three others with this design did find an effect.[55] Observational studies are similarly mixed; many find an association between breastfeeding and reduced risk of obesity, but others don't, especially when they compare outcomes in cultures with different social patterns of breastfeeding.[56] Focusing on the best quality observational studies, researchers have estimated that breastfeeding reduces a child's odds of obesity by about 13 percent, but given the observational study design, it's still not possible to say for sure whether breastfeeding *causes* a healthier body weight or this is just a correlation.[57] A direct effect of breastfeeding is certainly possible, given that breast milk helps to shape the baby's microbiome and contains hormones that affect regulation of appetite, growth, and adipose tissue.[58] But so many factors influence how a child grows, and children who were breastfed also are more likely to have access to healthy food and safe spaces to exercise and play, making it hard to tease out cause and effect in a longer term outcome like obesity.

Another proposed benefit of breastfeeding is that it might protect children from atopic or allergic diseases, including eczema, asthma, and food allergy. This is a reasonable hypothesis; atopic diseases are caused by a misfiring immune system, and breast milk contains immunologically active substances. However, the evidence in this area is also conflicting. Take eczema. This condition is characterized by inflamed, dry, scaly skin, and babies who suffer from eczema early in life are more likely to end up with other allergic diseases later. In the PROBIT study, children in the intervention group (with more breastfeeding) were about half as likely to have eczema at 12 months (3.3 percent in the intervention group vs. 6.3 percent in the control group) and again at 16 years of age, though eczema was quite rare in this older age group (0.3 percent in the intervention group vs. 0.7 percent in the control group).[59] Among observational studies, some conclude that breastfeeding reduces eczema, some find no effect, and some even find that breastfeeding is associated with greater incidence of eczema. A 2019 meta-analysis concluded that the evidence on this question is limited but that overall, it doesn't suggest a benefit of breastfeeding in reducing eczema.[60]

The evidence on asthma is similarly confusing. Overall, it suggests that breastfeeding is associated with less wheezing and asthma in the first few years of life, but less wheezing might be in part because breastfeeding can reduce respiratory illnesses. In the longer term, some studies conclude that breastfeeding protects against asthma.[61] However, this isn't seen in all studies. For example, a prospective cohort study of over 40,000 Norwegian children found no association between breastfeeding and asthma at age 7.[62] Likewise, the PROBIT study found no difference in asthma at ages 6.5 or 16 years. PROBIT also observed no effect of the breastfeeding intervention on the incidence of food allergies, a conclusion supported by meta-analyses on this question.[63]

Some research has also indicated that not being breastfed is linked to a slight increase in the risk of childhood leukemia and type 1 diabetes. These are relatively rare diseases, so most of the evidence on these outcomes comes from weaker case control studies. These diseases also generally develop long after breastfeeding is done, and there's not a clear mechanism for how breast milk could prevent them, so this evidence is less convincing.[64]

I know I just bombarded you with a lot of science, accompanied with plenty of qualifying words like "might," "mixed," and "conflicting." Sorry about that, but I think it is important to be clear about what the science does and doesn't tell us, because this can have an impact on our feeding choices and how we feel about them. Here, in summary, is what we know. During infancy, breastfeeding likely reduces a baby's risk of gastrointestinal, respiratory, and ear infections, and perhaps SIDS. Some studies also suggest breastfeeding might reduce the risk of eczema, wheezing, and asthma in early childhood, but not beyond. Later in childhood, kids who were breastfed may have a small increase in IQ and a reduced risk of obesity, but there is less certainty about these outcomes. There are lots of other proposed benefits, but the evidence for them is weaker, and studies are riddled with confounding factors.

It's worth adding here, too, that there's still a ton we don't know about breast milk. Lactation science has been chronically underfunded, and human milk is still a relatively mysterious biological substance. We're only beginning to understand all that breast milk contains, much less how these substances affect a baby in large and small ways. I find the emerging research on how breast milk shapes the infant microbiome—and how the microbiome shapes human health—to be particularly compelling, and it's possible that this growing field will reveal more benefits of breastfeeding. I hope such research will also pave the way for more support for new parents so that breastfeeding is more accessible to all, and for improvements to infant formulas for when breastfeeding doesn't work out.

BREASTFEEDING CAN BENEFIT MOM, TOO

Breastfeeding a baby represents a tremendous investment on the part of a mother's time and attention, but it's also a physiologic investment, requiring her body to rev up the milk-making cells of the mammary glands. Lactation requires an additional 450 to 500 kilocalories (this is the same unit of measure that's called simply "calories" on food labels) per day above and beyond normal caloric needs.[65] The metabolic demand of breastfeeding is also accompanied by altered levels of hormones, such as estrogen, oxytocin, and prolactin. Just as pregnancy is a different and unique physiological state, so is lactation, and this fact has led to a great deal of research on how breastfeeding might affect a mother's health in the short- and long-term.

Studies consistently find that breastfeeding, especially for longer durations, is associated with a reduced risk of breast and ovarian cancer for the mother, as well as a lower risk of hypertension (high blood pressure) and type 2 diabetes later in life.[66] For example, a 2019 meta-analysis estimated that breastfeeding for 12 months was linked to a 13 percent lower risk of hypertension and a 30 percent lower risk of diabetes.[67] These are impressive and important benefits, and the quantity and quality of evidence is at least as strong, if not stronger, for these maternal benefits as they are for many of the proposed infant benefits. However, these data come with all the same caveats that we've already discussed, because the evidence is from observational studies that can't indicate causation. As long as we live in a society where access to support for breastfeeding is inequitable, this will be an issue. Women who breastfeed are, on average, more privileged in lots of ways compared to women who don't, including having better access to health care, healthy food, and safe spaces to exercise, all factors that can affect their long-term health. Adding to the inequity, women with more health challenges at baseline may also struggle more with breastfeeding and be less likely to continue with it. Breastfeeding does seem to benefit a mother's health, but this is still an area of uncertainty and scientific debate.

Breastfeeding does usually delay the return of a mother's period, especially if she's breastfeeding exclusively, but it is by no means a reliable method of birth control.[68] It's not clear if breastfeeding helps with postpartum weight loss, because the increase in caloric demand necessary to produce milk is easily offset by an increase in appetite.[69] I know I've never been so hungry (or thirsty) as I was in the first few months of breastfeeding both of my babies, during which I often woke in the middle of the night with a growling stomach. It wasn't unusual for me to fuel a nighttime feeding with a 2:00 a.m. banana or granola bar.

ON EVIDENCE, UNCERTAINTY, AND TRUTH ABOUT SCIENCE

After sorting through all this science on the benefits of breastfeeding, I was struck by how messy and full of conflicting results it is. The scientists publishing this research are usually honest about the limitations of their work and careful in their interpretation, but somewhere between these studies and their translations into public health campaigns, this nuance can get lost in simplified "breast is best" messages that smooth over all the wrinkles and rough spots in the data.

The simplification of public health messages is understandable. After all, most of us prefer clear answers over uncertainty, hedging, and lengthy discussions of correlation versus causation. Yet this is real life, and it's undeniably complicated. I believe we can highlight the value of science while also acknowledging its limitations. Science is our ongoing pursuit to understand the truth of our own biology so that we can make smart choices at an individual and policy level. But part of the scientific process is questioning our assumptions and probing the evidence for weaknesses, and oversimplifying the evidence or exaggerating the benefits of breastfeeding can compromise public trust in science. If we're told that breastfeeding will solve all the woes of a chronically ill society (along with the message that every mother can breastfeed), then of course those who breastfeed can become judgmental of those who don't, and of course formula-feeding parents can end up feeling ashamed and defensive. There's plenty of solid data to support breastfeeding as beneficial. There's no need to exaggerate this. For many families, breastfeeding is a wonderful choice. For others, it isn't, and we can move on to talk about how to support all new parents and their babies. Honesty is essential in how we talk about the science and the barriers to breastfeeding; otherwise we unnecessarily increase the heavy burden of meeting the ideals of parenthood.

It's also worth pointing out that the hypothesized benefits of breastfeeding for long-term health are small in the scheme of things. Breastfeeding is one factor among many that will shape a child, which is why there's no apparent difference between cousins Cee and Amy Bell in their health or intelligence. If you can't or don't want to breastfeed, there are lots of other ways you can support your baby's brain development and healthy growth. However, such long-term benefits of breastfeeding could be more meaningful at a population level. This is especially true for more disadvantaged groups, such as those living in poverty or affected by systemic racism, who already face disparities in access to healthy food, safe spaces to exercise, and educational opportunities. As these communities are often the same ones who face more barriers to breastfeeding for reasons like lack of support in their workplaces, families and children would surely benefit from greater societal and political support for breastfeeding.

IF BREAST IS BEST, WHY DOESN'T EVERYONE DO IT?

Breastfeeding is good for babies and mothers, and science backs substantial benefits. Why, then, do so few women meet the recommendations of major health organizations to breastfeed exclusively until about 6 months, continuing, with the addition of solid foods, through at least the baby's first or second birthday?[70] According to UNICEF, just about 44 percent of infants worldwide are exclusively breastfed until 5 months.[71] In 2017, 84 percent of US moms initiated breastfeeding at birth, but only 58 percent were still breastfeeding at 6 months and 35 percent at 12 months.[72] These rates are a vast improvement over those of just a generation or two ago, but they still fall short of the goals that health experts have set for us.

In the United States, part of the problem is that we lack national policies that support new parents in caring for infants, including breastfeeding. Of the 41 high- and middle-income countries included in the Organisation for Economic Co-operation and Development and/or the European Union, only the US has no national policy requiring paid parental leave.[73] It wasn't until 2010 that, under the Affordable Care Act, employers were required to provide breaks and a clean and private space (i.e., not a bathroom) for breastfeeding employees to pump.[74] However, this law applies only to companies with 50 or more employees, and pumping breaks are unpaid, so they extend a mother's workday and time away from her children. Lack of economic and societal support for breastfeeding in the United States makes it awfully hard to breastfeed exclusively for six months, as much as many moms might love to do so.

But looking around the world, we can see that this isn't the whole story. Take Norway, for example. Norway doesn't allow formula advertising or free samples to be distributed in hospitals.[75] Nationally, every family has up to 46 weeks of fully paid parental leave or 56 weeks with 80 percent pay, and each parent is also allowed to take up to another year of unpaid leave.[76] Although 95 percent of Norwegian mothers initiate breastfeeding at birth, the proportion still breastfeeding at 6 months drops to 71 percent, and just 35 percent are breastfeeding at 12 months.[77] So, even with model societal support for breastfeeding, many Norwegian mothers aren't meeting the standards set by major health organizations.

If it were just about the health benefits of breast milk, I suspect that most mothers would breastfeed and breastfeed for longer durations. But clearly, it isn't that simple. Some moms, like Cheryl, just don't make enough milk. Research indicates that 10 percent to 20 percent of US women struggle to make enough milk in the first few weeks postpartum. In a Colorado study of first-time moms who were motivated to breastfeed and were provided with good lactation support, 15 percent were unable to make enough milk to support their infants' growth with exclusive breastfeeding after three weeks. A California study found that 19 percent of exclusively breastfed infants lost more than 10 percent of their body weight in the first three days of life, and for 42 percent of mothers, their milk hadn't "come in" by this time.[78] This amount of weight loss is associated with severe jaundice and dehydration, and nearly everyone agrees that it is an indication that the mother and baby need to be evaluated by a lactation professional who can provide help with breastfeeding, and that the baby may need to be supplemented, at least temporarily. If the mother isn't yet making enough milk to meet the baby's needs (whether through breastfeeding or pumping), the first choice is to supplement with donor human milk. If donor milk isn't available, then formula may be used, but most studies find that supplementation in the newborn period is linked with greater use of formula later in infancy and shortened breastfeeding duration.[79]

DO PACIFIERS INTERFERE WITH
BREASTFEEDING?

Pacifiers (or dummies or soothers, depending on your part of the world) have a long history of use for comforting and calming infants. However, they've also long been the subject of some controversy. What if they cause "nipple confusion," such that infants find them so soothing that they forget how to properly breastfeed, or if their use reduces nursing time so that the mother makes less milk? Doctors and lactation professionals have worried about pacifiers interfering with breastfeeding for years, and keeping pacifiers out of the mouths of babes was long part of the World Health Organization's "Ten Steps to Successful Breastfeeding." That organization softened its stance against pacifiers in 2018, in part because of a 2016 Cochrane review summarizing several randomized controlled trials finding that early pacifier use didn't compromise breastfeeding, a conclusion also supported by an RCT from Sweden published in 2020. In addition, a 2013 US study reported that when one hospital stopped providing pacifiers for newborns, rates of exclusive breastfeeding actually decreased, while formula use increased. This suggests that having a pacifier as an option for soothing a fussy newborn and allowing the breastfeeding mother to get a little rest could be helpful for breastfeeding. In addition to their calming effect on babies, pacifiers are also associated with a lower risk of SIDS, so the American Academy of Pediatrics recommends offering one at bedtime. The AAP does include the caveat that breastfeeding infants shouldn't be offered a pacifier until breastfeeding is firmly established. Based on the evidence, it's questionable whether this is necessary, but if you're breastfeeding and offering a pacifier early on, take care to also ensure that your baby is fed when hungry and given lots of opportunities to nurse to establish a good milk supply.

Sources: Å. Hermanson and L. L. Åstrand, "The Effects of Early Pacifier Use on Breastfeeding: A Randomized Controlled Trial," *Women and Birth* 33, no. 5 (2020): e473-82; S. H. Jaafar et al., "Effect of Restricted Pacifier Use in Breastfeeding Term Infants for Increasing Duration of Breastfeeding," *Cochrane Database of Systematic Reviews*, no. 8 (August 2016): CD007202; L. R. Kair et al., "Pacifier Restriction and Exclusive Breastfeeding," *Pediatrics* 131, no. 4 (2013): e1101-7.

Breastfeeding difficulties often persist beyond the immediate postpartum period, despite women's efforts to establish a full milk supply. A study led by Alison Stuebe of the University of North Carolina found that one in eight women (13 percent) had what the researchers called "disrupted lactation," meaning that they reported at least two of the following reasons for weaning: pain, low milk supply, and difficulty with infant latch. In this group of women, two out of three asked for help with breastfeeding from a health professional, but only one-quarter of them said that the help was actually helpful. Those with disrupted lactation breastfed for an average of five weeks, compared with seven months for the rest of the women in the study.[80]

There's some evidence that the magnitude of this problem is unique to Western developed countries. Maybe it is because breastfeeding wasn't the norm for several generations, so we're having to relearn both the practical techniques and how to best provide medical and societal support for mothers and infants. New mothers are learning about breastfeeding in an often-disjointed medical system, in which obstetricians focus on the mom, pediatricians on the baby, and lactation consultants on the breasts. We also know that delivering by cesarean, being a first-time mom, and maternal diabetes, obesity, stress, and older age are all associated with delays in milk coming in and more difficulty establishing breastfeeding, and these factors have increased in many Western countries over the past generation or two.[81] Studies in Peru and Ghana have found that in these settings, for the vast majority of women, their milk comes in within three days of birth, probably making for an easier start at breastfeeding.[82]

It's also worth pointing out that six months of exclusive breastfeeding is by no means a universal norm in human history, so perhaps it shouldn't surprise us that it's a standard that is hard to achieve today. In a survey of historical ethnographic records of 104 world cultures with descriptions of infant feeding practices, 93 percent mentioned "allomaternal nursing," or breastfeeding by a woman other than the infant's biological mother.[83] The context

WHAT WORKS TO INCREASE MILK PRODUCTION?

If you're worried you're not producing enough milk for your baby, seek help from your pediatrician and/or a lactation consultant right away. Your milk supply affects both your baby's immediate health and your longer-term breastfeeding relationship. If your baby is losing weight or not gaining well, your first priority is to ensure that he's getting enough calories and nutrients, which may mean supplementing with donor breast milk or formula. Meanwhile, you can work with a lactation professional to identify whether the issue is truly low milk supply or if it is another factor, such as the baby's latch or ability to remove milk.

The best way to increase milk production is to leverage the supply and demand nature of lactation. This means nursing frequently, whenever the baby is hungry. You might also try pumping after each feeding to remove any remaining milk, or adding an additional pumping session. These practices increase stimulation and promote full emptying of the mammary gland, which should lead to more milk production. However, know that while supply issues can often be overcome with these strategies and professional support, continued supplementation may be necessary.

There are a host of herbs, teas, and cookies marketed as "galactagogues" meant to boost milk supply. Common natural galactagogues include fenugreek, fennel, milk thistle, and stinging nettle. These botanical remedies have not been well studied for either efficacy or safety. A 2020 Cochrane review on this topic described the evidence on galactagogues as "extremely limited, very low certainty evidence." There's not good evidence that they work, and considering that there is nothing inherently safe about natural substances and the herbal supplement industry is poorly regulated, they shouldn't be assumed to be safe. If you're looking for a "natural" milk supply booster, a better approach may be focusing on nourishing yourself with good food, drinking plenty of water, and getting enough sleep. These self-care steps may or may not increase your milk supply, but they certainly won't hurt.

There are also several prescription galactagogues available. The most commonly used is domperidone, which is available around the world but not approved for use in the United States due to concerns that it may cause cardiovascular death. This risk may be overblown, as the drug is routinely prescribed to breastfeeding women in countries such as Canada and Australia, and it appears to be safe in women without a previous history of heart problems. Still, the evidence for this and other galactagogues is limited—a frustrating reality given how useful it would be to have a safe and effective medication to help mothers struggling with low milk supply. If you do use any galactagogue—natural or not—be sure to talk with your health care provider first.

Sources: S. C. Foong et al., "Oral Galactagogues (Natural Therapies or Drugs) for Increasing Breast Milk Production in Mothers of Non-Hospitalized Term Infants," *Cochrane Database of Systematic Reviews*, no. 5 (May 2020): CD011505, doi:10.1002/14651858.CD011505.pub2; L. E. Grzeskowiak et al., "What Evidence Do We Have for Pharmaceutical Galactagogues in the Treatment of Lactation Insufficiency? A Narrative Review," *Nutrients* 11, no. 5 (2019): 974, doi:10.3390/nu11050974.

for allomaternal nursing was most often that the mother was unable to nurse, didn't make enough milk, or died in childbirth, but it was also mentioned in records of some cultures as an option when the mother was ill or working away from home. In addition to help from other women with breastfeeding, ethnographic records also indicate that early supplementation with some sort of solid foods has been quite common worldwide.[84] "Contrary to the expectation of a prolonged period of breast-milk as the sole source of infant nutrition, solid foods were introduced before one month of age in one-third of the cultures, at between one and six months in another third, and was postponed more than six months for only one-third," wrote pediatrician scientist Betsy Lozoff in a 1983 paper entitled "Birth and 'Bonding' in Non-Industrial Societies," which summarized records from "186 geographically, linguistically and historically representative non-industrial societies."[85] In other words, the expectation that all mothers should be solely responsible for synthesizing all the nutrients their babies need for the first six months of life may be a relatively recent one in human history.

Even if scientists agreed that six months of exclusive breastfeeding was the optimal way to feed every baby (and they don't, though the majority agree that babies should wait at least until 4 months old to start solids, as we'll discuss in the next chapter), there's not much precedent for this practice being universally feasible.

Today, some of the women who end up having the hardest time with breastfeeding are among the most vulnerable during the postpartum period: those with postpartum depression, a common condition affecting approximately one in ten women.[86] While many women report that breastfeeding makes them feel more relaxed and less stressed, new moms struggling with depression report feeling more overwhelmed, stressed, and depressed during a feeding.[87] It may be that the neuroendocrine mechanisms underlying depression, on top of all the hormonal shifts of the postpartum period, predispose women at risk for depression to also be at risk for breastfeeding problems. Indeed, many studies find that feelings of depression and anxiety in the postpartum period are associated with breastfeeding problems and early weaning.[88] For a new mom who plans to breastfeed and wants desperately to do so, feeling like she's failing at what is supposed to be the natural way to feed her baby can be devastating, particularly against the backdrop of postpartum depression. Because of this, Stuebe urged health care providers to be aware of this connection and to look beyond breastfeeding as the end goal: "If, for this mother, and this baby, extracting milk and delivering it to her infant have overshadowed all other aspects of their relationship, it may be that exclusive breastfeeding is not best for them—in fact, it may not even be good for them."[89]

Survivors of childhood sexual abuse, thought to number 20 percent of women in North America, are also at risk for breastfeeding difficulties.[90] Some find that breastfeeding is a way to reclaim their bodies and identities as women, but others find breastfeeding disturbing and may experience panic attacks and flashbacks of abuse.[91] Women with a history of eating disorders can also struggle with breastfeeding, grappling with issues of body image, loss of control, and anxiety about attention on their bodies.[92] This shouldn't discourage these women, or those with a history of depression, from breastfeeding. Breastfeeding can still work beautifully. But these same women should also know that it might not go well, that this too is normal, and that a happy and healthy mother is much more valuable to her baby than any amount of breast milk.

While medical studies have focused on why we should breastfeed and how to get more women to do it, sociologists have been interested in hearing women's stories and learning how they feel about their infant feeding experiences. Their most compelling finding is that women's experiences are highly variable and rarely what the women expected. For some, like me, learning to breastfeed is a relatively straightforward process, and feeding is a sweet and relaxing routine of connection with the baby. However, negative experiences are common; in one study, two out of three women interviewed described breastfeeding as distorting, disrupting, painful, difficult, or disconnecting. Most women, regardless of their breastfeeding experience, agreed that it was harder than they thought it would be. Because they weren't prepared for this, those who faced serious difficulties establishing breastfeeding tended to blame themselves and reported feelings of failure and helplessness.[93]

These are stories that aren't being told in prenatal breastfeeding classes or promotion materials. Instead, the picture we are given is of a natural, mutually beneficial process, one in which mother and baby exist in harmony, each feeding an opportunity for an infusion of both health and love. A popular breastfeeding advice website features a page titled "Breastfeeding: It's So Easy" that claims, "Breastfeeding is just as easy for Mom as it is healthy for baby! What a divine design!"[94] A state health department's web page calls breastfeeding "the gift of feeling safe and loved."[95] When they mention challenges, breastfeeding promotion materials tend to offer quick reassurance that these are bumps in the road that can be solved with enough persistence and support.

It seems to me that there's a missed opportunity to educate new parents about breastfeeding challenges in prenatal classes and other promotion activities. The focus is on convincing us to breastfeed and on boosting our confidence, and perhaps advocates fear that more realistic information might be demoralizing. But new parents are also highly motivated to provide the best for their babies, and it would be better to prepare them for these challenges before they become emotional, exhausted, vulnerable new moms, rather than blindsiding them with these difficulties later. Research supports this more honest approach: women who have realistic expectations about breastfeeding are more likely to persevere through difficulties than women who are taken off guard by them.[96] At the very least, this type of breastfeeding education would help struggling mothers to feel less alone and would foster more empathy and a more caring dialogue between parents regardless of their ultimate feeding experiences.

WHERE TO FIND INFORMATION ABOUT MEDICATIONS AND BREASTFEEDING

When Cee was just a few months old, I was hit with one of the frustrating realities of breastfeeding. My wisdom teeth needed to come out, and the orthodontic surgeon told me that the anesthetic and pain medications needed for the procedure could harm my baby. When I asked him to tell me more about the risks and how long the drugs would be in my milk, he didn't have answers. To be on the safe side, he said, I should pump and dump for a full two weeks.

He said this as if it was no big deal, but I went home and cried. Cee was refusing to take a bottle, and the thought of pumping day and night only to dump my precious milk down the drain was heartbreaking. Luckily, after consulting my pediatrician and a breastfeeding toxicology hotline, the consensus was that I'd only need to pump and dump for eight hours. The surgeon, it seemed, was being overly cautious at best, and at worst, just couldn't be bothered to look up the data himself.

Most breastfeeding parents are faced with decisions about medication use at some point, and many are more complicated with greater ramifications than my own. Yet, we're often forced to make these decisions with little data. Breastfeeding parents have long been excluded from most drug trials, and for many medications, there aren't even studies to tell us something as basic as whether a drug is transferred into milk and in what quantity, let alone how it might affect the baby. Fortunately, this is starting to change, and researchers are increasingly recognizing this gap in knowledge and working to fill it. In the meantime, in addition to talking with your health care provider about these decisions, I recommend consulting these resources for information about safety of medications, supplements, and other substances like caffeine, alcohol, and cannabis:

- The National Library of Medicine's Drugs and Lactation Database, or LactMed, www.ncbi.nlm.nih.gov/books/NBK501922

- InfantRisk Center at Texas Tech University Health Sciences Center, which offers a phone hotline and online resources, www.infantrisk.com

Source: J. J. Byrne and C. Y. Spong, "'Is It Safe?'—The Many Unanswered Questions About Medications and Breast-Feeding," New England Journal of Medicine 380, no. 14 (2019): 1296–97.

FEEDING IS MORE THAN JUST FOOD

Feeding is love. It is one of the primary jobs of parenthood. In the first few weeks and months, we feed our new babies every few hours, day and night. It is one of the first, and constantly repeated, ways in which we communicate to them that we are here to meet their needs. By responding to our babies' cues, we show them that we're listening to what they have to say and that we can be counted upon to care for them with love and respect. This is the foundation of attachment, whether your baby is breastfed or fed expressed milk or formula from a bottle or a combination of these options.[97]

This much was apparent to my formula-fed niece, Amy Bell. Jordan, my brother, told me about a time when he and his infant daughter attended a meet-and-greet event for local political candidates at a neighborhood park. Jordan fed Amy Bell a bottle, and after she'd finished her milk, she started to drift off to sleep with the contentment of having a full belly and being in the safety of her father's arms. An older woman, probably about the age of Amy Bell's grandmothers, told Jordan that it almost looked like they could be breastfeeding, the way Amy Bell was snuggled so closely to his chest. He took that as a compliment.[98] Was that bottle of formula the same as a breastfeed? Of course not. But to Amy Bell, it conveyed the most important messages of love, trust, comfort, and connection.

This is ultimately what I most want to tell new parents about infant feeding. I cherish the memories of breastfeeding my children,

SUPPLEMENTS FOR INFANTS

Exclusively breastfed infants should receive a daily dose of 400 international units of supplemental vitamin D, which is important for bone growth, among other roles. Breast milk contains very little vitamin D, and because we diligently protect our babies' delicate skin from sunlight (as we should), they're unable to synthesize much of this important vitamin in their skin. You can purchase a liquid vitamin D supplement formulated just for babies and give it by placing a drop on your nipple before breastfeeding, adding it to a bottle of expressed milk, or dropping it directly onto your baby's inner cheek.

An iron supplement may be recommended for exclusively breastfed babies beginning around 4 months and continuing until they start eating iron-rich solid foods, but this is somewhat controversial (see chapter 2). If you live in an area with low concentrations of fluoride in the drinking water, your pediatrician and dentist may also recommend a fluoride supplement beginning around 6 months.

Formula-fed infants don't need dietary supplements, as infant formula is required by law to meet nutrient requirements for the first year. And once babies begin eating solid foods, in most cases, their nutrient needs can be met through a balanced diet. Multivitamin supplements aren't necessary for the vast majority of children at any age, so long as they're growing well and eating a varied diet.

Source: R. E. Kleinman and F. R. Greer, eds., *Pediatric Nutrition*, 7th ed. (Elk Grove, IL: American Academy of Pediatrics, 2014).

and I want every mother to be able to breastfeed if it's her choice. I believe breastfeeding is a reproductive right, and we should be supported in every way possible to establish breastfeeding and to feed our babies wherever and whenever we want. I also believe, and science supports, that women face a diverse array of very real barriers to breastfeeding. We need more investment in research to understand lactation and the properties of breast milk, in part so that we can better support breastfeeding mothers and in part so that we can design better formulas when a substitute is required or chosen. We need to appreciate each feeding—by breast or bottle—as a chance to build attachment and connection with our babies and to know that this is the greatest gift we can give them. The early days of parenthood are hard, and feeding is important, no matter what kind of milk the baby is drinking. We all deserve to be cheered on for the work we do.

9

GETTING STARTED WITH SOLID FOODS
When and How to Begin

There is nothing quite like a new baby to make older generations reflect on how things have changed since they were parents. After Cee was born, my mother-in-law unearthed boxes of keepsakes from my husband's baby days, among them his 1975 baby book. My favorite page is a carefully recorded list of early foods, titled "Growing Appetite." It begins with a mix of breastfeeding and formula but quickly adds rice cereal at 1 month, applesauce at 2 months, meat at 4 months, and egg yolk at 5 months. This was the precise protocol recommended by the pediatrician, and my husband's parents followed it faithfully. From about the 1950s through the 1990s, most infants in the United States, Canada, and Europe were fed in a similar way.[1]

But as we approached the transition to solid foods with Cee, nobody offered us a protocol, and the advice we were given was conflicting. Her pediatrician recommended starting solids between 4 and 6 months, but breastfeeding websites and books urged us to wait until at least 6 months. Some recommended spoon-feeding infant cereal and pureed fruits and vegetables, and others extolled the benefits of an approach called baby-led weaning, in which babies entirely feed themselves. Like many new parents, I was confused, and my fancy PhD in nutrition wasn't much help.

221

I fretted so much about Cee's transition to solids that I totally missed the joy of it. In hindsight, I realize that my worry led us to start off on the wrong foot with feeding. And feeding is at the heart of our relationships with our babies. It starts with how we breastfeed or bottle-feed, with respect for our baby's cues of hunger and satiety. As we begin offering solid foods, that back-and-forth conversation about feeding continues to be vital. It can't be based on a protocol or prescribed timeline. Yet, so much of the advice we receive about starting solids implies there's a way that works for every baby: what foods, in what form, and at what age.

In this chapter and the next, I tackle many of the questions that I had about feeding as a new parent. There are no set protocols here, just science-backed information on which to build the foundation of your confidence. This chapter focuses on when and how to start solid foods, and the next chapter explores what foods to offer.

WHY DO BABIES NEED SOLID FOODS?

Babies go through some incredible nutritional transitions in their first year of life. Before birth, their growth and development are fueled and nourished by simple nutrients: glucose, amino acids, and fatty acids, which cross the placenta from the mother's blood to the baby's blood. At birth, a newborn must rapidly adapt to getting nutrients from milk—high in lactose and more complex fats and proteins—through an inexperienced digestive tract. And then, when you begin adding solid foods to your baby's diet, yet another transition occurs to allow digestion of a wide variety of foods. You may start off feeding purees and mushy cereals, but by the end of the first year, your baby should be eating many of the same foods as the rest of the family. Scientists call this transition to solid foods "complementary feeding." Ideally, it takes place against a backdrop of continued breastfeeding, so the goal is to include solid foods that complement the nutrition provided by breast milk. (If your baby is predominantly formula-fed, don't worry, I'll be addressing considerations for complementary feeding with formula throughout the chapter.)

222

To understand why and when our babies need complementary foods, we first need to understand what breast milk provides. Breast milk is the evolutionary first food for babies, and it provides nearly all the nutrients that babies need for the first six months of life. (Notable exceptions are vitamin K, which is boosted through the injection at birth as discussed in chapter 3, and vitamin D, which should be provided to breastfed babies as an oral supplement as discussed in chapter 8.) But after about six months, several nutrients become a concern for an exclusively breastfed baby. The first of these—the nutrient most likely to become deficient in a diet of breast milk alone—is iron. Iron is like a nutritional bottleneck that affects when babies need solids and what types of foods are best.

As I discussed in chapter 2, babies are born with a certain endowment of iron, passed from their mothers during pregnancy. Babies need iron to support their rapid growth and development, and because breast milk is low in iron, most of breastfed infants' daily iron needs are met by slowly drawing down their iron stores. The iron endowment is generally depleted around 6 months of age, but depending in part on when the umbilical cord was clamped, iron stores may last for as little as 3 months or as long as 8 months.[2] One of the goals for complementary feeding of breastfed babies is that they be eating iron-rich solid foods before their birth endowment of iron is used up; otherwise, they'll need an iron supplement to fill the gap.

The picture is a little different for formula-fed babies. Formula is heavily fortified with iron, and it provides more than enough regardless of a baby's solid food intake. This is why breastfed babies are at greater risk for developing iron deficiency and even anemia during late infancy, particularly if they are slow to start solid foods.[3] This should not be interpreted as a shortcoming of breast milk but rather an indicator that it is important and natural for babies to begin eating solids by around 6 months. Iron deficiency, particularly when it is accompanied by anemia, is associated with long-lasting cognitive and behavioral deficits (see chapter 2). Appendix G provides a detailed explanation of how we calculate a baby's dietary iron requirement.

Iron isn't the only nutrient of concern for older breastfed infants. Zinc, a mineral important for normal brain development, growth, and immune function, is also limiting. The zinc concentration in breast milk declines sharply over the first several months of life, and by around 6 months, it isn't enough to meet the baby's needs.[4] For both iron and zinc, breast milk levels aren't improved if the mother takes supplements of these minerals.[5] Even in developed countries like Sweden and the United States, studies find that as many as 20 percent to 40 percent of 12-month-olds may have low iron or zinc, with breastfed babies at greatest risk.[6]

The period of 6 to 12 months is recognized as one of the most nutritionally vulnerable times in childhood. For their size, babies of this age have some of the highest nutrient needs of the lifespan, necessary to support growth and development.[7] For example, relative to the calories that they're consuming, 6- to 12-month-old infants need nine times as much iron and four times as much zinc as an adult man.[8] Besides iron and zinc, other nutrients can also become deficient in a diet of breast milk alone after about 6 months of age. Breast milk is an incredibly nutritious food, and it's amazing in lots of ways, but it isn't a complete diet for an older infant.

So, solid foods are important. And yet, their importance is often downplayed by folks repeating the catchy but misleading phrase "Food before one is just for fun!" The spirit of this slogan comes from a good place: to reassure parents who may be worried that breast milk isn't enough for their young infants and are feeling pressured to give their babies some "real" food. But many parents have instead interpreted this message to mean that breast milk provides all the nutrients that their baby needs for the first year of life, which just isn't true. The World Health Organization tirelessly promotes breastfeeding around the world, but it is also unequivocal about the necessity of solid foods: "Around the age of 6 months, an infant's need for energy and nutrients starts to exceed what is

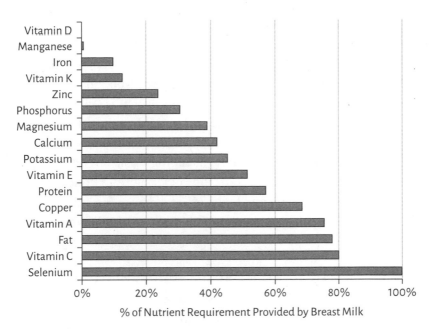

% of Nutrient Requirement Provided by Breast Milk

Percentage of nutrients provided by breast milk for a 6- to 8-month-old baby with average breast milk intake (600 ml/day). Note: The vitamin D concentration in breast milk can be increased if the mother takes a high-dose vitamin D supplement, but the data shown here assume that she is not. Always discuss supplement use with a health care provider, especially during lactation.

Sources: Breast milk data and most nutrient requirements from the World Health Organization and all other data from the Institute of Medicine in C. M. Chaparro and K. G. Dewey, "Use of Lipid-Based Nutrient Supplements (LNS) to Improve the Nutrient Adequacy of General Food Distribution Rations for Vulnerable Sub-Groups in Emergency Settings," *Maternal and Child Nutrition* 6, suppl. 1 (2010): 1–69.

provided by breast milk, and complementary foods are necessary to meet those needs."[9]

This is not to say that feeding can't be fun, and it isn't meant to scare you. It isn't that hard to meet your baby's nutrient requirements if you offer a variety of nutrient-dense foods, as we'll discuss in the next chapter. Most babies at this age love trying new foods, and it's fun to watch them explore.

If your baby is mostly or completely formula-fed, then you don't have to worry much about the nutritional bottlenecks discussed above. Formula is designed to meet the nutrient requirements of babies through the entire first year, and iron and zinc deficiency are rare among formula-fed infants.[10] However, it is still important to start solids in a timely manner. As you'll read in the following sections, there are long-term health issues associated with introducing solids too early or too late, including a risk of food allergies. And besides, this is an important time of learning for your baby—a chance to explore tastes and textures. So, if you're feeding formula, you can relax a bit about nutrition, but the rest of this information fully applies.

WHEN TO START SOLID FOODS: WHAT IS THE OFFICIAL ADVICE?

The official advice on starting solid foods depends on which official you ask. Again, the WHO recommends that all babies be exclusively breastfed—meaning no formula or solid foods—for the first 6 months of life.[11] Other health organizations, such as the American Academy of Pediatrics and the Canadian Paediatric Society, support this guideline but hedge a bit by adding words like "about" and "approximately," indicating that there's a little wiggle room around the 6-month mark.[12] Still others offer a broader age range for the introduction of solids. For example, the European Society for Paediatric Gastroenterology, Hepatology, and Nutrition (also known by the only slightly simpler acronym, ESPGHAN) said in a 2017 position paper: "Exclusive or full breast-feeding should be promoted for at least 4 months . . . and exclusive or predominant breast-feeding for approximately 6 months is considered a desirable goal. Complementary foods (i.e., solid foods and liquids other than breast milk or infant formula) should not be introduced before 4 months but should not be delayed beyond 6 months."[13]

While the experts debate exactly when babies should start eating solids, there's also plenty of variation in the recommendations of individual pediatricians. A 2020 survey of US pediatricians reported that 32 percent said exclusively breastfed babies should start solids at 4 months, 18 percent recommended solids at 5 months, and 48 percent recommended waiting until 6 months.[14] Timing of solids may seem like an academic debate, but there's a big difference between a 4-month-old and a 6-month-old, and to parents trying to make the best choices for their babies, the confusion about these recommendations has real-life implications.

Take college biology professor and single mother Valerie Wheat. Valerie exclusively breastfed her daughter, Caitlin Jo, from birth. But after four months, Valerie was not only going back to work but also starting a new job, and Caitlin refused to take a bottle. "She wanted nothing to do with a synthetic nipple," Valerie told me, and yes, she tried lots of different tricks and types of nipples. "She just screamed."[15]

Valerie's mom was caring for Caitlin Jo during the day, and it wasn't going well. Caitlin was hungry and let everyone know it. They started thinking about trying some solid foods. Valerie wrote to me, "My plan was to exclusively breastfeed for 6 months. I really wanted to wait even later than that, as I'd read on the internet that this was a minimum goal. . . . But here I was trying to start a new job with a baby that would scream for hours while I was gone." Finally, Valerie's mom started giving Caitlin some vegetable purees, which was a big help. Caitlin continued to breastfeed on demand when Valerie was home, and by the time Valerie shared her story with me, she described her daughter as a "strong and smart and amazing" 4-year-old. But this decision to start solids before 6 months caused Valerie a lot of anxiety and made her transition back to work more difficult.

A parent like Valerie, weighing the pros and cons of offering solid foods, might want to know more about the studies behind the recommendation for six months of exclusive breastfeeding. She might be interested in knowing that some researchers question its applicability to developed countries.[16] As the controversy on this topic suggests, there is complexity and nuance that can't be conveyed in a simple public health recommendation.

In the following sections, we'll look at how the timing of introducing solids might affect your baby's health in the short and long term, so that you can make your own decision.

TIMING OF SOLIDS AND IMMEDIATE HEALTH

To my knowledge, only a handful of randomized controlled trials, the highest quality study design, have investigated the optimal timing for the introduction of solid foods. The largest and most recent of these was conducted in the United Kingdom and published in the *New England Journal of Medicine* in 2016. Called the Enquiring about Tolerance (EAT) trial, it randomized 1,303 exclusively breastfed infants into two groups: one whose parents were asked to begin introducing them to solid foods between 3 and 4 months of age (with an emphasis on introducing common allergens such as peanut and egg, as we'll discuss in the next section) and the other whose parents were asked to wait until 6 months to begin offering solids. There was no difference between the two groups of babies in terms of how they grew, and most mothers in both groups (97 to 98 percent of them) continued to breastfeed regardless of when their infants started solid foods. That's reassuring; based on the EAT study, adding some solids into your baby's diet won't affect how well she grows or derail your breastfeeding relationship.[17]

At least three other RCTs have looked at how timing of starting solids (4 months or 6 months) affects immediate health. One was conducted in Iceland, with results published in 2012 and 2013.[18] The other two were conducted in Honduras in the 1990s, where you might think babies would be at greater risk for foodborne illness due to more challenges around potable water and refrigeration. However, the researchers took great care to reduce this risk by providing jarred commercial baby foods and advice on sanitary feeding practices.[19] The studies from both Iceland and Honduras found that starting solids at 4 months versus 6 months had no obvious effect on infant growth, indicating that both ways of feeding provide enough calories and nutrients to support normal growth. However, they all found that the babies who were exclusively breastfed until

6 months of age, without the addition of solids, had lower hemoglobin and iron stores, suggesting they may be at greater risk for iron deficiency. The Iceland study also tracked the babies through their third year, and found no differences in growth or the prevalence of obesity in toddlerhood.

What about risk of illness? In developing countries, six months of exclusive breastfeeding (compared with four months) decreases a baby's risk of gastrointestinal (i.e., diarrheal) and respiratory infections.[20] In some settings, the increased risk of diarrhea associated with starting solid foods is dramatic—as much as thirteenfold in the rural Philippines in the 1990s, for example.[21] In parts of the world where lack of access to clean water or refrigeration means that feeding solids puts babies at greater risk of exposure to infectious pathogens, the WHO recommendation to stick with exclusive breastfeeding for 6 months makes good sense.

In industrialized countries, however, the evidence is less clear. In the EAT study, parents in the early introduction group were a bit more likely to report that their babies had upper respiratory tract infections such as colds or ear infections between 4 and 6 months than those in the later solids group. This difference was small but significant, with about 46 percent in the early introduction group experiencing a cold-like infection compared with 40 percent in the later solids group, and there was no difference in the incidence of infections after 6 months. The early solids group was also more likely to experience vomiting and constipation between 4 and 6 months, but not diarrhea, lower respiratory tract infections, bronchiolitis, or other infections.[22] In the Honduran RCTs, where parents were counseled on sanitary feeding practices, there were no differences in diarrhea or other symptoms, including fever, cough, or nasal congestion.[23]

Large observational studies have also found that an earlier start at solids doesn't increase the risk of serious illness. A longitudinal study of 16,000 UK infants found that timing of the introduction of solids for babies—whether breastfed or formula-fed—had no impact on hospitalization for illness.[24] A similar study of more than

70,000 Norwegian infants found no differences in hospitalization for infections between those starting solids between 4 to 6 months versus those waiting until 6 months of age.[25]

Parents often hope that starting solids will somehow magically transform their babies into better sleepers. The EAT study asked participating parents about sleep and found a small improvement in the early solids group. At 6 months, early introduction parents said their babies were sleeping an average of 17 minutes longer each night and waking in the night about two fewer times per week compared with the later introduction group.[26] If you're an exhausted parent, you might take any small improvement in sleep, but this benefit alone is probably not a good reason to start solids. In addition, a couple of smaller, older studies didn't report improved sleep in babies starting solids earlier.[27]

Overall, I find the evidence on starting solids and immediate health reassuring. Some, but not all, studies show that an earlier start with solids might slightly increase your baby's risk of illness, but if this is the case, these seem to be minor bouts of diarrhea, vomiting, or colds, or discomforts like constipation. (Your baby's poop will definitely change when you introduce solids. This is normal, but it can take some time to get used to the evolving frequency and form of diaper deposits.) Those small risks might be offset by a lower risk of iron deficiency and a very small benefit in improved sleep for babies starting solids earlier than 6 months, but the evidence on the latter is mixed. And whether babies start solids on the earlier side or later side seems to have little effect on how they grow or their continued breastfeeding.

TIMING OF SOLIDS AND ALLERGY RISK

The food allergy world has undergone a seismic shift in the last few decades, resulting in radical changes to advice given to parents about introducing babies to allergenic foods such as peanuts, eggs, and fish. In the 1980s and 1990s, the working hypothesis was that food allergies were caused by early exposure to allergenic foods and that allergies could be prevented if mothers avoided eating these foods during pregnancy and breastfeeding and if babies didn't taste them until they were well into toddlerhood. By the end of the twentieth century, advice to avoid allergens—at least for those with allergies in their families—had become part of official recommendations in the US and UK.[28] But against the backdrop of this advice, the incidence of food allergies was increasing in Western countries, not decreasing. In the United States, for example, food allergies in children were estimated to have increased by 50 percent between 1997 and 2011, and parent-reported peanut allergies more than tripled between 1997 and 2008.[29] Clearly, this strategy of avoiding allergens wasn't working.

I can only imagine how parents of children who developed food allergies during this time must have felt—especially mothers, who had been told that prevention was dependent on their careful avoidance of food allergens throughout the long months of pregnancy and breastfeeding. We now know that this advice, while well intentioned, was the opposite of helpful. At best, it was an unnecessarily restrictive burden on mothers. At worst, it increased babies' chances of developing a food allergy.[30] That's heartbreaking; living with a food allergy means constant vigilance against the possibility of a severe allergic reaction, a mentally exhausting burden for both children and parents that affects their feelings of safety and ease in every situation from the school cafeteria to birthday parties and sports practice.

Hints that allergen avoidance might be hurting more than helping started appearing in observational studies in the early 2000s. One study found that children first exposed to wheat after 6 months had a fourfold increased risk of a wheat allergy.[31] Another found that children who first had cooked egg at 4 to 6 months had the lowest incidence of egg allergy, whereas those starting egg at 10 to 12 months had a sixfold increased risk.[32] Yet another study, led by researchers at Kings College London, reported that Jewish children in the UK had a tenfold higher incidence of peanut allergy compared with Israeli children. Peanut foods were avoided in late infancy in the UK, according to the advice given by experts at the

231

time, whereas they were a common part of the diet of the Israeli babies.[33] All these studies seemed to point to the idea that there might be an optimal window for exposure to common food allergens during which the baby's immune system can learn to tolerate novel food proteins. Introduce too late, and the immune system might only be able to react to the protein, instead of learning to tolerate it. As this scientific understanding developed, expert guidelines evolved as well. In 2008, the AAP stated that there was no evidence to suggest that waiting beyond 4 to 6 months to introduce allergens protects children from the development of food allergies, but it didn't specifically encourage introduction of these allergens within a certain time frame.[34] European, Australian, and Canadian pediatric officials put out similar advice.[35]

But the science did not stop there. Researchers recognized that we could only learn so much from observational studies, which are limited by those ever-present, ever-pesky confounding factors. They needed randomized controlled trials to really get to the bottom of this question.

The first of these studies to make a splash was the Learning Early About Peanut Allergy (LEAP) trial, led by the same Kings College researchers who reported the greater prevalence of peanut allergy in the UK than in Israel. The LEAP trial was designed to test the hypothesis that early introduction of peanut could prevent peanut allergy.[36] The researchers recruited 640 babies in the UK who already had severe eczema or an egg allergy, factors known to increase the chance of developing a peanut allergy. They randomly divided participants into two groups: a control group asked to avoid peanuts for the first five years of life, and an intervention group asked to introduce peanut protein to their babies between 4 and 11 months. The early introduction babies were given at least six grams of peanut protein each week, spread across at least three meals. Most babies ate their peanut protein in the form of Bamba, a peanut-corn puff snack product from Israel. Smooth peanut butter was used if a baby wasn't a fan of Bamba.

The results of the LEAP trial, published in 2015 in the *New England Journal of Medicine*, were impressive. Among infants who didn't show any sensitivity to peanut at the start of the study (judged by their reaction to a skin prick test with peanut protein conducted at baseline), 1.9 percent of those who started peanut early developed a peanut allergy, compared with 13.7 percent of those who had avoided peanut. That's an impressive 86 percent reduction in the incidence of peanut allergy! Even among the infants who showed some sensitivity to peanut at the start of the trial (indicating they were on the path toward developing an allergy), consuming peanut reduced the prevalence of a full-blown allergy to 10.6 percent of this group, compared with 35.3 percent in the avoidance group. At the end of the study, all participants were asked to avoid peanut for a year, but there was no increase in the prevalence of allergies, showing that the tolerance to peanut they developed in their early years was not temporary or contingent on continuing peanut.[37]

With the LEAP study, researchers were able to demonstrate for the first time that a food allergy could be prevented. This was incredibly exciting news, and it resulted in near-immediate changes to guidelines for introducing peanut protein to babies with risk factors for developing peanut allergy (moderate to severe eczema or an existing food allergy).[38] Now experts specifically recommend that these babies begin eating peanut protein in a safe form, such as thinned with breast milk or formula, as early as 4 to 6 months. The change in guidance was unusual, because it was based on only one study (the LEAP trial), and as we've discussed, we usually like to see studies replicated before we get too excited about their findings. This was different for a few reasons. First, the LEAP trial was a well-designed RCT with stunning results, indicating that early introduction could save children from the significant burden of living with a potentially fatal allergy, a finding also consistent with previous observational studies. Second, because the results of the LEAP trial were so clear and positive, it would be unethical to repeat the

study, because it would mean assigning some babies to avoid peanut, meaning that their participation in the research could cause
them harm.

A second RCT on allergen introduction was the 2016 EAT study,
which I've mentioned already. It was led by the same Kings College
investigators, with a similarly rigorous trial design. It began with
a group of 1,303 exclusively breastfed babies, and unlike the LEAP
trial, these babies weren't selected to be high-risk for developing
food allergy. One group of babies was asked to start eating solid
foods between 3 and 4 months, beginning with rice cereal, then
cow's milk yogurt, and then peanut, egg, fish, wheat, and sesame
in a randomly assigned order. Once foods were introduced into the
diet, parents were instructed to continue feeding four grams of protein from each food per week. That's equivalent to about one small
hard-boiled egg, one-third cup of yogurt, and three teaspoons of
peanut butter per week. The parents of the control babies were
asked to wait until 6 months to begin solid foods and then to introduce whatever foods they liked, with no special instructions. The
children were assessed for food allergies at 1 and 3 years of age.[39]

Was the EAT food introduction protocol effective at preventing
allergies? When the results were analyzed in the most rigorous way,
comparing food allergies in the two randomized groups (called an
intention-to-treat analysis), 5.6 percent of children in the early introduction group and 7.1 percent in the control group ended up
with an allergy to at least one food. Although fewer of the early
introduction children were allergic, this difference was not statistically significant; based on this analysis, early introduction did not
appear to be effective. However, the researchers also looked more
closely at how well the families were able to stick to their assigned
dietary protocol. It turned out that it was difficult for the early
introduction parents and babies to follow their food plan; only
43 percent of babies came close to eating all six foods in significant
amounts each week. When the researchers looked at this smaller
group of babies, the incidence of food allergies was just 2.5 percent,
significantly lower than the control group. This group also had zero

cases of peanut allergy compared with 2.5 percent of the control group. For egg, 1.4 percent of the early introduction group were allergic compared with 5.5 percent of the standard group. Infants who ate as little as 1.5 teaspoons of peanut per week (for at least four weeks, beginning by 5 months of age) had a tenfold reduced risk of developing peanut allergy compared to the control group. These differences were significant, so it seems that when the babies followed the early introduction feeding protocol (or their parents followed it, as the case may be), they enjoyed a level of protection against food allergies. However, this "per protocol" analysis is less rigorous, because there may have been confounding factors that affected both the early acceptance of solids and the incidence of allergies.

Several RCTs have also looked at early introduction of egg for the prevention of egg allergy. The results of these studies are a bit mixed and generally less dramatic than those of LEAP for peanut. However, taken together and with the results for egg from the EAT trial, they also show a protective effect of introducing cooked egg by around 6 months rather than waiting until a later age. There's some evidence from observational studies that early introduction of other allergens, such as milk, fish, and wheat, may also be protective against the development of these allergies, but we need more clinical trials to test whether this is true.[40]

Based on the evidence for peanut and egg from randomized controlled trials, guidelines from allergy experts around the world now recommend introducing these foods early on, although wording of this advice varies from country to country.[41] I like the 2019 Australasian guidelines because they're clear but also flexible: "When the infant is ready, at around 6 months, but not before 4 months, start to introduce a variety of solid foods. . . . Introduce peanut and egg in the first year of life in all infants, regardless of their allergy risk factors."[42]

The guidelines from the United States are more complex.[43] They stratify infants by their allergy risk, emphasizing that early introduction is most important for infants with greater allergy risk. The biggest risk factor for allergies is having persistent moderate to severe eczema in early infancy. This means the baby has dry, inflamed, scaly skin covering most of the body, and application of creams or topical steroids does little to improve symptoms. Eczema represents the first stage of what researchers and allergists call the "atopic (or allergic) march," meaning that eczema is usually the first in a progression of allergic diseases that may follow, including food allergy, asthma, and allergic rhinitis (otherwise known as hay fever). This doesn't mean that all babies with eczema will develop other allergic diseases or that babies without eczema will not develop these diseases, but this is a very, very common progression. The prevailing hypothesis is that if invisible bits of food proteins (on your hands, on household surfaces, or even the dust that inevitably collects around your home no matter how vigilant you are about vacuuming) enter a baby's body through tiny cracks in her inflamed skin, the resulting immune response can lead to food allergy. If, on the other hand, that baby first encounters the food protein in her digestive tract, she is more likely to develop tolerance, meaning that her immune system recognizes it as harmless.[44] If your baby has moderate to severe eczema or an existing food allergy, it's worth beginning solids early enough that peanut and eggs can be part of your baby's diet by around 6 months and definitely within the first year.

The US guidelines also suggest that these high-risk infants should first be screened for peanut allergy before introduction of peanut, though how this is handled in pediatric practices is variable.[45] Screening before peanut introduction is controversial in the international food allergy world, because screening tests represent an additional cost, aren't available everywhere, and often lead to overdiagnosis (diagnosing babies as allergic without adequate evidence). In addition, and perhaps most important, if parents wait to introduce peanut until they can get on a clinic's schedule for a screening test, this could lead to delays in introducing the baby to peanut, which could cause the baby to *develop* an allergy.[46] Of course, introducing a food like peanut to a baby who is high-risk for developing food allergy means that it's possible she will have an allergic reaction, and that can be scary. It helps to know that allergic reactions are usually milder in infants than in older children, and there are zero reports of a baby having a fatal allergic reaction to the first try of peanut.[47] In the next chapter, we'll discuss the safest ways to introduce peanut and other allergens to your baby.

All of this means that if your baby is high-risk for developing food allergies, begin the conversation about how and when to introduce solids with your pediatrician early on. And know that while research in this area is ongoing, and pediatricians' adoption of the recommendations vary, introducing peanut and egg earlier rather than later is the best way we know to prevent allergies to these foods.

PREVENTING FOOD ALLERGIES AND OTHER ATOPIC DISEASES

The effects of early diet on development of food allergy and other atopic diseases like eczema and asthma has been an area of intense research focus in recent years. Here's a summary of what we know so far:

- Avoiding certain foods during pregnancy or breastfeeding won't prevent food allergies in a baby—it only adds unnecessary restrictions to the mother's diet.

- Some studies have found that breastfeeding, especially exclusive breastfeeding for 3 to 4 months, is associated with a lower risk of eczema, wheezing, and asthma in early childhood, but it doesn't seem to prevent food allergies.

- Feeding partially or extensively hydrolyzed formula also doesn't seem to prevent food allergies, including in babies high-risk for allergies. If you're formula-feeding, you probably don't need to buy one of these special formulas, unless recommended by your child's doctor.

- Delaying the introduction of allergenic foods, like peanut, eggs, and fish, beyond 4 to 6 months of age won't prevent food allergies; instead, introducing these foods in the first year of life may prevent allergies, particularly in high-risk infants. The evidence is especially strong for early introduction of peanut.

Source: F. R. Greer et al., "The Effects of Early Nutritional Interventions on the Development of Atopic Disease in Infants and Children: The Role of Maternal Dietary Restriction, Breastfeeding, Hydrolyzed Formulas, and Timing of Introduction of Allergenic Complementary Foods," *Pediatrics* 143, no. 4 (2019): e20190281.

WANT TO KNOW WHEN TO START SOLIDS? ASK YOUR BABY.

Let's not forget that while the experts may still be debating the optimal age to start solids, there are real babies involved. They don't become instantly ready for solids the moment the clock strikes midnight on their 6-month birthday. Rather, they're all developing at different rates, with slightly different nutritional needs and preferences for tastes and textures.

This point was well made by UK pediatrician Martin Ward Platt in a 2009 editorial on "weaning," the British term for starting solid foods (while continuing breastfeeding or bottle feeding). He wrote, "The weaning debate has been largely predicated on the notion that there is some magic age at which, or from which, it is in some sense 'safe' or 'optimal' to introduce solids. Yet it is highly counterintuitive that such an age exists. In what other area of developmental biology is there any such rigid age threshold for anything? We all recognize that age thresholds are legal inventions to create workable rules and definitions, and have no meaning in physiology or development, yet when we talk about weaning we seem to forget this."[48] Given all the complex factors that I've discussed, a baby's unique development is probably the most important factor of all, and yet it is too often ignored.

Developmental readiness for solids is so important because it signals that babies are ready to be active participants in the feeding process. They need to have the oral-motor skills necessary to choose to open their mouth, close it over food, and move the food toward

> ### WEIGHING THE EVIDENCE FOR
> ### AGE-BASED SOLID FOODS RECOMMENDATIONS
> ### IN DEVELOPED COUNTRIES
>
> *Advantages of starting solids between 4 and 6 months of age:*
>
> - Lower risk of iron deficiency
>
> - Possible small improvement in nighttime sleep
>
> - Possible lower risk of food allergies, especially for peanut in babies at high risk for food allergies
>
> *Advantages of starting solids at 6 months (it is not recommended to wait much beyond this):*
>
> - Possible lower risk of colds and GI disturbance
>
> - Baby more developmentally ready for self-feeding, making feeding easier

the back of the mouth to swallow it without gagging. They also need to be able to tell us, in their own way, when they're ready for another bite and when they're done. This kind of back-and-forth communication is critical for beginning on the right foot with feeding.

What developmental milestones signal readiness to start solids? First, babies need to have the strength and gross motor skills to hold their heads upright and with control, and to be able to sit upright, if with a little support from your lap or a high chair. This happens in most babies between 4 and 6 months.[49] Babies born prematurely often approach developmental milestones at their corrected age and sometimes on their own timetable altogether, so talk with your pediatrician about developmental readiness if your baby was premature or developmentally delayed.

To understand the importance of your baby being upright for feeding, feeding expert Ellyn Satter recommends that you try eating a bowl of yogurt with your chin down on your chest or looking to the side.[50] It feels funny to us adults, and we have the benefit of already being skilled at maneuvering food in our mouths and knowing how to swallow. Babies are learning all of this by trial and error, and starting solids before they can comfortably sit upright makes their job more difficult and less fun.

Besides, if your baby can't sit upright, you can't look one another in the eye while feeding solid foods. How will your baby tell you that she's ready for another bite, or that she's done? Face-to-face interaction is essential. At about the same time that babies begin sitting up, they often show interest in watching other people eat and start grabbing for foods. This is normal development, not necessarily an indication that they need more calories. They're probably most interested in watching the bigger people in their lives and in exploring objects in their world using their mouths. But if they're showing all these signs, and they're 4 months or older, they're probably also ready to try some solids.

When you do start solids, watch your baby carefully to see how she responds to your offer of a spoonful of food. If she's ready, she'll lean forward and open her mouth, and she'll accept a bite without pushing it right back out with her tongue (although she

---

SIGNS OF DEVELOPMENTAL READINESS FOR SOLID FOODS

- Baby is at least 4 months old.
- Baby can sit upright and hold head up to face you.
- Baby shows interest in eating.
- If you offer baby a bite, she leans forward and opens her mouth with interest.
- Baby can close her lips over a spoon, scrape the food off, and move most of it from the front to the back of her mouth to swallow. Or, she can self-feed soft finger foods.
- Baby can signal to you when she's had enough by closing her mouth or turning her face away. (This is also a great time to teach your baby a little sign language. Communicating using signs such as "more" and "all done" can be empowering for babies and decrease frustration for them and their caregivers.)

---

may still make a big mess!), showing that she's lost the tongue thrust reflex present in younger babies. If she can do all of these things and then opens her mouth for another bite after swallowing the first, she's probably developmentally ready to eat solids.[51] If she struggles with any of these steps or just doesn't seem to be interested or enjoying the process, that's a signal to put the food away and try again in a few weeks.

As your baby gets stronger, she'll be more interested in feeding herself. She'll try to grab the spoon from your hand, and she'll rake foods forward on a tray and try picking them up. She'll point at foods that she'd like to try and push them away when she's all done. She'll quickly outgrow purees, and she may prefer to feed herself if you let her. You can progress to offering lumpier textures and chunks of soft finger foods. Most babies are able to grasp foods and self-feed by 7 to 8 months, if not sooner.[52] The more you let your baby do for herself, the more confident you both will be in her ability to lead the way with feeding.

This is a time of rapid development, and babies are open to tasting lots of foods at this age, so try not to get into a dull cereal and puree rut. A careful study of babies' chewing efficiency showed that the biggest leap in oral skills with solid textures occurred between 6 and 10 months, although babies continued to improve their chewing skills for several years.[53] Babies who eat foods that require chewing also have higher nutrient intakes than those fed purees, probably because purees have more water, which dilutes the nutrients in every bite.[54] Furthermore, among a large, longitudinal UK cohort of babies, those that didn't start eating lumpy solids until 10 months or later were more likely to have feeding difficulties at 15 months and 7 years of age.[55]

If your baby is slow to make the transition from purees to finger foods, the important thing is to keep giving her low-pressure opportunities to learn. Offer some finger foods but also provide enough softer foods to satisfy her appetite. She'll explore when she's ready. If your baby doesn't seem to be showing signs of developmental readiness or interest in starting solids—whether pureed or chunky—and she's older than 6 months, please do talk to your child's pediatrician. He or she may want to assess growth and development and check your baby's iron status. You don't want to push your baby to eat before she's ready, and you don't want any of your own anxiety about feeding to spill into your interactions with your baby. Knowing that she's doing okay in her development and nutrition can help you relax about the feeding process.

BE RESPONSIVE IN YOUR FEEDING

When Cee was a baby, I studied the data on age-based recommendations and noticed that she was sitting up and reaching for food, so I started offering her some solids at around 5 months of age. I dutifully mixed rice cereal with breast milk and offered Cee a bite. She moved it around in her mouth and then burst into tears. Determined that the problem was just the pasty cereal, I pureed some sweet potatoes and mashed some avocado. Cee loved watching me make these colorful foods, but again, tasting them only led to more distress. Whatever I put on Cee's spoon, and whenever I gently cajoled her to open her mouth to try a bite, she emphatically rejected my offers by closing her mouth and turning her head away. Meanwhile, a good friend with a baby around the same age was busy making large batches of homemade purees, and her baby was having such a blast with eating that my friend worried he was eating too much. (In hindsight, neither of us should have worried; I now know that both of our babies were normal, just different.)

After about six weeks of half-hearted dabbling in pureed food, our family went on a vacation in Hawaii. Determined to relax, I decided that offering Cee her customary spoonful of solids (almost always rejected) every day was too much trouble. But then a funny thing happened. One day I was sitting on the beach eating a banana, and Cee reached out for it and grabbed a piece. She ate more banana in one sitting than all the solids, combined, in her life so far. At a restaurant in the evening, she reached for a soft roll and devoured it.

That week on vacation was a breakthrough for us. Cee discovered the joy of eating, and I learned that she really wanted to feed herself. I should have picked up on those signals much earlier, but Cee caught up in no time. Back home, she was ready to try any food that we put on her tray, as long as she could fully control the actual eating part. By 8 months, she was eating three square meals a day, with a voracious and adventurous appetite.

All babies are different. Some love being fed purees, and others prefer to feed themselves. Cee was a baby who preferred to feed herself. But as I studied the research on feeding, I wondered about another possibility: perhaps my pressure, my insistence that she try a tiny taste of food each day, even when she wasn't interested, put a bad taste in her mouth about spoon-feeding. I wasn't being responsive in my feeding. I was paying more attention to the research and rules about starting solids than to my baby, who was trying to tell me that she wasn't quite ready.

My experience with introducing solids to Max was totally different. I offered him his first taste of solids around 4.5 months. He was able to comfortably sit up in my lap and had been making a game of trying to grab food off my plate and get it into his mouth, so I put a bit of mashed sweet potatoes on a spoon and offered him a taste. He enthusiastically opened his mouth for the first bite but then pushed most of it right back out, demonstrating that he hadn't quite grown out of the tongue thrust reflex. He fussed a little and showed no interest in trying another bite. A few days later, I offered him a bit of oatmeal thinned with breast milk, and he had the same response. So, I stopped offering him food and just enjoyed the simplicity of breastfeeding for a few more weeks. Max continued to join us at the table, where he learned other things about food—that it's enjoyable, social, and something to be shared with those you love. Then, one day at lunch, about three weeks after his first try at sweet potatoes, he grabbed at my fork as I attempted to eat a bit of reheated pot roast. I gave a small, juicy portion a few pulses in the food processor and offered him a bite. He ate like a pro and kept opening his mouth for more bites, even fussing a little when I was too slow to offer him the next spoonful. Letting him lead the way and following his cues made feeding a more joyful and relaxing experience for both of us.

I thought about my contrasting experiences with Cee and Max when I read the EAT study. While the results were promising in terms of allergy reduction, the fact that so many of the families assigned to early introduction of solids struggled to follow the protocol tells us something important about developmental readiness and the importance of responsive feeding. The parents in the early introduction group were asked to follow a complex schedule of feeding six different foods, all in amounts of at least four grams per week, with the first foods introduced as early as 3 months. Less than half of the participating families could follow this protocol. That's probably because many (and perhaps most) babies are not developmentally ready for solids before 4 months, and the pressure of trying to follow the study's instructions may have turned meals into a struggle. At the beginning of the study, parents of the early introduction babies reported that their babies often gagged on the foods or spit them out, or they seemed to not enjoy the taste. The researchers describe the parents as having a "growing sense of defeat." One caregiver wrote this of feeding their 24-month-old: "Becoming fussy with food. Struggling to get food into her, both intervention foods and others. No two days are the same at present."[56] This fussiness about what and how much to eat is absolutely normal and familiar to any parent of a baby or toddler. It must have been hard for these study parents, doing their best to be good research participants, to follow this protocol.

I appreciated the advice of Dr. David Fleischer, head of allergy and immunology at the University of Colorado Denver School of Medicine, when I interviewed him for an article I wrote for the *New York Times* on this topic. He acknowledged that babies develop at different rates, and he said he doesn't want families to stress about introducing foods at a precise time in a precise amount. "We don't want to medicalize this process," he said. Offer foods to your baby—including common food allergens like peanut, egg, and dairy—and let them eat them often, but don't stress about getting a certain amount in every week.[57]

When you introduce solids to your baby, you're beginning a long and hopefully healthy relationship with food as a source of nourishment. Just as important as how and when we begin complementary feeding is how we proceed. From the first bite of food and continuing as your baby grows, being responsive in your feeding is most important. Just as with breast- or bottle-feeding, don't push her to eat if she isn't ready or isn't hungry, and don't expect her to finish some arbitrary portion of food if she's signaling to you that she's full. Be sure that she is an active participant every step of the way. Babies are good at self-regulation, and nobody knows better than your baby if her belly is full.[58] This ability to self-regulate appears to decline in the toddler years, maybe because parents have convinced their children that their signals of hunger and satiety aren't that important. That's the message a child receives if she declares that she's all done (in whatever language she's using at her age), and the parent says, "How about one more yummy bite?"

Research clearly shows that pressure tactics and feeding don't mix. Pressure comes in many forms. It can mean prompting, like the example just given, or praise ("What a good girl for finishing your broccoli!"), rewards for eating, or coercion, like sneaking a bite of food into your baby's mouth while she's distracted. Over time, pressure during feeding seems to reduce a child's ability to self-regulate food intake and often increases pickiness.[59] In these days of rising rates of childhood obesity, early feeding practices can support babies in healthy growth. A fascinating study found that when mothers were responsive in their feeding of solids, their babies seemed to self-correct their growth trajectories in late infancy. Babies that had gained weight quickly in early infancy showed slower growth between 6 and 12 months, and those that were growing slowly began to gain more. On the other hand, babies whose mothers were more controlling in feeding did the opposite: those that were fatter at 6 months continued getting fatter, and those that were smaller at 6 months stayed small.[60] When it comes to how much to eat, baby knows best.

To feed responsively, begin by creating a supportive environment, giving your baby a comfortable place to sit, facing you, with few distractions, so that both of you can focus on the task at hand. Bringing your baby to the family table where everyone else is enjoying food is usually the best way to create a supportive environment. You offer food that is developmentally appropriate and nutritious. Your baby tells you if she's hungry or full, if she'd like to eat faster or take a break. You respond appropriately, and your baby experiences the satisfaction of knowing that you trust her, and she can trust her own body's signals.[61]

IS BABY-LED WEANING A BETTER WAY?

There's growing interest in an approach to introducing solids called baby-led weaning (BLW), in which babies completely skip spoon-fed purees and instead begin feeding themselves from the very start of complementary feeding. In BLW, the baby joins the family at the table and begins to eat what she can of pieces of whole foods, usually prepared to be relatively soft and stick-shaped for ease of grasping. BLW proponents recommend waiting until babies are 6 months old to begin solids so that they have the motor skills necessary for self-feeding, and they claim that BLW encourages greater independence and confidence in babies, develops their hand-eye coordination and chewing skills, decreases picky eating, and improves self-regulation of energy intake, leading to a decreased risk of developing obesity.[62] But critics, including many health care professionals, worry that BLW might increase the risk of choking and make it difficult for babies to consume enough calories and nutrients if they're dependent on self-feeding.[63] What does the evidence say? Is BLW a better way to approach the transition to solids; or, put another way, is there any harm in feeding soft purees with a spoon?

When I finished writing the first edition of this book in 2014, the evidence on BLW was very limited. It was based solely on observational studies and, like so much of parenting science, was difficult

246

to interpret because of confounding factors. Data from the UK indicates that families who choose BLW tend to be led by married women with higher levels of education and occupation, more of whom are stay-at-home mothers not engaged in paid work, and more of whom breastfeed. Any observed benefits of BLW in observational studies might therefore be due not to BLW but to these confounding factors.[64] Concerns about risks of BLW were also largely speculative, so I wrote in the first edition that we needed randomized controlled trials to test the claims of benefits and risks of BLW.

Happily, at the time of this writing, we now have two randomized controlled trials of BLW, one conducted in New Zealand and the other in Turkey.[65] Both included a BLW-like intervention group (called "Baby-Led Introduction to SolidS," or BLISS) in which parents were counseled to wait until 6 months to introduce solids, let their babies self-feed, offer foods rich in iron and calories that are easy to pick up and manipulate, and avoid foods that pose a heightened choking risk. The babies were assessed at 12 months and compared to a control group who started solids with a traditional spoon-fed approach. Reassuringly, both the New Zealand and Turkish studies found no differences in iron intake or incidence of iron deficiency.[66] They also reported no greater incidence of choking in the BLISS babies, a finding that is backed by observational studies.[67] The New Zealand study did report that the BLISS infants gagged more at 6 months than the control infants, but by 8 months, they were gagging less than the control group. Gagging is a reflex that closes off the back of the throat and pushes the food back toward the front of the mouth. Although it can be scary for parents, gagging is a helpful defensive mechanism against choking, so it's not surprising that gagging was common in the BLISS infants when they were just starting solid foods and learning to self-feed. The fact that the BLISS babies were gagging less than control infants by 8 months indicates that they had become more adept at feeding themselves. However, it's worth pointing out that the parents in these trials received extensive education about how to decrease their babies' risk of choking, so families beginning BLW without the benefit of that type of counseling might not experience the same level of safety.[68] Regardless, babies can choke on foods of any texture, including milk, so be sure you know how to respond.

One of the main claims about BLW is that it decreases the risk of obesity in children, because it emphasizes letting the baby eat at her own pace and trusting her to decide for herself when she's had enough. But the New Zealand and Turkish studies had contradictory results when it came to infant growth.[69] The Turkish study found that BLISS infants weighed less at 12 months (average weight of 10.4 kg) compared with the spoon-fed infants (average of 11.1 kg).

PREVENTING AND RESPONDING TO CHOKING

More than 12,000 children end up in the emergency room for food choking incidents in the United States each year, and 62 percent are under 4 years old. Take these steps to prevent choking and be sure you're prepared to respond:

- Your baby should be sitting upright and always supervised during mealtimes.

- Avoid feeding common choking hazards: nuts and seeds, hot dogs, chunks of meat or cheese, whole grapes, hard candy or gum, popcorn, globs of peanut butter, and other round and firm foods. (See page 250–251 for more foods to avoid.)

- Know the difference between gagging and choking. Gagging is a reflex that closes off the back of the throat and pushes food back to the front of the mouth; baby should recover quickly and then be able to breathe and talk. Choking means that the baby's airway is blocked, and it may cause the baby to cough, splutter, or just be silent, which makes it extra scary—and extra important that children are supervised while eating.

- Know the Heimlich maneuver and CPR for babies, children, and adults. The American Heart Association offers community and online courses (www.heart.org).

Source: M. M. Chapin et al., "Nonfatal Choking on Food among Children 14 Years or Younger in the United States, 2001–2009," *Pediatrics* 132, no. 2 (2013): 275–81.

The New Zealand study found no difference in body mass index at 12 months, although the BLISS infants had a nonsignificant tendency to be *heavier*, not lighter. So, it's not clear how BLW or spoon-feeding affects body weight. My guess is that it has less to do with the texture and presentation of foods offered and more to do with whether the baby is pressured to eat more than she wants, which can happen in both a spoon-feeding or self-feeding setting. It may also be affected by the energy density of foods offered. In the New Zealand trial, parents were specifically counseled to offer high-calorie foods to address concerns about inadequate energy intake in BLW, and that emphasis might have also influenced parents to encourage their babies to eat a bit more.

While the New Zealand study didn't find that BLW made a difference to the way babies grew, it did find that the BLW infants were less fussy or picky about food at 12 months, though not at 24 months, and they seemed to enjoy food more.[70] And while there weren't any major differences in the nutritional value of their diets, the BLW babies ate a greater variety of foods at 7 months and more variety of fruits and vegetables at 24 months.[71] In other words, BLW may offer some benefits in terms of more enjoyable mealtimes and encouraging more adventurous eating, which is great! BLW doesn't seem to increase the risk of iron deficiency or choking, but it also doesn't consistently protect infants from becoming overweight or obese.

It's also worth noting that no study has randomized one group of babies and parents to BLW and the other to spoon-feeding and given both groups counseling and support regarding responsive feeding and nutritious food choices. And no study has included a group counseled to feed some purees and some finger foods. I suspect that a study with this design would find that any of these approaches can work well for families and support babies in learning about a variety of foods and trusting their own satiety signals. In my opinion, looking at feeding as a binary choice of either starting with spoon-feeding or starting with self-feeding puts too much emphasis on the tools and textures of feeding solids and not enough on the responsiveness of the parent or caregiver. Regardless of how

---

**BABY-LED WEANING SAFETY PRINCIPLES,
AS TESTED IN THE BLISS TRIAL**

Before researchers in New Zealand began the BLISS trial of baby-led weaning, they thought carefully about how to minimize the risk of choking for study participants. They developed the following guidance, which may differ from baby-lead weaning advice you read from other sources. Babies in the BLISS group had no greater risk of choking compared with those spoon-fed pureed foods.

General principles:

- Test foods before they are offered to ensure they are soft enough to mash with the tongue on the roof of the mouth or are large and fibrous enough (e.g., strips of meat) that small pieces do not break off when sucked and chewed, especially in the early months of starting solids.

- Avoid offering foods that form large crumbs in the mouth.

- Make sure that the foods offered are at least as long as the child's fist, on at least one side of the food.

- Make sure the infant is always sitting upright when he or she is eating, never leaning backward.

---

you feed, you should be responsive to your baby's signals of hunger and satiety. In this sense, all feeding should be baby-led.

I think that following BLW by the book (i.e., never feeding your baby with a spoon) adds unnecessary restrictions to starting solids, limiting timing and types of foods. For one, your baby probably won't be developmentally ready to feed herself until 6 months or even a bit later. That's fine for most babies, but if your baby is at high risk for allergies, you may want to prioritize earlier introduction of solids. BLW also limits your baby's first foods to those that she can handle and gum up on her own, taking food like yogurt and oatmeal—usually convenient, nutritious options—off the table. I suggest a more relaxed approach that allows you to start with purees if it seems appropriate for your baby and then advance quickly to new textures. You will help your baby with many things in life.

- Never leave your baby alone with food; always have an adult with the child when he or she is eating.
- Never let anyone except your baby put food into her mouth; the infant must eat at her own pace and under her own control.

Foods to avoid when introducing solids to your baby:

- Very small foods such as nuts, grapes, sweets, and fruit with stones (unless you've removed the stones)
- Raw vegetables
- Raw apple (whole or sliced)
- Underripe or hard fruit
- Citrus fruits (oranges, mandarins) unless each segment has been peeled
- Whole nuts (smooth peanut butter and other nut butters are fine)
- Popcorn
- Sausages, carrots, and any other similar food cut into rounds or "coins"

Source: L. J. Fangupo et al., "A Baby-Led Approach to Eating Solids and Risk of Choking," *Pediatrics* 138, no. 4 (2016): e20160772.

Feeding solids may or may not be one of them, but there's no shame in giving her a hand if she needs it. That's just responding to her needs, which is good parenting.

Since Cee resisted spoon-feeding from the start, we essentially did BLW without knowing that it had a name and a devout following. It worked well for us. With Max, we started with spoon-feeding, which he enjoyed for a few weeks. But by 6 months, he was self-feeding most of the time, with an occasional spoon-fed session when we were traveling or eating out and didn't have the benefit of a high chair with a tray where he could make a mess. One reason why I liked letting him self-feed was that I found it hard to give Max my full attention for responsive spoon-feeding (in part because I was also caring for Cee) and he sometimes grew impatient with me or me with him. It was easier, more relaxed, and more enjoyable for everyone if Max fed himself, while the rest of us ate our own food. I remain a little skeptical about BLW for its strict rules and claims of lifelong benefits, which just aren't borne out in the evidence. Still, I appreciate how it facilitates responsive feeding and emphasizes the value of shared, enjoyable meals.

Of course, there's one big question we haven't even tackled yet: what foods should you give your baby? I devote the entire next chapter to exploring appropriate complementary foods.

RISE OF THE FOOD POUCHES

While baby-led weaning has gained popularity, there's also an opposing feeding trend: baby food pouches. These are usually fruit- and vegetable-based purees, but they often incorporate other ingredients, and their low-mess, grab-and-go, shelf stable nature makes them a convenient option for parents. My children certainly ate their share when they were little. But feeding and development experts caution against relying too much on food pouches for developmentally normal babies. For one, sucking a puree from a pouch uses very similar oral skills as drinking from a bottle, and eating this way gives the baby fewer opportunities to strengthen oral and fine motor skills by eating from a spoon, advancing to lumpier textures, and self-feeding finger foods. For this reason, it's better to squeeze pouch-packaged food onto a spoon before offering it to your baby. Sucking food from a pouch also lacks many of the sensory aspects of food exploration for babies, including seeing and smelling the food, touching it, rubbing it in their hair, and so on—and research shows that this full sensory experience helps infants and toddlers accept new foods. Finally, pouched purees tend to be sweeter than other commercial baby foods and almost always blend a sweet fruit or vegetable with more bitter vegetables. Increased sugar can lead to cavities, and the dominance of sweet taste in the diet can interfere with learning to like other flavors. So, use food pouches on occasion for their convenience, but don't let them become a mainstay of your child's diet.

Source: A. Callahan, "The Truth About Food Pouches," *New York Times*, April 17, 2020.

10

EAT, GROW, AND LEARN

The Best Foods for Babies

Eve, a new mom in Littlehampton, England, was preparing to offer her baby solid foods for the first time. Like many new parents, she wasn't quite sure how to start, and she turned to the internet for advice. She posted her question on the Facebook page of *Natural Mother Magazine*, a busy page with 30,000 followers at the time.[1] Eve wrote: "I am hell-bent on giving him the best start in life, so he will be fed organic and ideally fresh local produce if it kills me." She goes on to say that she has heard that baby rice cereal is "a bad option," but that leaves her at a loss about what to start with instead. "One source said the first food should be egg yolk, and another said raw liver! Please HELP!"

Responses poured in from parents around the world, and the recommendations for first foods read like a holiday feast. Smashed banana, pumpkin, and avocado. Carrots, potatoes, and pears. Pureed lamb and rabbit. Bone and meat broth. Quinoa, amaranth, and oats. Egg yolk scrambled with breast milk and organic butter. And, oh yes, liver—cooked or raw, your choice.

The *Natural Mother* demographic is just one slice of today's parenting population, but their feeding advice to Eve mirrors the current shift toward greater emphasis on whole, or unprocessed, foods. Surely that pasty, processed cereal isn't an optimal first food for a baby. (Spoiler: It's probably not. But it can be part of a balanced baby diet.)

Throughout human history, how and what we feed our babies has varied tremendously over time and across cultures. Our most recent traditions—the way our parents fed us—are based on refined infant cereals and pureed fruits and vegetables, but go back another few generations, and you'll find an entirely different set of traditions. Dr. L. Emmett Holt's classic text *Diseases of Infancy and Childhood* was published in 11 editions between 1897 and 1953 and illustrates a radical shift in advice over that period. Early editions recommended feeding beef juice, thin cereal porridges, and custards, and specifically avoiding vegetables until 3 *years* of age. By 1953, Holt recommended introducing a variety of foods, including vegetables, by 5 months.[2] How we've fed infants over the course of time hasn't been rooted in particularly strong scientific evidence but rather in evolving traditions and cultural norms.

Where does this leave us as new parents, trying to feed our babies well? If we try to crowd-source feeding advice, as Eve did, we find vastly different answers depending on the crowd we ask. Who is right? Can we see some evidence, please?

In this chapter, I ignore the trends and identify some of the best foods for babies based on the science of infant nutrition. To do this, we start by taking a step back and looking at the bigger picture. Breast milk or formula will remain a major source of calories and nutrients for your baby as you introduce solids, so the foods that you choose should fill the nutritional gaps between what breast milk can provide (see the graph in chapter 9) and what your baby needs. Because formula is fortified with minerals and vitamins, getting these nutrients from solid food is less critical to a predominantly formula-fed baby.

But meeting nutrient needs is just one of three main goals of complementary feeding. A second goal is to introduce your baby to a wide variety of foods, with different tastes and textures and from all the different food groups. Dietary diversity supports your baby in learning about food, improves nutritional adequacy, and may support microbiome development and lower the risk of allergies. The third goal is to introduce babies to potentially allergenic foods, because as we discussed in the last chapter, earlier introduction may decrease the risk of food allergies.

FIRST, AN EVOLUTIONARY PERSPECTIVE ON INFANT FEEDING

In the United States and other Western countries, we rely heavily on iron-fortified infant cereal to meet the nutrient needs of older infants, but the popularity of baby cereal is declining. The percent of parents who reported that fortified infant cereal was part of their 6- to 12-month-old's daily diet has trended downward—from 76 percent in 2002, to 65 percent in 2008, to 52 percent in 2016.[3] That's likely a reflection of parental preference for less processed foods, more parents adopting a baby-led weaning approach, and a few rounds of bad press for baby rice cereal. And some babies, like Cee, simply don't like baby cereal—understandable, given its cardboard-like taste. But fortified cereal has only been around for about a half-century or so. How did babies get enough iron before we had fortified cereals? Surely our ancestors and less industrialized societies can teach us a thing or two about feeding babies without processed foods.

Because of the high nutritional needs of older infants and the risk of malnutrition in this age group around the world, child nutrition experts work hard at figuring out how best to feed babies using traditional and locally available foods. But when they look at a diet of on-demand breastfeeding, plus legumes, eggs, fish or chicken, green vegetables, and a staple grain each day, they find that babies manage to get only about 30 to 50 percent of their daily requirement for iron and fall short on zinc as well.[4]

The reality is that many babies around the world are fed thin, grain-based gruels and don't have access to fortified foods or supplements, so it's no wonder that nutritional deficiencies and faltering growth are exceedingly common in babies and young toddlers in poor countries.[5] In developed countries, iron-fortified cereals probably save many babies from deficiencies. According to the WHO, "Average iron intakes of breastfed infants in industrialized countries would fall well short of the recommended intake if iron-fortified products were not available."[6] Indeed, prior to the widespread use of today's fortified cereals, iron deficiency was much more common in young children in the United States.[7] (If you're wondering how we know that babies need so much iron, see appendix G for a detailed explanation of how the recommended iron intake is estimated.)

This is puzzling, isn't it? How is it that breast milk—this beautiful, nearly complete food for young infants—suddenly becomes nutritionally inadequate in late infancy, and we can't make up the shortfall using traditional foods? Have babies always run the risk of iron deficiency, throughout our evolutionary history? (The same might be asked of vitamins K and D, also low in breast milk but today routinely supplemented through the vitamin K shot and oral vitamin D supplements.)

Dr. Kathryn Dewey, professor of nutrition at the University of California, Davis, and a long-time breastfeeding and complementary feeding researcher, has been trying to answer this question. As she wrote in a 2013 review paper, the answer may lie in the human history of 10,000 to 15,000 years ago, during a time before agriculture, when we were hunter-gatherers reliant on foods caught or harvested from the wild. Wild game, fish, shellfish, and insects dominated the diets of hunter-gatherers, making up 45 percent to 65 percent of calories, and these would have provided iron and zinc.[8] The rest of the diet came from wild plants, including leaves, flowers, nuts, seeds, roots, and fruits, many of which would have provided vitamin K. This preagricultural diet would have been high in many of the nutrients that are essential to babies' growth and development, and adults probably prechewed these otherwise tough foods to make the nutrients available to their babies.[9] Baby-sized portions of a hunter-gatherer diet, along with continued breastfeeding, would nicely meet the needs of infants. They fall a little short in iron by 6 to 8 months, but this difference might easily be made up by delayed cord clamping, which would have been the norm at hunter-gatherer births.

The preagricultural diet was also probably higher in vitamin D and omega-3 polyunsaturated fatty acids, in part because of the regular consumption of fish. Many wild plants are also relatively high in omega-3s, and these are incorporated into the meat of wild game. As humans domesticated plants for agriculture, seeking higher yields and better stability for storage, there was a gradual shift in our food supply toward more omega-6 fatty acids and less of the more healthful omega-3s.[10] Of particular importance for babies is the omega-3 docosahexaenoic acid (DHA), which is necessary for vision and brain development.[11] DHA is found in breast milk, but its concentration is dependent on the mother's diet, and with the exception of fish and pasture-raised eggs, modern complementary foods contain little DHA.[12]

Maybe our hunter-gatherer ancestors were onto something when it came to feeding babies, but before you pick up a spear and head out the door to look for some wild game for your baby, or start digging around for insects at your neighborhood playground, let's put this into a modern perspective. We aren't hunter-gatherers. Even if we wanted to be, there isn't enough wild game for all of us to go back to hunting 50 percent of our food. And it would put too much of a strain on the environment to increase animal agriculture so we could eat much more meat or aquaculture so we could eat more fish. I personally like relying on local farmers to provide my family with delicious fresh vegetables, and I like beans and whole grains. However, I do think that taking an evolutionary perspective can help us to make sense of the nutritional bottlenecks in infancy and to make smart choices with all our modern options.

WHY MEAT AND FISH MAKE GOOD BABY FOODS

Here's something that hunter-gatherer parents almost certainly got right: they fed their babies meat. Including a daily serving of meat in your baby's diet can help meet the recommended intake for both the iron and zinc.[13] One reason that meat is such a valu-

Baby-friendly sources of iron

FOOD	SERVING SIZE	IRON (MG/SERVING)
Heme sources (25% to 35% absorbed)		
Home-cooked foods	30 g (*~1 oz*)	
Chicken liver		3.3
Beef liver		1.8
Beef (ground)		0.7
Sardines and clams (canned)		0.5–0.8
Tuna (canned)		0.5
Turkey		0.4
Chicken thigh		0.4
Salmon		0.2
Commercial baby food—meats	71 g (*2.5 oz jar*)	0.5–1.0
Whole egg (*>90% of iron is in the yolk*)	1 (*large*)	0.8
Nonheme sources (~5% absorbed)		
Blackstrap molasses	1 Tbsp	3.6
Home-cooked foods	~¼ cup (*prepared, weight as below*)	
Lentils	45 g	1.5
Spinach, cooked	45 g	1.4
Black beans	45 g	1.3
Other beans	45 g	0.5–1.0
Whole wheat bread	36 g (*1 slice*)	0.9
Quinoa	43 g	0.6
Green peas, cooked	40 g	0.6
Oatmeal	60 g	0.4
Rice, pasta, bulgur, barley	40 g	0.3–0.4

Apricots, dried	40 g	1.1
Raisins	40 g	0.7
Fortified cereals		
Infant cereal	15 g *(dry)*	6.3
Fortified oatmeal, instant*	60 g *(prepared)*	2.8
Fortified breakfast cereals*	~30 g *(dry)*	6–12

Source: US Department of Agriculture, Agricultural Research Service, Food-Data Central, accessed January 4, 2021, https://fdc.nal.usda.gov.

Note: Although many nonheme sources have moderate amounts of iron, low bioavailability makes it difficult for infants to get enough iron from plant foods.

* Fortified cereals not made specifically for infants, such as instant oatmeal and cold breakfast cereals, are often fortified with iron. The iron in these cereals may be less bioavailable than in infant cereals, but these are still a good option.

able food for babies is that it contains heme iron (i.e., iron bound to hemoglobin or myoglobin), and heme iron is absorbed relatively efficiently from the digestive tract into the bloodstream. In these foods, about 25 to 35 percent of the iron is absorbed for use in the body—a measure called bioavailability.[14] Plant foods such as legumes, grains, and vegetables contain nonheme iron, which has a much lower bioavailability, often 5 percent or less.[15] However, there are many dietary factors that can increase or decrease the absorption of nonheme iron.

Not only is the heme iron in meat highly bioavailable, but it also improves the absorption of nonheme iron included in the same meal.[16] Meat is easily digested and makes an ideal first baby food if pureed or slow-cooked. And yet, in the United States, while about three out of four babies aged 6 to 9 months old are eating grains, vegetables, and fruits on a daily basis, just 17 percent are eating meat.[17] The popularity of meat as a baby food has increased over the last 15 years, probably because the AAP and other pediatric organizations recommend meat as a good first food for babies, especially breastfed babies.[18] Yet, it's clearly still not a favorite.

OPTIMIZING IRON ABSORPTION

Absorption of nonheme iron, the form found in plant foods, is highly variable and depends on other components present within the same meal. Planning your baby's meals with this in mind can help optimize iron absorption.

The following food components decrease the absorption of nonheme iron when included in the same meal:

- Phytates, found in high levels in whole grains, legumes, seeds, and nuts (but you can reduce phytates by soaking, sprouting, or fermenting foods)
- Calcium, including in dairy products
- Soy products
- Phenolic compounds, found in tea, coffee, and chocolate (I've added these just for the sake of completeness, but I doubt you feed them to your baby)

To *increase* nonheme iron absorption, include any of the following in the same meal:

- A good source of vitamin C (at least 25 mg; see the table on page 269).
- A source of heme iron (meat, poultry, fish)

Liver is often recommended as a good food for infants, because it is one of the best sources of bioavailable iron and zinc. It has the additional advantages of being relatively inexpensive, easy to prepare, and well-liked by many babies. However, liver also accumulates potentially toxic levels of vitamin A and other fat-soluble compounds, so there is at least a theoretical concern about the safety of routinely feeding it to babies.[19] If your baby enjoys liver, consider limiting it to one or two servings per week. Raw liver poses a risk for foodborne illness, so be sure to cook it before serving. (Self-proclaimed nutrition "experts" on the internet may claim that raw liver is beneficial; they're wrong.)

Fish is also a good source of bioavailable iron and zinc. Sardines and some shellfish, like mussels and clams, are particularly good sources of iron. Fatty fish species are rich sources of omega-3 fatty acids, vitamin D, and vitamin B_{12}. For all these reasons, salmon was one of my children's first solid foods, and it remains one of their favorite foods to this day.

Observational studies also consistently find that babies who eat fish earlier in life have lower rates of atopic diseases such as eczema, asthma, hay fever, and food sensitization. For example, a prospective study of more than 4,000 Swedish infants found lower risks of these atopic diseases in infants that started eating fish between 3 and 8 months of age compared to those introduced at 9 months or later.[20] In addition, the study found a dose-response relationship between eating fish and atopic protection, meaning that consuming greater amounts of fish was associated with greater levels of protection from atopic diseases.

The tricky thing about fish is that it can contain concerning levels of mercury. US experts recommend sticking with just one or two age-appropriate servings of fish per week for young children and 8 to 12 ounces per week for breastfeeding mothers.[21] The good news is that many popular fish species are relatively low in mercury and are safe choices, and experts say that so long as you avoid the high mercury species, the nutritional benefits of fish consumption outweigh the risks.[22]

FEEDING YOUR BABY EGGS AND DAIRY

Egg yolk is an excellent first food for babies. After all, it's a concentrated source of nutrients meant to support the earliest stages of development, albeit for a chick. Egg yolk is high in fat and a good source of iron. Since these nutrients are concentrated in the yolk, and babies just starting solids eat only a small amount each day, the yolk is the most valuable part of the egg. It's easy to separate out the egg yolk before cooking or from a hard-boiled egg, and it's already a nice, soft texture for feeding. You can whisk a little cooked

CHOOSING FISH WISELY

Eating fish means balancing its nutritional benefits with the risks of mercury consumption. This is important for everyone, but especially for pregnant and lactating women, infants, and young children. Mercury poses a greater risk to these groups, but the same groups also stand the most to gain from fish's brain-nourishing omega-3 fatty acids.

Best choices: these seafood species are relatively low in mercury, and I've added the amount of long-chain omega-3 fatty acids (DHA and eicosapentaenoic acid, or EPA) provided per 100 grams so that you can select species with higher levels of omega-3s. (This not a comprehensive list by any means.)

- Salmon (1,150 mg of omega-3 fatty acids for wild Alaskan Chinook or king; 1,866 mg for farmed Atlantic)
- Sardines (1,480 mg)
- Rainbow trout (587 mg)
- Crab (549 mg)
- Catfish (364 mg)
- Tuna, canned light (281 mg; albacore and yellowfin contain more mercury)
- Flounder (245 mg)

Avoid these fish species due to their high mercury levels:

- King mackerel
- Marlin
- Orange roughy
- Shark
- Tilefish
- Bigeye tuna

Sources: US Food and Drug Administration, "Advice About Eating Fish: For Women Who Are or Might Become Pregnant, Breastfeeding Mothers, and Young Children," accessed September 29, 2020, www.fda.gov/food/consumers/advice-about-eating-fish; A. S. Bernstein et al., "Fish, Shell-fish, and Children's Health: An Assessment of Benefits, Risks, and Sustainability," *Pediatrics* 143, no. 6 (2019): e20190999, doi: 10.1542/peds.2019 –0999.

egg yolk into some baby oatmeal or thin it with breast milk or formula for spoon-feeding, and older babies can feed it to themselves (or at least smear it around their high chair tray).

There's a little confusion around egg as an iron source. Egg contains both heme and nonheme iron, but studies have shown that whole egg inhibits iron absorption. This is probably due to the egg white protein rather than the yolk.[23] A randomized controlled trial found that feeding four egg yolks per week between 6 and 12 months (in addition to a well-balanced diet) resulted in a small improvement in iron status.[24] Thus, egg yolk alone seems to be at least a decent source of iron. As your baby gets older and eats greater quantities of other iron-rich foods, you can start feeding whole egg.

Eggs are also a good source of omega-3 fatty acids. In breastfed infants, levels of DHA in red blood cells have been shown to decline between 6 and 12 months, most likely because of a decreasing intake of DHA from breast milk. Because our evolutionary diet was probably much higher in omega-3s, it is reasonable to think that we should try to maintain DHA levels during this period of rapid brain development. The trial mentioned above found that feeding four regular egg yolks per week maintained red blood cell DHA during late infancy, and feeding omega-3–enriched eggs actually increased DHA levels.[25] Of course, fatty fish is an even better source of DHA, but unlike fish, eggs can be eaten daily without any concerns about mercury.

Purchasing omega-3–enriched eggs for your baby may be a good choice. These are made by feeding hens a diet naturally high in omega-3s (more like what wild birds might eat), usually in the form of flax or fishmeal. These eggs are particularly high in α-linolenic acid, which boosts the total omega-3 count listed on the package but isn't the most beneficial fatty acid on its own. DHA is also increased, and although the amount varies substantially with the hens' diet, omega-3–enriched eggs usually provide at least 100 mg of DHA, more than double that found in a typical supermarket egg.[26] One study found a significant improvement in visual acuity of infants fed 83 mg of DHA from egg yolk each day from 6 to 12 months.[27] An even better choice may be eggs from pasture-raised hens, which are naturally higher in DHA than eggs from conventional grain-fed hens.[28] The problem here is that your local grocery store may or may not carry eggs from real pasture-raised hens—those that have been able to eat grass, seeds, and insects to their heart's content. In the United States, the label "free range" on poultry products means only that the hens have access to the outdoors, which could just be a strip of concrete.[29] The term "pasture-raised" is currently unregulated, so your best bet is to buy eggs from a local farmer (check your farmers' market) or to raise your own.

If you're worried about your baby getting too much cholesterol from eggs, don't be. In the randomized trial in which babies were fed four egg yolks per week, this amount did not affect plasma cholesterol. Besides, breast milk is naturally high in cholesterol, and this is probably a good thing for babies.[30] Egg yolks are also rich in the nutrient choline, which is important for brain development in early childhood.[31]

Between 6 and 12 months, dairy products can be included in your baby's diet, but avoid giving your baby cow's milk. Cow's milk doesn't provide the balanced nutrition found in breast milk and infant formula. It's also low in iron, and filling up on cow's milk leaves less room for foods that provide iron and other minerals.[32] Wait until your baby is 12 months old to begin offering cow's milk as a regular beverage. However, dairy foods like whole milk yogurt and cheese are good sources of fat and calcium, and they can be incorporated into your baby's diet along with other solid foods.

After 12 months, your baby's iron needs decrease (because she's not growing as fast as she did in the first year), and she should be eating more iron-rich foods, so serving plain, pasteurized cow's milk with meals is recommended as a good source of vitamin D, calcium, and other nutrients. Whole cow's milk is usually the best choice for 1-year-olds, because children at this age need fat to support brain and body growth. However, your pediatrician may recommend reduced fat milk if you have a family history of heart disease or your toddler shows other risk factors for developing obesity.[33]

Formula companies market "toddler milks" or "growing up milk" for children 12 months and up, but the American Academy of Pediatrics and other experts don't recommend these products. They often have added sugar, and it's more beneficial—and totally feasible—for toddlers to meet their nutrient needs from regular foods. Likewise, plant-based milks such as soy, rice, oat, or almond milk are not recommended for babies under 12 months; they come nowhere close to the nutritional value of breast milk or formula, and using these products as a substitute may cause malnutrition. After 12 months, plant-based milks can be used for toddlers with a dairy allergy or intolerance, with careful attention to labels to select a product low in added sugar and with calcium and vitamin D levels similar to cow's milk. However, if cow's milk is tolerated by your child and acceptable to your family, it generally provides the best nutrient profile and is least expensive.[34]

I sometimes hear from parents who take issue with my emphasis on animal-derived foods for babies. I get it. For all their nutritional value, meat, fish, eggs, and dairy foods all come with some amount of environmental baggage, in addition to concerns like animal welfare and occupational safety for workers. In general, animal protein sources are more resource-intensive from farm to fork than plant proteins, and cutting meat consumption is one way that individuals can trim their personal carbon footprint.[35] As a parent, I desperately want my children and grandchildren to be able to live in a world with clean air, a stable food supply, and healthy wilderness areas—without increasingly intense and terrifying hurricanes and wildfires, among the many other consequences of climate change. So, we've decreased meat consumption in our family, and we're a lot pickier about what we buy. We spend more to purchase pasture-raised beef and eggs, which also happen to come with the added benefit of having greater levels of omega-3 fatty acids.[36] For seafood, I rely on the Monterey Bay Aquarium Seafood Watch program for guidance on choosing sustainable sources (seafoodwatch.org).

All of that said, if anyone should be eating animal-derived foods, it's growing babies. In addition to their high requirements for iron and zinc, it's recommended that babies consume 30 to 40 percent of their calories from fat to support growth and brain development, and it's very hard to meet that recommended intake with plant-based foods alone.[37] Although whole grains and legumes, including soy, contain a reasonable amount of iron, its bioavailability is very low. Most adults in Western countries eat far more protein than they need, and it would benefit the planet if we all ate less meat. But for babies and their disproportionately high nutrient needs, small servings of animal-derived foods go a long way toward meeting their needs.

If it's important to you, your baby can be vegetarian, but you'll need to plan carefully. Including full-fat dairy products and eggs can provide enough fat, but your baby may still fall short on iron and zinc. For these nutrients, you'll need to look to fortified cereals. According to the WHO, "Vegetarian diets cannot meet nutrient needs at this age unless nutrient supplements or fortified products are used."[38] I talk more about fortified cereals in the next section.

On the extreme end of vegetarianism are vegan and macrobiotic diets. Macrobiotic diets emphasize whole grains, legumes, nuts, seeds, seasonal fruits, and fermented foods, and avoid meat, eggs, and dairy products. A study in the Netherlands found that babies and children raised on a macrobiotic diet had ubiquitous nutrient deficiencies, stunted growth, muscle and fat wasting, and slower psychomotor development.[39] A review of vegetarian diets for children noted that "the more restricted the diet and the younger the child, the greater the risk for deficiencies."[40] If you are considering such restrictions on your child's diet, consider consulting with a registered dietitian to be sure you're covering all the nutritional bases, which may mean using nutritional supplements.

A ROLE FOR INFANT CEREALS
AND OTHER GRAINS

Cereals are traditional first foods for babies around the world, and in the developed world, iron-fortified infant cereals have been a nutritional cornerstone for babies for several generations. However, if you're incorporating foods like meat and fish into your baby's daily diet, he probably doesn't need fortified cereals. Likewise, fortified cereals aren't necessary for formula-fed babies, because formula includes more than enough iron to meet babies' needs through the first year. Still, fortified cereals can be useful, especially for breastfed babies. In this and the following sections, I discuss the advantages and disadvantages of fortified cereals, as well as grains in general, and address some of the modern myths about grains.

Let's start with what is in the typical infant cereal. The standard baby rice cereal is mostly rice flour—essentially a finely ground white rice. It's a refined grain, meaning that the bran and germ of the grain have been milled away, along with most of the nutrients, leaving just the starchy endosperm. (Brown rice is an example of a whole grain, since it still has the bran and germ intact.) Added to the rice flour is a bunch of supplementary vitamins and minerals, including iron and zinc, in part to replace those that were removed in refining, but also to make rice cereal a more nutrient-dense food to meet the specific needs of babies. In effect, rice cereal is a nutritional supplement carried by otherwise nutrient-poor refined flour, though reconstituting it with breast milk or formula adds protein and fat to make the meal more complete.

There's no doubt about it: baby cereal is a processed food. Why not serve our babies whole foods—foods our great-grandmothers would recognize, with more interesting tastes and textures? That is, after all, how we hope our babies will eat as they grow into children and adults.

This argument may have some merit, but let's consider the advantages of fortified cereals. Most obviously, fortified cereals are a good source of iron. Just two servings of baby cereal a day can nearly meet the recommended intake for iron, and studies show that fortified cereal prevents iron deficiency in breastfed babies.[41] For example, one study found that in babies receiving a fortified cereal, just 2.5 percent developed iron deficiency. In contrast, in a control group of babies fed solids completely at the parents' discretion, 14 percent became iron-deficient.[42]

Meat may be a better and more natural source of iron, but because so few babies eat meat regularly, fortified cereals play a vital role in preventing iron deficiency and anemia among the vulnerable 6- to 12-month-old age group. And compared with meat, cereals are often a more practical choice. They're inexpensive, convenient, and safe. They are stable to store at home or on the go, and you can mix up just a tablespoon or two at a time, which is perfect for babies just starting to eat small amounts of solid foods. It is easy to adjust the texture, allowing you to start with very soupy cereal or make it progressively thicker as your baby's oral motor skills develop. I even incorporated fortified cereals into things like pancakes and muffins to increase the iron content in some of Cee's favorite finger foods. Cereals can also be mixed with breast milk or formula, providing a familiar taste bridge from milk to solids. One study found that breastfed babies were more likely to enjoy infant cereal when it was made up with breast milk, and the same is probably true for formula if it is the familiar milk for the baby.[43]

There is a very real concern about high levels of arsenic in rice products, including infant cereals. Although I think rice cereal and crackers can be included in your baby's diet occasionally, it's a good idea to feed different types of grains, including oats, barley, and wheat, all of which come in fortified versions. In addition to reducing arsenic exposure, this gives your baby more variety in taste and texture. (See appendix H for more information about arsenic in rice.)

If you do feed your baby commercial infant cereal, look for a brand fortified with both iron and zinc. (In the United States, almost all are fortified with iron, but not all companies have adopted zinc fortification, and fortification practices vary in other countries.) Serve infant cereal with a good source of vitamin C, because it enhances the absorption of nonheme iron severalfold.[44] Some cereals are fortified with vitamin C; otherwise, pair it with a vitamin C–rich fruit or vegetable. In addition to infant-specific cereals, many other hot and cold cereals found in your grocery store are fortified with iron. However, the iron source used in these cereals is less bioavailable than that used in infant cereal.[45] If cereal is your baby's major source of iron, infant cereals are a better choice.

Good sources of vitamin C for babies

FOOD	VITAMIN C (MG/SERVING)
Fruits (raw)	
Kiwifruit	34
Citrus fruits (*oranges, clementines*)	15–25
Strawberries	22
Pineapple	20
Mango	15
Honeydew melon	7
Vegetables	
Bell pepper (*raw, any color*)	30–50
Broccoli (*cooked*)	30
Kale (*cooked*)	23
Cauliflower (*cooked*)	16
Sweet potato (*baked, mashed*)	12

Source: US Department of Agriculture, Agricultural Research Service, FoodData Central, accessed January 4, 2021, https://fdc.nal.usda.gov.

Note: Vitamin C amounts are given for a one-quarter-cup serving of chopped fruit or vegetable (about 40 to 50 grams). Aim to include at least 25 mg of vitamin C with a meal containing nonheme iron.

WHAT ABOUT WHOLE GRAINS?

Whole grains are generally nutritionally superior to their refined counterparts. The whole grain includes not only the starchy endosperm but also the bran and the germ, which are naturally rich in vitamins, minerals, fiber, and phytochemicals (chemical compounds produced by plants, some of which are beneficial). They also include some protein and healthy fats, resulting in a nicely balanced package of nutrients. Whole grains are even reasonably high in iron. However, like legumes and nuts, whole grains are also high in chemical compounds called phytates, and these bind iron during digestion, inhibiting absorption. Phytates are concentrated in the bran of cereal grains, and the higher the level of phytates, the lower the iron bioavailability.[46] Thus, from an infant nutrition standpoint, whole grains may be a trade-off. They're better nutritionally in lots of ways, but refined cereals are usually a more bioavailable source of iron for babies.

Many baby food companies are nonetheless taking advantage of the popularity of whole grains and marketing whole-grain fortified infant cereals, although it isn't clear what effect phytate levels may have on iron bioavailability in these products. A 2013 survey of phytates in infant foods deemed the whole-grain cereals marketed in the United Kingdom and Denmark to have phytate levels "unsuitable for infants and young children."[47] However, a small US study compared the iron status of babies fed a regular refined cereal and a whole-grain version, both fortified with iron.[48] Although the whole-grain cereal had nearly five times the phytate level of the refined version, there was no difference in babies' iron status in the two groups. That's encouraging, but this question needs to be studied in more depth.

Some parents avoid commercial cereal products altogether and make their own whole-grain cereals. Of course, these aren't fortified with iron, but if your baby has other good sources of iron, homemade whole grains are a nutritious and well-liked food for babies. You can take some steps at home to reduce the phytate levels in whole grains and legumes. Soaking them and then rinsing with fresh water before cooking can decrease phytates; one study found that a six-hour soak in warm water decreased phytate levels by about half.[49] Germination of grains and legumes prior to cooking can similarly reduce phytates, and fermentation results in as much as 90 percent lower phytate levels.[50] Of course, all of these strategies take your time and energy, as well as a certain degree of dedication. And they remind me that while we might strive to avoid "processed foods," some processing—whether by soaking whole grains or refining them—can also have benefits when it comes to availability of nutrients.

BUT I HEARD THAT BABIES CAN'T DIGEST STARCH!

Adding to cereal's popularity slump, there's a funny rumor circulating around "crunchy" parenting websites that babies can't digest starch. Hence, some parents are choosing to avoid grains and other starchy foods (think root vegetables, winter squash, beans, and some fruits) until their children are 1 or 2 years of age. There is a truthful origin to this claim, but it has been grossly misconstrued.

Starch is made up of long, branching chains of glucose. When we eat starch, we need to break up those chains to liberate the glucose, making it available for absorption into our bloodstream so that it can be used as an energy source for cells. An enzyme called amylase, secreted both in saliva and from the pancreas into the small intestine, is responsible for most of our starch digestion. It turns out that newborns have little to no pancreatic amylase activity, and although this activity increases slowly over the first months of life, it doesn't reach adult levels until well into childhood.[51]

This deficiency in pancreatic amylase among babies puzzled the scientists researching it in the 1960s and 1970s. For one thing, babies appeared to digest starch just fine. When researchers fed starch to infants just a few months old, very little of it came out in their diapers.[52] And the infants didn't have symptoms of carbohydrate malabsorption, like diarrhea, nausea, cramping, bloating, and gas. (Think of what happens if someone who is lactose intolerant—lacking the enzyme to break down lactose—drinks milk.) These symptoms weren't apparent in young babies eating starchy infant cereals, which in the United States in the 1970s were usually introduced by 1 to 2 months of age.[53] And this approach to infant feeding wasn't unique to the US. Ethnographic reports are filled with examples of starchy first foods for young infants around the world: millet flour at 3 months in Tanzania, corn porridge at 3 months in Zimbabwe, beans and rice at 4 months in Brazil, a little butter and flour at 3 days in Bhutan, rice mash at 3 weeks in Nepal, and prechewed taro root at 2 weeks in the Solomon Islands.[54] If all these little babies were eating starch, how were they digesting it without pancreatic amylase?

Babies seem to have a few strategies for starch digestion. For one, they make a lot of saliva, as is on display in the drool-soaked collars of onesies everywhere, and their saliva contains lots of amylase enzyme. By 6 months of age, concentrations of salivary amylase in babies are near adult levels.[55] This amylase starts to break down food starch as babies gum food around in their mouths, and it also seems to survive the trip through the acidic environment of the stomach and to continue its work in the more neutral small intestine.[56]

There is also a lot of amylase in human breast milk, 25 times more than that found in raw cow's milk.[57] It is highest in colostrum and decreases slowly during infancy, as the baby's salivary and pancreatic amylase levels increase.[58] Like salivary amylase, breast milk amylase appears to survive the acidic stomach, in part because it is protected by other proteins in breast milk.[59] For this reason, it might be beneficial to use breast milk to thin baby cereal, and amylase has been shown to be stable in breast milk even after freezing and thawing.[60] Finally, another enzyme, called glucoamylase, helps with starch digestion in babies. Glucoamylase is made by cells lining the walls of the small intestine, and it is very active in infants.[61]

Even after all that amylase activity, some starch does escape the small intestine undigested, passing on to the colon.[62] This happens to some extent in adults too, and it isn't necessarily a bad thing. The beneficial oligosaccharides (short chains of sugars) found in breast milk, as well as dietary fiber from plant foods, also pass through the small intestine undigested. Bacteria in the colon ferment these undigested carbohydrates, all as part of the symbiotic relationship between us and our gut microbes. The microbes benefit from this food supply, and as is becoming more and more apparent, the microbes benefit us as well. The end products of microbial fermentation in the colon are short-chain fatty acids, which can improve nutrient absorption, enhance gut health, and even be used as a source of energy for both the microbes and their human hosts.[63] Including complex carbohydrates, such as starch and fiber, in the diets of older babies and toddlers might help to encourage the development of a healthy gut microbiome.[64]

When I hear about parents choosing to avoid grains and other starchy foods for the first year or two of their babies' lives, I feel concerned, for a couple of reasons. For one thing, as I noted in the previous chapter, if wheat is anything like peanut and egg, introducing it in late infancy may prevent the development of a wheat allergy. For another, I worry about our culture's ongoing obsession with restrictive diets. Barring allergies and intolerances, eating a variety of foods from all the food groups pretty much ensures that you'll meet your nutrient needs without even trying, and I think this is a valuable practice to teach to our kids. Eating a diverse diet allows us all to relax and enjoy our food with the people we love, babies included.

A VARIETY OF VEGETABLES AND FRUITS

It's also important to include fruits and vegetables in your baby's diet. For one thing, many fruits and vegetables are good sources of vitamin C, which increases the absorption of nonheme iron as much as twofold to sixfold. Including a fruit or vegetable high in vitamin C in a meal with nonheme iron sources like cereals, beans, and whole grains, can help your baby get more iron out of every bite (see page 269).[65] Fruits and vegetables are also good sources of trace minerals, folic acid, and B vitamins, as well as fiber, which encourage regular poops and the development of healthy gut bacteria.

Beyond nutrition, there is a benefit to exploring lots of fruits and vegetables during infancy. For one thing, babies this age are open to trying new foods, and they readily accept most flavors.[66] It's worth taking advantage of the open-minded period in infancy, because it won't last forever. At some point in their second year of life, most babies become more skeptical of new flavors and accept fewer new foods, especially bitter vegetables. Trying lots of vegetables and fruits during the "honeymoon" phase of eating in late infancy may not fully prevent their rejection later, but it might help.[67] Research shows that babies who are fed a greater variety of fruits and vegetables are more likely to accept novel ones when offered, and those who eat more vegetables before their first birthday end up liking and eating more vegetables later in childhood.[68] If that pattern holds, it might benefit your child across the lifespan. For adults, a diet rich in fruits and vegetables is not only associated with better nutritional quality, but also a healthier body weight and lower risk of chronic diseases such as heart disease and some cancers. And it's just plain fun to eat with a baby who joyfully eats everything, from broccoli to Brussels sprouts.

Infants are born with a preference for sweet taste, so they usually enjoy sweet fruits and vegetables like applesauce, carrots, and sweet potatoes on the first or second try. Not surprisingly, they are more hesitant about the bitter taste associated with many green vegetables. However, study after study has shown that with repeat exposures—as many as 10 small tastes, a little each day for a week or two—babies will learn to like bitter vegetables.[69] Without putting pressure on your baby, continue to offer tastes and model enjoyment of these same foods yourself. This is easy to say but hard to do. None of us like to offer something that is rejected time and time again, but just consider "palate development" another part of your baby's education. It may help to mix vegetables with familiar and well-liked foods like breast milk, formula, or cereal.[70]

There is some recent evidence that starting your baby on vegetables before fruits can enhance liking of vegetables.[71] Several randomized controlled trials have tested starting solids with a two-week period focused solely on trying a variety of vegetables and holding off on fruits and other foods except for basic infant cereals. After that two-week experimental period, babies ate more vegetables, including an unfamiliar one (artichoke puree in this study) compared with babies who had eaten fruit during the trial period.[72] It's not clear if this early focus on vegetables has a lasting impact on babies' food preferences, or if including other foods like meat or eggs in the early days of solids would change the results. Still, these studies suggest it might be worth waiting to introduce sweet fruits for a few weeks to give your baby plenty of time to experience the taste of vegetables without competition from more palatable fruits.

Also, be aware that some babies are more sensitive to bitter tastes than others, and some might still refuse certain foods even after many tastes.[73] A UK study of twins demonstrated that more than 50 percent of the variation in food preferences was explained by genetics.[74] If your baby seems skeptical of everything green, resist comparing him to the foodie babies grinning through faces smeared with vegetables in your social media feed. Food preferences are just as much about nature (i.e., genetic differences) as about nurture. It's okay to blame genetics and bring out the applesauce, while continuing to give your baby plenty of opportunities to taste, see, and smell a variety of other foods that you enjoy.

THE VALUE OF DIETARY DIVERSITY

One of the goals of complementary feeding is to introduce your baby to a variety of foods from all the food groups. Benefits of dietary diversity in infancy include balanced nutrient intake and taste and texture learning, but recent research also indicates an additional perk: reduced risk of food allergies. In a study published in 2020, researchers followed a cohort of 969 children born between 2001 and 2002 in the Isle of Wight in the UK, tracking their introduction to 21 different solid foods and then testing them for

SHOULD YOU CHOOSE ORGANIC OR CONVENTIONAL FOODS?

Organic farming practices are usually better for the environment and for farm workers and their families. Organic produce also generally has lower levels of synthetic pesticide residues, and studies have shown that children consuming an organic diet had lower levels of metabolites of these pesticides in their urine. However, there's no evidence that the pesticide levels found on conventionally grown produce are dangerous to children's health. In the United States, an annual pesticide monitoring program consistently finds that levels are hundreds to millions of times lower than limits set by the US Environmental Protection Agency. And commercial baby food, whether organic or conventional, carries very little to no pesticides. Organic produce costs more, is no more nutritious than conventional produce, and can also be contaminated with organic pesticides (although not synthetic, these are not necessarily less dangerous). Buying organic supports organic farming systems, but it is unlikely to affect your child's health.

Likewise, there's little difference in the nutritional profile of organic and conventional milk and meat, and both are safe to consume. Choosing certified organic milk and meat does ensure that antibiotics weren't used in their production, thus reducing animal agriculture's contribution to the growing problem of antibiotic resistance. However, you'll also find conventional products labeled as "raised without antibiotics."

There is one thing we know for sure: a diet rich in fruits and vegetables, however they are grown, has many health benefits. The best nutrition is found in the freshest produce, grown in your own garden or purchased from local farms. Buying local also gives you the benefit of talking directly with farmers about their farming practices, supporting your local economy, and showing your kids where their food comes from.

Sources: J. Forman, J. Silverstein, and the AAP's Committee on Nutrition and Council on Environmental Health, "Organic Foods: Health and Environmental Advantages and Disadvantages," *Pediatrics* 130, no. 5 (2012): e1406; C. K. Winter and J. M. Katz, "Dietary Exposure to Pesticide Residues from Commodities Alleged to Contain the Highest Contamination Levels," *Journal of Toxicology* 2011 (2011): 589674, doi:10.1155/2011/589674.

food allergies at ages 1, 2, 3, and 10 years.[75] They defined dietary diversity in several different ways, including how many food groups, total foods, fruits and vegetables, and common allergens that the babies had tried by 3, 6, 9, and 12 months of age. (At the time of this study, advice in the UK was to introduce solids at 4 months, but 33 percent of infants had started eating foods by 12 weeks of age.) No matter how the researchers looked at it, greater dietary diversity at 6, 9, and 12 months (but not 3 months) was associated with a lower risk of food allergies in the first 10 years of life. For example, for each additional food introduced by 6 months, the odds of developing a food allergy was reduced by 22 percent. Greater fruit and vegetable variety at 6 and 9 months was associated with a 23 and 17 percent reduction in food allergy, respectively. And for each additional allergenic food introduced in the first 12 months of life, children had a 33 percent reduced risk of developing a food allergy in the first decade of life.

Other studies have found similar patterns, including a 2014 study of children in Austria, Finland, France, Germany, and Switzerland, which found that greater dietary diversity in the first year of life was associated with a lower risk of both asthma and food allergies up to age 6.[76] Why might variety prevent allergic diseases from developing? That's not clear, but several mechanisms have been proposed, including promoting greater gut microbial diversity, improved intake of nutrients like omega-3 fatty acids or fiber, and more opportunities to develop immune tolerance to food proteins.[77] Whatever the reason, feeding your baby lots of different foods seems to be a good thing, and it certainly can't hurt.

HOW TO INTRODUCE COMMON FOOD ALLERGENS

As we discussed in chapter 9, the more we learn about food allergy development, the more it seems that it's best for babies to begin eating common food allergens in the first year. The evidence is most clear for peanut and egg, and from what we know of other food allergens, there is no benefit to delaying them. So, if these foods are part of your family's regular diet, you can go ahead and make them part of your baby's diet, too. Early introduction of egg and peanut is probably most beneficial for babies at high risk of food allergies, defined as those with severe eczema and an existing food allergy; if that's your baby, talk with your pediatrician to make a plan for how you'll introduce these foods.[78]

Your baby's first foods should be ones that aren't usually allergenic, like fortified oatmeal, vegetable purees, or pureed meat.

How to introduce common food allergens

COMMON FOOD ALLERGENS	BABY-FRIENDLY SERVING IDEAS
Peanuts and tree nuts	• Thin smooth peanut or other nut butter with reconstituted baby cereal, fruit/vegetable puree, or yogurt • Bamba or similar peanut puff product • Spread thin layer of nut butter on toast and cut into strips for baby to grasp
Cow's milk	• Plain whole cow's milk yogurt • Spread cream cheese on toast and cut into strips
Shellfish and fish	• Cook and flake, mash, or puree
Eggs	• Mash cooked egg yolk into cereal, yogurt, or fruit/vegetable puree • Bake whole egg into low-sugar cookies, biscuits, or muffins • Scrambled, hard-boiled, or omelet
Wheat	• Infant wheat cereal or regular cooked wheat cereal • Cereal such as Weetabix or Cheerios (softened if needed) • Well-cooked pasta • Toast, crackers, etc. (as age-appropriate)
Soy	• Plain soy milk yogurt • Soft tofu
Sesame	• Add hummus (containing tahini) to yogurt or fruit/vegetable puree • Spread hummus on toast and cut into strips

Introduce only one new food at a time so that if your baby has a reaction, you'll know the culprit. Pediatricians have traditionally recommended waiting three to five days between each new food, but there was never any evidence to support this practice, and it's been questioned recently as research reveals the value of early dietary diversity. Most allergic reactions are mediated by immunoglobulin E (IgE) and occur within minutes to two hours of ingesting the food, while non-IgE reactions may occur between one and four hours of ingesting the food.[79] This time course means that it's wise to introduce new foods earlier in the day, and then you'll know long before bedtime if your baby tolerates it well. You'll also want to try to introduce common allergens when your baby is feeling well, so that you don't wonder if a runny nose or bout of diarrhea was caused by a new food or an existing infection.[80]

The most common signs of an allergic reaction in infants are a new rash, hives, vomiting, and lip or facial swelling. Respiratory symptoms such as wheezing, coughing, and difficulty breathing are more common in older children but can occur at any age. Babies tend to have milder allergic reactions than older children, but don't hesitate to seek medical attention if you think your baby is having an allergic reaction.[81] Be aware that acidic foods such as citrus and tomatoes can cause contact irritation and redness. These symptoms are common and most likely don't represent an allergic reaction.[82]

One of the easiest allergens to introduce is cow's milk, because whole milk yogurt makes an easy baby food.[83] When you're ready to introduce peanut, thin a bit of smooth peanut butter with warm water and then add it to a familiar fruit or vegetable puree or infant cereal. Offer your baby a small taste of this mixture on the tip of a spoon, placing it on the tongue or inside lip (not on the skin). Then wait for 10 minutes and watch for any signs of reaction. Starting with this tiny taste means that if your baby does have a reaction, it will likely be mild. And assuming there is no sign of reaction, you can continue feeding a few more teaspoons of the peanut butter mixture. Use other nut butters to introduce tree nuts, and take care not to give babies choking hazards like globs of nut butters or whole nuts.[84] If your baby is eating finger foods, you can offer peanut puffs like Bamba (these can also be moistened to soften), or spread a thin layer of nut butter on a stick of toast. I've included ideas for introducing other common allergens in the table on page 278.

SKIP THE SUGAR AND SALT, AND SERVE UP SPICE INSTEAD

A 2016 survey of US babies found that 34 percent of 6- to 12-month-olds consumed desserts, sweets, or sweetened beverages at least once a day.[85] This is concerning. Sugary foods displace much-needed nutrients during this period of rapid growth and development, and they promote the development of cavities. Babies like sweet foods, and feeding them sweets only increases their preference for them.[86] A preference for sweet taste may have been evolutionarily beneficial in an environment where sweetness signaled a good, safe source of calories.[87] But these days, our babies are usually raised in environments where calories are plentiful, and we should lead by example to introduce them to the complex tastes of a variety of foods. Don't hesitate to feed fruits, which are naturally sweet but also come in a package that includes beneficial fiber, vitamins, and minerals. But for babies under 1 year, avoid feeding foods with added sugar, except in small amounts as an occasional treat.

There's also no reason to give babies juice, even 100% fruit juice; whole fruits provide more nutrients. The American Academy of Pediatrics recommends avoiding juice entirely before 12 months, and beyond that, offering no more than 4 to 6 ounces per day. Juice should always be given in a cup, not a bottle. Bottles make it too easy for a toddler to drink a lot of juice, and this is associated with greater risk of cavities.[88] (Pediatricians might make an exception to the no-juice-for-baby rule for temporary use to relieve constipation or other medical issue.)[89]

Finally, avoid honey completely during the first year of life. The toxin that causes botulism is found in honey, even when baked into foods, and honey consumption has been associated with infantile botulism.[90]

Likewise, there's no reason to add salt to your baby's food. A Dutch study put some babies on a low-salt diet for the first six months of life, and at 15 years of age, these children had lower blood pressure than those in a control group, despite having similar salt intake at that age.[91] I started adding small amounts of salt to Cee's vegetables soon after her first birthday, around the time she started showing a little bit of pickiness and rejecting some vegetables. In my opinion, a little bit of salt does wonders for vegetables, but

---

THE INS AND OUTS OF COMMERCIAL BABY FOODS

It's easy to make your own baby food. All you need is a blender or food processor, or even just a fork for mashing. But what if you're short on the time or the desire to make your own? Are store-bought foods a good option?

It depends on the product. If you choose simple purees that contain only fruits or vegetables, then store-bought foods are just fine, though more expensive than what you could make in your own kitchen. However, be wary of ingredients like "puree concentrate" or "fruit juice concentrate." Although these ingredients are made from real fruits, they are processed to remove water and often fiber, which ends up concentrating the sugars. Check labels carefully.

Baby food companies like you to think that you need to introduce foods to your baby in predetermined "stages," which linger in various pureed variations for way too long. Most babies need pureed foods only for a few months, if at all (some skip them entirely), and you should follow your baby's lead to advance to more complex textures and self-feeding.

The real rip-off in baby foods is the meals and snacks marketed for older babies and toddlers. These often have added sugar, salt, and filler ingredients. For example, I found a turkey stew meal that includes an ingredient called "cooked white turkey meat chopped and formed," which, as is clarified in parentheses, contains not only turkey meat and broth but also modified cornstarch, tapioca starch, and salt. These meals are expensive and nutrient-poor, and they don't help your baby learn to eat real food.

---

babies don't need it and will readily accept most veggies without it. Having the ability to control sugar and salt content is one reason to make your own baby food, but with careful label reading, you can find good options among commercial baby foods.

So, hold the salt and skip added sugar during this stage of exploring new and different tastes, textures, and flavors. However, this is a great time to introduce spices to your baby's palate. As far as I can tell, there aren't any studies on feeding spicy foods to babies, but given the variety of flavors fed to babies around the world, it's hard to imagine that offering spicy food is a bad thing. Just start with small amounts and be observant; your baby will let you know if the flavor is too strong for her.

THE MOST IMPORTANT PART OF FEEDING: IT ISN'T THE FOOD

In this chapter, I've summarized the foods that are most nutritionally beneficial to growing babies. In an ideal world, I think babies do best eating meat, eggs, whole milk dairy products, a variety of grains and legumes, and lots of different fruits and vegetables. However, I live in the real world, just like you, and I don't even follow my own advice all the time. For example, even though meat may be a better source of iron, I still don't hesitate to tell busy parents that fortified cereals are a great way to ensure that their baby gets enough iron—because it's true; these cereals work just fine and are generally more convenient than meat. And while some parents find joy in preparing homemade foods for their babies, others don't, or just don't have time. There's no shame in shortcuts.

We humans are flexible omnivores; over the ages and around the world, we have thrived on very different diets. The nutritional principles in this chapter can help you figure out the right foods for your baby, but in practice this will look very different from household to household, depending on dietary preferences and traditions. The goal is to bring your baby to the family table and explore a variety of nutrient-dense foods that fit your life.

I also want to leave you with a note of caution: beware of making nutritional perfectionism your goal. Even if you're committed to serving up the best foods every day, your baby may have his own ideas about what that means. You might be determined that your baby should eat salmon, for example, and he might turn up his nose at it. You have to honor that. Keep offering tastes and modeling happy eating of good foods, but don't push your baby to eat something he doesn't want. If you're worried about specific nutrients, find alternative sources and talk to your pediatrician. And then relax, and enjoy feeding and eating with your baby.

GOALS OF COMPLEMENTARY FEEDING

1. *Offer nutrient-dense foods to meet nutrient needs.*
   - Meat, fish, and fortified cereals provide iron and zinc.
   - Fish, eggs, and dairy provide healthy fats, vitamins, and minerals.
   - Vegetables and fruits provide fiber, vitamins, and minerals.
   - Limit added sugar and salt, and avoid honey.

2. *Introduce a variety of foods.*
   - Let your baby explore many tastes and textures.
   - Veggies before fruit and an emphasis on vegetable variety in infancy promotes more adventurous eating.
   - Dietary variety is associated with reduced risk of allergies.

3. *Make common food allergens a part of your baby's diet. Feed allergens early and often to reduce risk of food allergies.*

4. *Avoid nutritional perfectionism, and teach your baby that food is one of the great pleasures of life, especially when shared with those you love.*

EPILOGUE

The room was hushed. I watched on the ultrasound monitor as strokes of gray gave way to a dark space—a gestational sac. It looked empty at first, but within seconds, an oblong smudge came into view at the edge of the darkness. And then, within that smudge, came a little flutter, barely perceptible but persistent. "There's the heartbeat," the ultrasound tech said. "It probably just started beating today, or yesterday." I was pregnant, but just barely.

This news came as I was writing the last chapter of this book. I pushed through waves of nausea, fatigue, and anxiety to finish writing and editing the manuscript. All the while, as I struggled with the many words in the book, I chanted just two, over and over, in my head: "Be there. Be there. Be there." Sometimes I'd place a hand on my flat belly, look down from my computer, and repeat, "Be there. Please." It wasn't very scientific, but it was all I had.

As I write this, on the day that I'll send this manuscript to the publisher, I'm about 14 weeks pregnant. It's still there. The journey to this pregnancy has been just as long as the journey of this book. The two have been intertwined, and both have taken me to the intersection of parenting and science.

On the day I signed the contract committing to write the book, almost two years ago, my period was one day late. A couple of days later, a home pregnancy test confirmed that I was pregnant. Cee would have a little brother or sister at just about the sibling interval we had hoped for. And I would tackle this book with the looming deadline of a due date and lots of personal motivation to answer all of my own questions before the arrival of another baby.

But that wasn't how it turned out. That pregnancy ended in miscarriage, a profound and intangible loss. What I mourned the most was the vision of the family I wanted: the baby born in summertime, the doting big sister that Cee would be, and the personal growth for my husband and me as we adapted from parenting one to two. With the loss of that pregnancy and two more miscarriages that followed, there also came a feeling of loss of control. I couldn't control the processes in my own body, the timing of our next baby, or the age gap between our children. Things were not going to turn out as I had planned. It was humbling and disheartening.

This is a magnification of what parenting is every single day. I don't know anyone who finds that having a baby is exactly what they envisioned. Some parts may turn out as we had hoped, but others will be much harder, and a few will be surprisingly easy. We can't pick and choose the challenges, and we can't always predict how we will react to the stress and uncertainty of parenting. And none of us will experience it in the same way. This fact was front and center in my mind as I wrote this book, and it gave me more empathy for all the challenges and successes we each have with parenting.

Science continued to be a refuge for me as I worked on the book, even as I recognized its limitations. I could set aside my personal struggles and lose myself in a fascinating world of babies and parents, seen through the lens of science. It gave me a greater appreciation for the complexities of this task of parenting and for the many ways that good parenting takes shape across different families.

Now I get the absolutely best reward I could hope for. If all goes well, I'll have a new baby to care for by the time this book is published. I'll get to watch that baby grow and develop and fit into our family. Maybe I'll even get to use a few of the things that I learned in the process of writing the book. What is certain is that this baby, like all new babies, will bring new challenges—and *lots* more questions.

June 2014

UPDATE

Reading those words is like opening a time capsule from my life and pulling out a moment shaped by longing, hemmed with grief, and washed in cautious hope. If you've read this updated edition of *The Science of Mom*, you know that things worked out. Max was born in December 2014, and I frantically worked through edits on the manuscript while he fed and slept. By the time the book was published, he was eating solid foods and *almost* sleeping through the night. It's a well-worn parenting cliché that the early months fly by, but it's true. I was just grateful that I could enjoy Max's infancy so fully, having researched most of the tough questions before he was born. It's not that it was easy, or that I got everything right—far from it. But writing this book taught me as much about what we don't know as what we do know, and acknowledging the messiness of both parenting and science helped me let go of any ideas I had about what caring for a baby should look and feel like. I hope that reading this book has done the same for you.

January 2021

APPENDIXES

APPENDIX A

Ingredients in the Newborn Vitamin K Shot

In chapter 3, I discuss the evidence for giving a vitamin K shot at birth. Despite its proven benefits, some parents have opted out of giving their newborns this shot. When asked why, one of the common concerns is that the shot contains "toxins."[1] I wanted to find out if there is any reason to fear the ingredients in the vitamin K shot, so I dug into the pharmacology and toxicology literature looking for answers. After careful evaluation of each ingredient, I've concluded that each one serves an important role in the efficacy and safety of the shot, and none pose toxicological concerns in the amounts used.

Anytime you want to know whether a chemical is safe or effective, it is critical to look at the amount used, or the dose. A life-saving drug could be worthless if you didn't take enough of it, and it could also be toxic if you took too much. For the vitamin K shot, there are toxicological concerns with several of the ingredients, and these concerns are listed on the package insert for the vitamin K shot. However, in all cases, these were based on incidents using large, often continuous, intravenous doses of these ingredients, quite different from the one-time intramuscular dose of the vitamin K shot.[2]

Two types of vitamin K shots are commonly used. Both contain phytonadione, another name for vitamin K_1, but they contain different "inactive" ingredients. Most hospitals use the preservative-free version[3] for newborns, so let's start with the ingredients in that one:

- *Propylene glycol* (10.4 mg) acts as a solvent to keep the vitamin K in solution. (Vitamin K is fat-soluble, so just as oil and water don't mix, it can't simply be dissolved in water or saline for the injection.) Propylene glycol is commonly used in foods, supplements, and other medications, and in the amounts used, it is safe. And don't confuse propylene glycol with ethylene glycol, a much more toxic chemical used in antifreeze. According to the World Health Organization, propylene glycol is safe to consume in amounts up to 25 mg/kg of body weight per day. The 10.4 mg of propylene glycol in the vitamin K shot equals about 3.3 mg/kg for a 7-pound newborn.[4]

- *Polysorbate 80* (10 mg) is made from a plant-based sugar alcohol (sorbitol) and a fatty acid (oleic acid). It's often used in ice cream to make it smoother,[5] and it serves a similar purpose in the vitamin K shot. It is an emulsifier, helping fat-soluble vitamin K stay in solution. Polysorbate 80 was probably the culprit when an intravenous vitamin E product proved to be toxic in premature babies (an incident included on the package insert for the vitamin K shot), but these babies received more than 70 mg/kg daily for weeks and even months. The one-time vitamin K shot's 10 mg of polysorbate 80 is about 3 mg/kg for a 7-pound baby, and there is no reason to believe that this amount is harmful to newborns.[6]

- *Sodium acetate anhydrous* (0.17 mg) helps to maintain a neutral pH in the vitamin K shot. There are no toxicity concerns with this small amount. This ingredient does contain a small amount of aluminum, which is noted on the package insert, but the amount is no more than 0.05 µg (a µg is 1/1000th of a milligram). At birth, a newborn's body already contains 8,000 times this amount of aluminum.[7]

- *Glacial acetic acid* (0.00002 ml) is a weak acid and the main component of vinegar. It is used to adjust the pH and has no safety concerns as used in the vitamin K shot.[8]

A second type of vitamin K shot is less commonly used for newborns, but it is also safe.[9] It contains the following ingredients:

- *Benzyl alcohol* (4.5 mg) prevents bacterial growth in the vitamin K shot. The WHO sets the safe daily intake of benzyl alcohol at no more than 5 mg/kg of body weight, and the amount contained in the shot comes to about 1.4 mg/kg for a 7-pound newborn. The vitamin K package insert warns that benzyl alcohol can cause toxicity in newborns, but this requires much larger, daily, intravenous amounts (more than 99 mg/kg/day).[10]

- *Polyethoxylated castor oil* (35 mg) acts as an emulsifier and solvent to keep vitamin K in solution and is used in many other drugs for this purpose. Very rarely, this ingredient has caused an anaphylactic reaction in patients receiving large doses by intravenous infusion, but there are no reported cases of this effect in newborns receiving the intramuscular vitamin K shot with this ingredient.[11]

- *Dextrose monohydrate* (19 mg) is a fancy name for glucose, the simple sugar that circulates in our blood and fuels our cells. Much larger doses are routinely given to newborns who have low blood sugar. There are no safety concerns with this ingredient.[12]

A third product, called Konakion MM, is licensed for both oral and injectable use in Europe, Australia, and New Zealand. First introduced in 1994 in Switzerland, this product contains glycocholic acid (a bile salt) and lecithin (a phospholipid) to disperse the fat-soluble vitamin K into small droplets, similar to the mixed micelles (hence the MM in the name) that are part of the normal digestion of fats and fat-soluble vitamins. The idea behind this preparation was that it would be more absorbable via the oral route, even for babies with liver disease and limited bile salts, but it hasn't turned out to be much more effective than the other oral preparations at preventing late vitamin K deficiency bleeding (VKDB) in these babies.[13]

The package inserts for all three types of vitamin K products note that they can cause jaundice (hyperbilirubinemia), and this is often mentioned in anti–vitamin K articles. However, these cases occurred in babies receiving 10 to 20 mg doses of a synthetic, water-soluble form of vitamin K, which is no longer used. Jaundice has not been observed in babies who received the recommended dose of 1 mg or less.[14]

APPENDIX B

Why the Hepatitis B Vaccine Is Recommended at Birth

The World Health Organization recommends that newborns receive their first dose of the hepatitis B vaccine soon after birth, and preferably within 24 hours.[1] In the United States, the recommendation is for newborns weighing at last 2,000 grams to get their first dose either within 12 hours or 24 hours, depending on risk factors. A second dose is given between 1 and 2 months and a third dose between 6 and 18 months of age. (Newborns weighing less than 2,000 grams should wait until hospital discharge or 1 month of age to receive their first dose of vaccine, because it's less effective in these tiny babies.)[2]

The hepatitis B virus (HBV) infects the liver. An acute HBV infection causes nausea, vomiting, jaundice, loss of appetite, and abdominal pain, but most people recover without lasting effects. Much more serious is a chronic HBV infection. Although a person may be asymptomatic for years (and thus not know that he or she is carrying the disease, so inadvertently infecting others), chronic HBV infections may eventually cause cirrhosis or liver cancer and are responsible for about 3,000 deaths each year in the United States. Unfortunately, babies and young children are at very high risk of developing chronic infections because they are unable to clear the virus. Ninety percent of infected infants develop chronic infections, and of these, 25 percent will die prematurely due to complications of the disease.[3]

HBV can be transmitted through blood, semen, vaginal secretions, and saliva. Some people mistakenly assume that sexual contact is the only way that HBV can be transmitted from one person to the next, but this is not the case. Most HBV-positive moms pass the virus on to their newborn babies, although vaccination at birth will prevent the majority of these infections. For this reason, women should be tested for HBV during pregnancy so that their babies can be vaccinated and treated for HBV soon after birth.[4] However, the women at greatest risk of being HBV-positive are less likely to have prenatal care, and infection can also occur between the prenatal test and the time of giving birth.[5]

There are other ways for babies to be exposed to HBV. The virus can live for more than seven days at room temperature; it can easily be passed from one person to the next on a washcloth or toothbrush. It has been passed from one child to another through biting in a day care setting.[6] I thought about HBV when, as a toddler, Cee started "discovering" litter such as candy wrappers and empty water bottles at the park. The birth dose of HBV vaccine protects babies from the start, should they be exposed to the virus.

The HBV vaccine is highly effective, inducing immunity to HBV in 98 percent of infants who complete the series.[7] Because it prevents chronic liver infections, which cause liver cancer, the HBV vaccine is an anticancer vaccine. Before the vaccine, about 300,000 people, as many as 24,000 of them children, were infected with HBV each year in the United States.[8] With the universal vaccination of infants, recommended in 1991, the incidence of acute hepatitis B in children less than 12 years old has decreased by 94 percent, and the incidence in the overall population has decreased by 75 percent.[9] Chronic HBV infections are more difficult to track because they are often asymptomatic. However, since they can take decades to cause illness, the greatest benefits of HBV vaccination—reduction in chronic infections—may not yet have been detected.[10]

The HBV vaccine is very safe. It can cause minor soreness at the site of injection and a low-grade fever. Very rarely, it can cause a severe allergic reaction (1 in 1.1 million doses), but if this happens, a health care provider can rapidly respond.[11] Based on the evidence for the safety of the HBV vaccine and the risk of infection in early infancy, it makes sense for babies to be vaccinated at birth.

APPENDIX C

Not Too Many Vaccines Too Soon

When my parents were born, both in 1948, the only vaccines available and recommended were for smallpox and a combined shot for diphtheria, tetanus, and pertussis. That was it—protection from four diseases. By the time I was born in 1980, the measles, mumps, and rubella (MMR) and the polio vaccines had been added to the schedule. Smallpox had been successfully eradicated, and the vaccine was no longer needed. I was immunized for seven diseases. In 2020, as I write this, the recommended schedule provides protection from 14 diseases, requiring as many as 38 doses in the first two years of life.[1] (We are still waiting and looking forward to a time when children can be immunized against a fifteenth disease—COVID-19.) Your baby will often get several shots at a time, although combination shots have helped to reduce the total number needed. The sheer number of needles you see at a well-baby doctor's visit might make you wonder: can your little baby handle so many vaccines, in such quick succession, at such a young age?

As parents, we are most aware of the number of needles we see, but a more important measure of the vaccine "load" is the number of unique antigens—proteins or polysaccharides that stimulate an immune response. Over the past few decades, as new vaccines have been developed, they have been refined to contain fewer antigens at

295

Antigen load in vaccines recommended for children under 2 years of age in the United States, 1900–2020

	1900	1960	1983	2020
Disease protection provided by recommended schedule	Smallpox	Smallpox Diphtheria Tetanus Pertussis Polio	Diphtheria Tetanus Pertussis Polio Measles Mumps Rubella	Diphtheria Tetanus Pertussis Polio Measles Mumps Rubella Hib* Varicella Pneumococcus Hepatitis A Hepatitis B Rotavirus Influenza
Total number of diseases prevented	1	5	7	14
TOTAL NUMBER OF ANTIGENS	~200	~12,268	~12,077	285–327†

Sources: J. M. Glanz et al., "Association between Estimated Cumulative Antigen Exposure through the First 23 Months of Life and Non–Vaccine-Targeted Infections from 24 through 47 Months of Age," *JAMA* 319, no. 9 (2018): 906–13; P. A. Offit et al., "Addressing Parents' Concerns: Do Multiple Vaccines Overwhelm or Weaken the Infant's Immune System?" *Pediatrics* 109, no. 1 (2002): 124–29; American Academy of Pediatrics, Committee on Control of Infectious Diseases, "Immunization Against Poliomyelitis," *Pediatrics* 26, no. 2 (1960): 331–32; Centers for Disease Control and Prevention, "Schedule-Related Resources: Prior Immunization Schedules," Immunization Schedules, last updated February 2020, https://www.cdc.gov/vaccines/schedules/hcp/schedule-related-resources.html.

Note: The two vaccines with the largest number of antigens were smallpox and the whole-cell pertussis vaccine. Since global eradication of smallpox, the vaccine is no longer used. The whole-cell pertussis vaccine contained about 3,000 antigens and required four doses before age 2. In 1999, it was replaced with the acellular vaccine, containing only parts of the pertussis pathogen and just 2 to 4 antigens.

* Haemophilus influenzae type B.

† Several types of vaccines are licensed for some vaccinations, so the number of antigens depends on which vaccine is received.

smaller doses, just enough to give an immune response. When I was a child, immunization against seven diseases required exposure to more than 12,000 antigens. Today's recommended schedule protects babies from 14 diseases, and it does so with only about 300 antigens. Advances in science have given us the benefit of greater protection from infectious diseases *and* smaller, safer vaccines.

When a baby is given a vaccine, her immune system responds to those antigens, but this is only one of many tasks that it is handling on that day. From the moment of birth, a newborn baby is bombarded with bacteria and viruses, and she generates a range of effective immune responses to sort the good from the bad and to survive in a germy world. Research has demonstrated that vaccines don't overwhelm a baby's immune system, whether one or five are given in a day. For example, when a child already battling an ear infection, upper respiratory tract infection, or diarrhea is vaccinated, she can mount just as robust an immune response to the vaccine as a perfectly healthy child, and with no greater risk of an adverse reaction. Her immune system can handle it. And when combination shots are given, the immune response to each vaccine is no different from when the vaccines are given separately.[2]

If the recommended immunization schedule overwhelmed infants' immune systems, we would expect vaccinated babies to be less capable of responding to other infectious diseases. A randomized controlled trial in Germany tested this hypothesis, dividing 496 newborn babies into two groups, one receiving five vaccines at 2 months, and the other delaying those vaccines until 3 months.[3] Between 2 and 3 months of age, the unvaccinated babies were *more* likely to have symptoms of illness such as vomiting, coughing, runny nose, and rash, suggesting that the vaccinated babies' immune systems were strengthened in a nonspecific way that protected them from everyday sorts of pathogens. Likewise, a 2018 study conducted in the United States looked at how many vaccine antigens children were exposed to in the first two years of life and how likely they were to end up in the emergency room or hospital sick with other infections (not targeted by vaccines) between ages

2 and 4. Comparing children who received the protection of the full vaccine schedule with those who were partially or completely unvaccinated, there was no difference in their likelihood of coming down with another illness.[4]

A 2013 study specifically looked at the concern that the number of vaccines in the modern immunization schedule may be associated with a higher risk for autism. It tallied the total number of antigens in the vaccines given to children with and without autism, and it found no relationship between the antigen "load" and the development of autism.[5] Another study found that children who received all of their vaccines on time in the first year of life scored the same or better on neuropsychological outcomes compared with children who had delayed or fewer immunizations.[6] Finally, when the Institute of Medicine evaluated the safety of the entire childhood immunization schedule, it found no evidence that the recommended schedule is linked to autoimmune diseases, asthma, hypersensitivity, seizures, learning or developmental disorders, or attention deficit or disruptive disorders.[7]

The concern that we give too many vaccines too soon is unfounded, but it has led some parents to vaccinate on a delayed schedule, spreading out shots to reduce the number given at one time or waiting until their baby is older for some shots. There are a few problems with this. First, there's no evidence that delaying or spacing out vaccines offers any benefit or is any safer. And, on the flip side, delaying vaccines has known risks. The recommended schedule is based on expert assessment of the research on vaccine safety and efficacy, and it is specifically designed to vaccinate children when they are able to respond appropriately to the vaccine and when they are most vulnerable to the disease. Delaying vaccines increases the amount of time that your child is susceptible to getting sick and passing a disease on to a more vulnerable person, such as a newborn baby or an immune-compromised cancer patient.

During the 2019 New York City measles outbreak, Dr. Jennifer Lighter, a pediatric infectious diseases physician and epidemiologist at Hassenfeld Children's Hospital at NYU Langone, observed firsthand the risk of delaying a child's immunizations as she helped lead her hospital's response to the outbreak. In an opinion article in the *New York Times*, she wrote that none of the children she had treated were completely unvaccinated. Rather, their parents had only delayed their vaccines, including the MMR shot that would have protected them against measles, because of personal preferences. That choice not only put their own children at risk, but it likely stoked the fires of the outbreak as it infected hundreds of others.[8]

As children grow and develop, so do their immune systems. It may seem intuitive that a child could respond better to a vaccine if it is given at an older age, but this is an overly simplistic assumption. For example, febrile seizures are a known and rare side effect of the MMR vaccine, occurring in about 1 in 3,000 vaccinated children. Febrile seizures aren't dangerous and don't cause long-term damage to the child, but they are understandably scary to parents. A 2013 study of more than 840,000 children found that compared with those vaccinated at the recommended time (12 to 15 months), children that got the MMR shot at 16 to 23 months had double the risk of a seizure.[9] In other words, delaying the MMR shot actually *increased* the risk of side effects. This could be because the older age group did indeed have a more rigorous immune response to the vaccine, but if this increases side effects as well, then later vaccination isn't necessarily the better option. Giving the MMR shot at the recommended time ensures an appropriate immune response—enough to provide immunity to measles, mumps, and rubella—at an age for which the side effects are well studied. Deviating from the schedule puts your child in uncharted territory for both safety and efficacy of the vaccine.

Finally, spacing out your child's vaccines has some practical implications. It means more trips to your doctor's office for shots, and if you're trying to split up combination shots, it increases the total number of shots given. That could mean more overall stress for your baby.[10] Each visit to the doctor's office also increases your baby's risk of coming into contact with another sick child who could make her ill. In other words, spacing out your baby's vaccines just adds up to more stress, more risk, and no known benefit.

Historical changes in vaccine-preventable diseases

DISEASES VACCINATED AGAINST BEFORE 1980	PRE-VACCINE ANNUAL AVERAGE	
	Cases	*Deaths*
Diphtheria	21,053	1,822
Measles	530,217	440
Mumps*	162,344	39
Pertussis	200,752	4,043
Poliomyelitis, paralytic	16,316	1,879
Rubella	47,745	17
Smallpox	29,005	337
Tetanus	580	472

DISEASES VACCINATED AGAINST BETWEEN 1980 AND 2014	PRE-VACCINE ANNUAL AVERAGE	
	Cases	*Deaths*
Hepatitis A	117,333	137
Hepatitis B, acute	66,232	237
Invasive Hib†	20,000	1,000
Invasive pneumococcal disease‡	63,067	6,500
Varicella	4,085,120	105

Sources: S. W. Roush, T. V. Murphy, and Vaccine-Preventable Disease Table Working Group, "Historical Comparisons of Morbidity and Mortality for Vaccine-Preventable Diseases in the United States," *JAMA* 298, no. 18 (2007): 2155–63; W. Atkinson, S. Wolfe, and J. Hamborsky, eds., *Epidemiology and Prevention of Vaccine-Preventable Diseases*, 12th ed. (Washington, DC: Public Health Foundation, 2012).

in the United States, pre- and post-vaccine

POST-VACCINE REPORTS OR ESTIMATES, 2006		PRE-POST % REDUCTION	
Cases	Deaths	Cases	Deaths
0	0	100%	100%
55	0	100%	100%
6,584	1	96%	97%
15,632	9	92%	>99%
0	0	100%	100%
11	0	100%	100%
0	0	100%	100%
41	4	93%	99%

POST-VACCINE REPORTS OR ESTIMATES, 2006		PRE-POST % REDUCTION	
Cases	Deaths	Cases	Deaths
15,298	18	87%	87%
13,169	47	80%	80%
<50	<5	>99%	>99%
41,550	4,850	34%	25%
612,768	18	85%	83%

*2006 was an unusually bad year for mumps due to outbreaks in college dormitories. Most years, there are only about 20 mumps cases.

†Haemophilus influenzae B; post-vaccine estimates are for 2005.

‡Post-vaccine estimates are for 2005.

APPENDIX D

Vaccines and Autism

The purported link between vaccines and autism is probably the vaccine-related concern that has garnered the most attention in the media in recent years. Such a link has been thoroughly investigated by scientists around the world, and study after study has found no evidence that vaccines cause autism. Still, this concern is often cited by parents as a reason why they hesitate to vaccinate their children.[1] So, let's take a closer look.

There are two historical origins of theories about vaccines and autism. The first is a 1998 paper published in the *Lancet* by Andrew Wakefield, a gastroenterologist then based in London.[2] The paper was a case series of 12 children, all of whom had symptoms of digestive problems and concerns about their neurodevelopment, many (but not all) of the children having been diagnosed with autism. (Recall from chapter 1 that case reports and case series provide the lowest quality of scientific evidence.) The paper didn't provide any evidence for a link between the MMR vaccine and children's medical symptoms, but it did allude to this possibility, and Wakefield voiced his concern about the MMR shot in press conferences following its publication. This one paper was successful in getting a disproportionate amount of media attention given its scary (albeit weak) findings, and fear about the MMR vaccine led parents to opt out of the MMR vaccination, particularly in the UK. Unfortunately, measles outbreaks have followed. In 1998, when Wakefield published his paper, there were 56 cases of measles in England and Wales. Fifteen years later, in 2013, there were 1,843 measles cases, many of them among older kids and teens who didn't receive the vaccine during the autism scare. Several children have died of measles in recent outbreaks in the United Kingdom and Ireland.[3]

A number of concerns arose about Wakefield's research, and an investigation found him guilty of ethical, medical, and scientific misconduct. Wakefield was stripped of his medical license, and the *Lancet* finally retracted his paper in 2010.[4]

A second autism-related matter focused on the use of the preservative thimerosal in vaccines. Thimerosal prevents bacterial contamination of multi-dose vaccine vials, an important role in maintaining their safety. But thimerosal contains ethylmercury, and there was some concern that the total amount of thimerosal in the childhood vaccination schedule could cause neurological problems. In 1999, the US Public Health Service and the American Academy of Pediatrics asked that thimerosal be removed from childhood vaccines (which meant switching to more expensive single-dose vials), not because there was any evidence that it was a problem, but because they thought they didn't have enough evidence to say for sure that it wasn't.[5] Subsequent research has shown that the ethylmercury in thimerosal is much less toxic than the methylmercury found in fish. Ethylmercury is metabolized and cleared by the body much faster, most of it being excreted in the stool, and the amount used in vaccines did not pose a risk to children's health. Regardless, thimerosal is no longer used in childhood vaccines in the United States, except for some types of flu vaccine.[6]

Both hypotheses—that autism was in some way related to the MMR vaccine or to thimerosal—have been thoroughly investigated and thoroughly rejected. These studies have been conducted around the world, from Canada to California and Finland to Japan, and they've looked at millions of children in multiple types of study designs. The Institute of Medicine, Cochrane, and others have carefully reviewed these studies and found no link between vaccines and autism.[7] A 2014 meta-analysis combined the results of all the high-quality studies of vaccines and autism published up to that point, including nearly 1.3 million children, and found no relationship between autism and MMR, thimerosal, mercury, or vaccines in general.[8] A more recent study from Denmark, published in 2019 in *Annals of Internal Medicine*, followed a cohort of more than 650,000 children born in the country between 1999 and 2010. It found that children who received the MMR vaccine were no more likely to be diagnosed with autism than children who hadn't gotten the shot.[9] In addition, a US study published in *JAMA* in 2015 looked at more than 95,000 children and found no link between the MMR vaccine and autism. This study also specifically looked at children with an older sibling with autism, because this family history increases the risk of diagnosis in younger siblings. Again, in these higher risk children, receiving the MMR vaccine did not increase the likelihood of having autism.[10]

We don't know exactly what causes autism, but we do know that genetics plays a big role, with as many as 102 different genes linked to the disease, according to a 2020 paper published in the journal *Cell*.[11] Environmental factors such as parental age, maternal infection during pregnancy, and pregnancy complications may also contribute.[12] Whatever the cause, most evidence to date indicates that autism is part of a person's neurological wiring before birth. For example, a 2014 study published in the *New England Journal of Medicine* showed that children with autism have atypical organization in the layers of cells in the cortex of the brain, changes that must have occurred during fetal development.[13] A 2013 paper published in *Nature* reported that differences in social interaction begin to appear in babies later diagnosed with autism as early as 2 months of age, long before children receive their first MMR shot (around their first birthday).[14]

The vast amount of research on vaccines and autism—all finding no relationship—should have put these fears to rest years ago, but some parents still insist that their children's autism is related to vaccines. This is understandable. Children receive a lot of vaccinations during the first two years of life, and parents begin to notice the signs of autism during this time, even though biologically, the differences that make a child autistic have most likely been present in that child from before birth. It's human nature for parents to look for some explanation or something to blame to help them make sense of a change in their child's behavior, and statistically, some parents are bound to notice these changes soon after a vaccination. But what parents are noticing here is a correlation, not evidence of causation. We need science to evaluate causation. We need careful, systematic study of many variables in many people. When scientists have looked at the autism question in this way, it's clear that there is no relationship between autism and vaccines.

It's good to know that vaccines don't cause autism. But, in all, this is a very sad story. A few scary stories planted seeds of fear, which then spread like wildfire on the internet. Immunization rates went down, leaving kids vulnerable to disease and leading to outbreaks. Lots of energy and money were spent investigating a link between vaccines and autism, a hypothesis that never had much evidence supporting it in the first place. Those resources would have been much better spent on research to understand autism or on helping families support their autistic children.

APPENDIX E

Vaccines and SIDS

Another longstanding and particularly terrifying concern about vaccines is that they might increase a baby's risk of dying of SIDS. Like the autism myth, the SIDS concern persists because of the association in time between vaccines and SIDS. Most SIDS deaths occur between 2 and 4 months of age, when infants typically receive several rounds of immunizations, and statistically, there is a reasonable chance that a baby who died of SIDS was recently immunized. For parents looking for a way to explain the inexplicable, vaccines might seem like a plausible culprit.

But as we've already discussed, noticing a correlation in time between two events (recent immunization and SIDS) does not mean that one caused the other. To investigate the possibility that vaccines might increase the risk of SIDS, researchers have used case control studies comparing the immunization history of babies who died of SIDS to babies who did not. A 2007 meta-analysis combined the results of nine case control studies and found that, in fact, immunization was associated with a *reduced* risk of SIDS.[1] It's not clear why this might be, and not all studies have found this protective effect.[2] It's possible that vaccinated babies are protected from infections, and respiratory illness is sometimes associated with SIDS. Or it may be the result of what researchers call the "healthy vaccine effect," caused when parents delay vaccines when their babies are ill, such that those receiving vaccines are healthier from the start and thus less likely to succumb to SIDS.

Other studies have searched huge numbers of medical records for any association between vaccines and SIDS deaths and found none. For example, one study examined 350,000 births in California in the 1990s looking for a correlation between the hepatitis B vaccine and neonatal deaths; it could find no such link.[3] Another looked at the records of 14,000 infants receiving the combined shot containing vaccines for diphtheria, tetanus, pertussis, polio, and Hib and found no cases of SIDS linked to the shot.[4]

The research on this question has been consistent and clear: there is no evidence that vaccinating your baby increases the risk of SIDS, and it's even possible that it could give your baby a little extra protection. You can rest easy with the choice to vaccinate your baby.

While we're on the topic of vaccines and sleep, here's a helpful heads up: vaccines have been shown to affect babies' sleep patterns. A 2011 study of 70 2-month-old babies found that, on average, the babies slept 69 more minutes in the 24 hours after getting their shots compared with the 24 hours before.[5] The sleepy baby effect wasn't universal, however, as 37 percent of the babies in this study slept less. As usual, babies are unpredictable and don't all follow the same script!

APPENDIX F

Aluminum in Vaccines

Small amounts of aluminum salts are present in some vaccines. They are used as adjuvants, substances that help to stimulate the immune response to a vaccine, often allowing smaller quantities of antigen or fewer doses to be used. Without aluminum, some vaccines are less effective, meaning that more people fail to develop immunity in response to the vaccine. Aluminum may also reduce adverse reactions to vaccines by slowing the release of antigens from the muscle, where the vaccine is injected, into the bloodstream. Aluminum salts have been used as adjuvants in vaccines for more than 75 years, and like every ingredient in the vial, they play an important role.[1] However, some parents are worried about the cumulative effect of aluminum in vaccines. What does the science say?

Aluminum is all around us. It's the most abundant metal in the earth's crust, found in our drinking water, our food, and the air we breathe. It's also used in products like sunscreen and antiperspirant, and in antacids and other medicines. At birth, a newborn already has some aluminum in his body (~0.4 mg), and this "body burden" builds slowly across the lifespan with exposure to aluminum from a variety of sources. By 6 months, an infant will have consumed 10 mg of aluminum if breastfed, 40 mg if fed regular formula, and 120 mg if fed soy-based formula. Starting solid foods means even more aluminum.[2]

It's true that too much aluminum can have harmful effects on health. For example, studies have shown that preterm infants fed intravenously for weeks at a time can have impaired neurodevelopment because the feeding solutions often contain aluminum and their underdeveloped kidneys limit their ability to excrete the mineral.[3]

But as with any chemical, we have to look at the *amount* of the dose and the *route* of exposure to assess its toxicity. Over the first year of life, an infant immunized according to the recommended schedule will receive, at most, 4.2 mg of aluminum from vaccines, with no more than 1.2 mg at a time. The aluminum salts used in vaccines are insoluble, so they dissolve and enter the bloodstream very slowly after injection.[4] Most of the aluminum that is absorbed into the blood is quickly filtered by the kidneys and excreted in the urine. A small amount contributes to the body burden, mostly stored in bone, but this is well below the safety limits established for infants.[5]

Several recent studies have investigated the effects of vaccines on infants' aluminum levels and neurodevelopment. A 2013 study published in *JAMA Pediatrics* measured blood aluminum levels in 15 infants born preterm, at an average of 27 weeks gestational age, before and after they received their regular 2-month shots. Despite these babies' small size and prematurity, with an average body weight of just five pounds, there was no detectable increase in their blood aluminum levels after receiving their vaccines on schedule.[6] A 2018 study published in *Academic Pediatrics* found no correlation between aluminum received in vaccines, blood or hair aluminum levels, or infant development in 9- to 13-month-old babies.[7]

Many parents have been misled about aluminum in vaccines by Dr. Robert Sears, whose popular book encourages parents to space out shots using one of his recommended alternative schedules. Dr. Sears cites concerns about too much aluminum as one of his reasons for promoting an alternative schedule. However, he based his aluminum calculations on studies of intravenous aluminum in hemodialysis patients and severely premature infants, both of which have impaired kidney function.[8] Intravenous administration of aluminum acts very differently from an intramuscular injection, as used for vaccines, because the aluminum in an IV injection is already dissolved and hits the bloodstream all at once.[9] Dr. Sears's aluminum calculations failed to account for this distinction, not to mention that he based them on patients whose natural pathway for aluminum excretion was compromised. There is no indication that the aluminum in vaccines is dangerous and no reason to spread out vaccinations to reduce the amount of aluminum given at one time. (Plus, there are good reasons *not* to space out vaccinations; see appendix C.)

APPENDIX G

How We Know Babies Need So Much Iron

I've discussed iron a lot in this book. Iron nutrition is one of the most compelling reasons to delay cord clamping (chapter 2), start solid foods by 6 months (chapter 9), and choose iron-rich complementary foods for your baby (chapter 10). If you're like me, you might wonder how we know that babies need so much iron. How do we determine the recommended iron intake for babies, and how certain are we of its accuracy? These are great questions, and since iron is so important to babies, I thought I'd dissect the calculations that go into dietary recommendations for this mineral.

The World Health Organization says that babies aged 6 to 12 months need to absorb 0.93 mg of iron from their food (or supplements) each day to meet their bodies' needs.[1] How did the experts on the WHO committee arrive at this number? To start, they looked at how much a baby grows during this period, because growth means an increase in blood volume, requiring iron to make more hemoglobin. Tissues, including the developing brain and the muscles working overtime as your baby learns to crawl, also grow in size and need more iron. For normal growth and development, the average baby needs about 0.55 mg of iron per day. In addition, 0.17 mg of iron is lost in feces, urine, and dead skin every day and must be replaced. Add these two numbers together, and that brings us to 0.72 mg of iron needed each day by the average baby.

But this number is just an average. Some babies will need less iron and some will need more, depending on factors like genetics, body size, and growth rate. We want all babies—not just "average" babies—to get enough, so the WHO recommends 0.93 mg of absorbed iron per day for babies aged 6 to 12 months, which is estimated to meet the needs of 95 percent of all babies.

This number, however, is *absorbed* iron—the iron that actually crosses from the digestive tract into the blood to be used by the body. Iron absorption, or bioavailability, is highly variable, depending on the food source and other components of the diet. The best iron bioavailability is found in heme sources such as meat, poultry, and fish; about 25 to 35 percent of the iron in these foods will be absorbed into the blood.[2] Nonheme iron found in plant foods has much lower bioavailability, often 5 percent or less.[3] Other foods included in the same meal can also affect the bioavailability of nonheme iron (see the box "Optimizing Iron Absorption" on page 260).[4]

Iron bioavailability in breast milk is between about 15 and 50 percent, depending on the research methods used to measure it and the babies studied. Babies who are exclusively breastfed or iron-deficient are more efficient at absorbing iron from breast milk; those receiving an iron supplement or solid foods are less efficient.[5] The bioavailability of the iron added to infant formula is estimated at about 10 percent.[6]

To return to the WHO's estimated iron requirement, we must consider bioavailability of the total diet to estimate how much dietary iron is needed. For example, if the average bioavailability of a baby's diet is 10 percent, she'll have to consume a total of 9.3 mg of food iron to meet the goal of 0.93 mg of absorbed iron. If she gets most of her iron from plant foods, she'll need much more. If she eats lots of meat and breast milk, she'll need less.

I like the way the WHO shows that the iron requirement is dependent on the bioavailability of the baby's diet because it allows you to base your baby's target iron consumption on the type of diet

World Health Organization's recommended iron intakes for infants 6 to 12 months of age based on bioavailability in food

DIETARY BIOAVAILABILITY	15%	12%	10%	5%
Type of diet	More heme sources ◄──► Vegetarian diet			
Recommended iron intake (mg/day)	6.2	7.7	9.3	18.6

Source: Joint FAO/WHO Expert Consultation on Human Vitamin and Mineral Requirements and WHO Department of Nutrition for Health and Development, *Vitamin and Mineral Requirements in Human Nutrition*, 2nd ed. (Geneva: World Health Organization, 2004).

Note: With higher dietary bioavailability (as from heme sources), less dietary iron is required. A vegetarian diet has about 5 percent bioavailability, whereas a diet with frequent servings of meat has a bioavailability of 15 percent or more.

your baby is eating. However, depending on where in the world you live, you may see other values for iron requirements, usually simplified to single recommendations to avoid overwhelming parents with the bioavailability discussion. For example, for babies 6 to 12 months, US experts recommend 11 mg iron per day, and European Union experts recommend 8 mg per day.[7] This is not because babies in the United States need more iron than those in Europe but rather because each region's expert committees decided to use slightly different approaches or assumptions in their calculations. The discrepancy shows us that nutrition is not an exact science, but still, you can see that the recommendations are in the same ballpark. The European Society for Paediatric Gastroenterology, Hepatology, and Nutrition (ESPGHAN) describes the theoretical dietary iron requirement of 6- to 12-month-olds as 0.76 mg iron per kg body weight, assuming dietary bioavailability of 10 percent.[8] That may be a helpful calculation, especially if your baby is much smaller or larger than average, as it gives you a more individualized recommendation based on body weight.

When you understand how the iron requirement is calculated, you can see that because it is meant to cover the majority of babies, it is intentionally an overestimate for most. A smaller-than-average baby or one growing at a slower rate might need much less iron. This explains why some babies do fine with exclusive breastfeeding beyond 6 months or eating complementary foods that provide little iron, but what works for one baby might be inadequate for another.

APPENDIX H

Why We Should Worry About Arsenic in Rice Cereal

Rice cereal has been a popular first infant food for several generations because it is easily digested, unlikely to cause an allergic reaction, and makes a good vehicle for iron fortification. However, we now know that there's a major downside to rice and rice-based products: they often contain high levels of inorganic arsenic. Arsenic is a naturally occurring element that is present in the earth's crust, and thus in our soils and groundwater. However, we've added more arsenic to our environment through mining, fuel burning, and pesticide use. Because rice grows in flooded paddies, it tends to accumulate a lot of arsenic, though how much depends on local concentrations. For example, arsenic levels are especially high in rice grown in the southern United States on land that was formerly cultivated for cotton, with a legacy of heavy use of arsenic-containing pesticides.[1]

Exposure to too much arsenic has been linked to cancer, skin lesions, heart disease, diabetes, and neurodevelopmental toxicity.[2] Of course, as is true for all chemicals, it's the dose that makes the poison. A little bit of arsenic is a part of life; it's naturally (but also unnaturally) present in our food and water, and it's unrealistic to think that we'll eliminate it from our lives. The challenge is in defining how much is too much. That's especially hard to study for children, given that the effects of chronic early-life arsenic exposure may only show up years later. But there is reason to think that current exposure levels for children are affecting their health. For example, a 2014 study reported that children in Maine with greater levels of arsenic in their drinking water had lower IQ scores by 5 to 6 points, compared to children with lower arsenic levels in their drinking water.[3] Other studies have found that food sources contribute just as much, if not more, inorganic arsenic as drinking water in the United States.[4]

High levels of arsenic in rice are especially worrisome for infants. Infants may eat several servings of rice cereal per day, and because of their small body size, this level of exposure is about three times that of adults on a body weight basis.[5] And while smaller amounts of arsenic are present in drinking water and other foods, among babies who eat rice cereal, more than half of their daily arsenic intake comes from this food alone.[6] One US study found that 12-month-olds who ate rice cereal or rice snacks (such as puffs, rusks, or crackers) had two to three times the urinary concentrations of arsenic compared to those who didn't eat rice products at all.[7]

Until recently, there were no federal standards for arsenic levels in food in the United States or the European Union.[8] That has started to change in the last decade, in large part because of consumer and child health advocacy groups publishing their own analyses of arsenic in apple juice and baby food and calling on government agencies to investigate and regulate arsenic in food.[9] In 2013, the US Food and Drug Administration's analysis found an average of 1.8 micrograms (µg) of inorganic arsenic per serving in baby rice cereal. Since then, arsenic levels have been reduced, at least in part because manufacturers have sourced their ingredients from regions with lower environmental arsenic levels. When the FDA repeated their analysis of rice cereal in 2018, they found an average of 1.3 µg inorganic arsenic per serving, though levels as high as 2.1 µg per serving were measured.[10] Similarly high levels of arsenic have been found in baby rice cereal products from Australia and Europe. Interestingly, some of the lowest levels are found in China, a good thing since rice is such a dietary staple there.[11]

Brown rice usually has more arsenic than white rice, because arsenic is concentrated in the bran, which is removed in the polishing process that makes white rice. In the FDA analyses, certified organic rice had no less arsenic compared with conventionally grown rice. Similar levels were also found in regular white and brown rice, so homemade baby rice cereal won't reduce arsenic exposure.[12]

In 2020, the FDA recommended to the food industry that baby rice cereal should contain no more than 1.5 μg inorganic arsenic per serving or 100 parts per billion (ppb), though this is a voluntary standard that is not enforceable by the FDA.[13] The agency also doesn't claim that this is a safe level, just that it is achievable through good manufacturing processes and that it will reduce the risk of cancers and neurodevelopmental effects. Advocacy groups say the voluntary standard doesn't go far enough.[14] However, the European Union adopted the same standard in 2015, so there is some level of international consensus for it.[15] Based on the FDA's 2018 analysis, 24 percent of samples had inorganic arsenic levels greater than 100 ppb.[16]

Here's the bottom line: Arsenic is bad for babies, and rice products are high in arsenic. Feeding your baby small amounts of rice products is fine—those magical baby puff snacks were a lifesaver for my family (and neighboring passengers) on several long airplane trips when my kids were little. But there's no reason to make rice cereal one of your baby's primary foods; simply choose other iron-fortified cereals, like oatmeal, barley, and wheat, and you'll slash your baby's arsenic exposure. And as my children grew, they started eating regular cooked rice with dinner a few times per week, and I'm not worried about that level of intake, but we also incorporate other grains, like quinoa, barley, and wheat pasta, into our meal rotation. Arsenic exposure is most concerning for babies who eat several servings of rice cereal per day because their caregivers haven't heard about the arsenic problem, or it's a staple at their day care. It could also be a problem for children and adults with celiac disease or a wheat allergy, as gluten-free products tend to use a lot of rice-derived ingredients.

The story of arsenic in rice illustrates some of the most important nutrition advice for everyone, babies included: dietary diversity is important. Eating a balanced diet with a variety of foods from every food group provides better nutrition and protects you from problems that may pop up with diets too focused on any one food.

NOTES

1. SHOW ME THE SCIENCE

1. A. Gopnik, "Scientific Thinking in Young Children: Theoretical Advances, Empirical Research, and Policy Implications," *Science* 337, no. 6102 (2012): 1623–27.

2. Editors of the *Lancet*. "Retraction—Ileal-Lymphoid-Nodular Hyperplasia, Non-Specific Colitis, and Pervasive Developmental Disorder in Children," *Lancet* 375 no. 9713 (2010): 445, doi:10.1016/S0140-6736(10)60175-4.

3. E. Dumas-Mallet et al., "Poor Replication Validity of Biomedical Association Studies Reported by Newspapers," *PLOS ONE* 12, no. 2 (2017): e0172650.

4. OCEBM Levels of Evidence Working Group, *Oxford Centre for Evidence-Based Medicine 2011 Levels of Evidence* (Oxford: Centre for Evidence-Based Medicine, 2011), https://www.cebm.ox.ac.uk/resources/levels-of-evidence/ocebm-levels-of-evidence; University of Cincinnati Libraries, "Evidence-Based Clinical Practice Resources," accessed December 8, 2020, https://guides.libraries.uc.edu/ebm/ebmcategories; D. Coggon, G. Rose, and D. J. P. Barker, "Epidemiology for the Uninitiated," *British Medical Journal*, accessed June 24, 2014, http://www.bmj.com/about-bmj/resources-readers/publications/epidemiology-uninitiated.

5. T. G. Ong et al., "Probiotics to Prevent Infantile Colic," *Cochrane Data-base of Systematic Reviews*, no. 3 (2019): CD012473, doi:10.1002/14651858 .CD012 473.pub2.

6. G. Du Toit et al., "Randomized Trial of Peanut Consumption in Infants at Risk for Peanut Allergy," *New England Journal of Medicine* 372 (2015): 803–13.

7. G. Du Toit et al., "Early Consumption of Peanuts in Infancy Is Associated with a Low Prevalence of Peanut Allergy," *Journal of Allergy and Clinical Immunology* 122, no. 5 (2008): 984–91.

8. Du Toit et al., "Randomized Trial of Peanut Consumption in Infants at Risk for Peanut Allergy."

9. C. Doctorow, "Correlation between Autism Diagnosis and Organic Food Sales," *Boing Boing* (blog), January 1, 2013, http://boingboing.net/2013/01/01 /correlation-between-autism-dia.html.

10. J. Wright, "Autism Rates in the United States Explained," *Spectrum*, September 3, 2020, https://www.spectrumnews.org/news/autism-rates-united -states-explained; G. S. Fisch, "Nosology and Epidemiology in Autism: Classification Counts," *American Journal of Medical Genetics: Part C, Seminars in Medical Genetics* 160C, no. 2 (2012): 91–103; K. M. Keyes et al., "Cohort Effects Explain the Increase in Autism Diagnosis among Children Born from 1992 to 2003 in California," *International Journal of Epidemiology* 41, no. 2 (2012): 495–503.

11. R. Gilbert, "Infant Sleeping Position and the Sudden Infant Death Syndrome: Systematic Review of Observational Studies and Historical Review of Recommendations from 1940 to 2002," *International Journal of Epidemiology* 34, no. 4 (2005): 874–87.

12. P. Franco et al., "Arousal from Sleep Mechanisms in Infants," *Sleep Medicine* 11, no. 7 (2010): 603–14.

13. A. Lundh et al., "Industry Sponsorship and Research Outcome," *Cochrane Database of Systematic Reviews*, no. 2 (2017): MR000033.

14. H. K. Hughes, M. M. Landa, and J. M. Sharfstein, "Marketing Claims for Infant Formula: The Need for Evidence," *JAMA Pediatrics* 171, no. 2 (2017): 105–6; S. A. Abrams, "Is It Time to Put a Moratorium on New Infant Formulas That Are Not Adequately Investigated?" *Journal of Pediatrics* 166, no. 3 (2015): 756–60.

15. S. Vosoughi, D. Roy, and S. Aral, "The Spread of True and False News Online," *Science* 359, no. 6380 (2018): 1146–51.

16. D. A. Broniatowski et al., "Weaponized Health Communication: Twitter Bots and Russian Trolls Amplify the Vaccine Debate," *American Journal of Public Health* 108, no. 10 (2018): 1378–84.

2. BIRTH DAY, FIRST DAY

1. A. C. Yao, M. Moinian, and J. Lind, "Distribution of Blood between Infant and Placenta after Birth," *Lancet* 294, no. 7626 (1969): 871–73; D. Farrar et al., "Measuring Placental Transfusion for Term Births: Weighing Babies with Cord Intact," *BJOG: An International Journal of Obstetrics and Gynaecology* 118, no. 1 (2011): 70–75; A. C. Katheria et al., "Placental Transfusion: A Review," *Journal of Perinatology* 37 (2017): 105–11.

2. T. Raju, "Timing of Umbilical Cord Clamping after Birth for Optimizing Placental Transfusion," *Current Opinion in Pediatrics* 25, no. 2 (2013): 180–87, doi:10.1097/MOP.0b013e32835d2a9e; P. M. Dunn, "Dr Erasmus Darwin

(1731–1802) of Lichfield and Placental Respiration," *Archives of Disease in Childhood: Fetal and Neonatal Edition* 88, no. 4 (2003): F346–48, doi:10.1136/fn.88.4.F346.

3. C. M. Chaparro, "Timing of Umbilical Cord Clamping: Effect on Iron Endowment of the Newborn and Later Iron Status," *Nutrition Reviews* 69, suppl. 1 (2011): S30–36, doi:10.1111/j.1753-4887.2011.00430.x.

4. Camila Chaparro, telephone interview with the author, August 2, 2013.

5. C. M. Chaparro et al., "Effect of Timing of Umbilical Cord Clamping on Iron Status in Mexican Infants: A Randomised Controlled Trial," *Lancet* 367 (2006): 1997–2004, doi:10.1016/S0140-6736(06)68889-2.

6. Raju, "Timing of Umbilical Cord Clamping after Birth for Optimizing Placental Transfusion"; Chaparro, "Timing of Umbilical Cord Clamping: Effect on Iron Endowment of the Newborn and Later Iron Status."

7. R. D. Baker and F. R. Greer, "Diagnosis and Prevention of Iron Deficiency and Iron-Deficiency Anemia in Infants and Young Children (0–3 Years of Age)," *Pediatrics* 126 (2010): 1040–50, doi:10.1542/peds.2010-2576.

8. Chaparro et al., "Effect of Timing of Umbilical Cord Clamping on Iron Status in Mexican Infants: A Randomised Controlled Trial."

9. S. J. McDonald et al., "Effect of Timing of Umbilical Cord Clamping of Term Infants on Maternal and Neonatal Outcomes," *Cochrane Database of Systematic Reviews*, no. 7 (2013): CD004074.

10. A. Kc et al., "Effects of Delayed Umbilical Cord Clamping vs Early Clamping on Anemia in Infants at 8 and 12 Months: A Randomized Clinical Trial," *JAMA Pediatrics* 171, no. 3 (2017): 264–70.

11. American College of Obstetricians and Gynecologists (ACOG) Committee on Obstetric Practice, "Committee Opinion No. 543: Timing of Umbilical Cord Clamping after Birth," *Obstetrics and Gynecology* 120, no. 6 (2012): 1522–26.

12. A. Callahan, "Doctors No Longer Rush to Cut the Umbilical Cord," *New York Times*, March 2, 2017; ACOG Committee on Obstetric Practice, "Committee Opinion No. 684: Delayed Umbilical Cord Clamping after Birth," *Obstetrics and Gynecology* 129, no. 1 (2017): e5–e10.

13. O. Andersson et al., "Effect of Delayed versus Early Umbilical Cord Clamping on Neonatal Outcomes and Iron Status at 4 Months: A Randomised Controlled Trial," *BMJ* 343 (2011): d7157, doi:10.1136/bmj.d7157.

14. O. Andersson et al., "Effect of Delayed Cord Clamping on Neurodevelopment at 4 Years of Age: A Randomized Clinical Trial," *JAMA Pediatrics* 169, no. 7 (2015): 631–38.

15. J. S. Mercer et al., "Effects of Delayed Cord Clamping on 4-Month Ferritin Levels, Brain Myelin Content, and Neurodevelopment: A Randomized Controlled Trial," *Journal of Pediatrics* 203 (2018): 266–272.e2.

16. B. Lozoff et al., "Long-Lasting Neural and Behavioral Effects of Iron Deficiency in Infancy," *Nutrition Reviews* 64, no. 5, pt. 2 (2006): S34–43; J. C. McCann and B. N. Ames, "An Overview of Evidence for a Causal Relation between Iron Deficiency during Development and Deficits in Cognitive or Behavioral Function," *American Journal of Clinical Nutrition* 85, no. 4 (2007): 931–45; C. Algarín et al., "Iron Deficiency Anemia in Infancy: Long-Lasting Effects on Auditory and Visual System Functioning," *Pediatric Research* 53, no. 2 (2003): 217–23, doi:10.1203/01.PDR.0000047657.23156.55; M. Roncagliolo et al., "Evidence of Altered Central Nervous System Development in Infants with Iron Deficiency Anemia at 6 Mo: Delayed Maturation of Auditory Brainstem Responses," *American Journal of Clinical Nutrition* 68, no. 3 (1998): 683–90; B. Lozoff, E. Jimenez, and J. B. Smith, "Double Burden of Iron Deficiency in Infancy and Low Socioeconomic Status: A Longitudinal Analysis of Cognitive Test Scores to Age 19 Years," *Archives of Pediatrics and Adolescent Medicine* 160, no. 11 (2006): 1108–13; E. L. Congdon et al., "Iron Deficiency in Infancy Is Associated with Altered Neural Correlates of Recognition Memory at 10 Years," *Journal of Pediatrics* 160, no. 6 (2012): 1027–33, doi:10.1016/j.jpeds.2011.12.011; T. Shafir et al., "Iron Deficiency and Infant Motor Development," *Early Human Development* 84, no. 7 (2008): 479–85, doi:10.1016/j.earlhumdev.2007.12.009; B. Lozoff et al., "Poorer Behavioral and Developmental Outcome More Than 10 Years after Treatment for Iron Deficiency in Infancy," *Pediatrics* 105 (April 2000): E51.

17. K. G. Dewey and C. M. Chaparro, "Session 4: Mineral Metabolism and Body Composition Iron Status of Breast-Fed Infants," *Proceedings of the Nutrition Society* 66 (August 2007): 412–22, doi:10.1017/S002966510700568X.

18. M. M. Black et al., "Iron Deficiency and Iron-Deficiency Anemia in the First Two Years of Life: Strategies to Prevent Loss of Developmental Potential," *Nutrition Reviews* 69, suppl. 1 (2011): S64–70, doi:10.1111/j.1753-4887.2011.00435.x; C. Cao and K. O. O'Brien, "Pregnancy and Iron Homeostasis: An Update," *Nutrition Reviews* 71, no. 1 (2013): 35–51, doi:10.1111/j.1753-4887.2012.00550.x.

19. Baker and Greer, "Diagnosis and Prevention of Iron Deficiency and Iron-Deficiency Anemia in Infants and Young Children (0–3 Years of Age)."

20. American Academy of Pediatrics (AAP) Section on Breastfeeding et al., "Concerns with Early Universal Iron Supplementation of Breastfeeding Infants," *Pediatrics* 127, no. 4 (2011): e1097, doi:10.1542/peds.2011-0201A; O. Hernell and B. Lönnerdal, "Recommendations on Iron Questioned," *Pediatrics* 127, no. 4 (2011): e1099–1101, doi:10.1542/peds.2011-0201C.

21. K. G. Dewey et al., "Iron Supplementation Affects Growth and Morbidity of Breast-Fed Infants: Results of a Randomized Trial in Sweden and Honduras," *Journal of Nutrition* 132 (November 2002): 3249–55.

22. M. Domellöf et al., "Iron Requirements of Infants and Toddlers," *Journal of Pediatric Gastroenterology and Nutrition* 58, no. 1 (2014): 119–29.

23. Baker and Greer, "Diagnosis and Prevention of Iron Deficiency and Iron-Deficiency Anemia in Infants and Young Children (0–3 Years of Age)"; Domellöf et al., "Iron Requirements of Infants and Toddlers"; P. M. Gupta et al., "Iron Status of Toddlers, Nonpregnant Females, and Pregnant Females in the United States," *American Journal of Clinical Nutrition* 106, suppl. 6 (2017): 1640S–46S.

24. H. Rabe et al., "Effect of Timing of Umbilical Cord Clamping and Other Strategies to Influence Placental Transfusion at Preterm Birth on Maternal and Infant Outcomes," *Cochrane Database of Systematic Reviews*, no. 9 (2019): CD003248.

25. J. S. Mercer et al., "Effects of Placental Transfusion on Neonatal and 18 Month Outcomes in Preterm Infants: A Randomized Controlled Trial," *Journal of Pediatrics* 168 (January 2016): 50–55.e1.

26. McDonald et al., "Effect of Timing of Umbilical Cord Clamping of Term Infants on Maternal and Neonatal Outcomes"; Andersson et al., "Effect of Delayed versus Early Umbilical Cord Clamping on Neonatal Outcomes and Iron Status at 4 Months"; N. Rana et al., "Delayed Cord Clamping Was Not Associated with an Increased Risk of Hyperbilirubinaemia on the Day of Birth or Jaundice in the First 4 Weeks," *Acta Paediatrica* 109, no. 1 (2020): 71–77; E. K. Hutton and E. S. Hassan, "Late vs. Early Clamping of the Umbilical Cord in Full-Term Neonates: Systematic Review and Meta-analysis of Controlled Trials," *JAMA* 297 (2007): 1241–52, doi:10.1001/jama.297.11.1241.

27. McDonald et al., "Effect of Timing of Umbilical Cord Clamping of Term Infants on Maternal and Neonatal Outcomes"; Hutton and Hassan, "Late vs. Early Clamping of the Umbilical Cord in Full-Term Neonates"; S. E. Purisch et al., "Effect of Delayed vs Immediate Umbilical Cord Clamping on Maternal Blood Loss in Term Cesarean Delivery: A Randomized Clinical Trial," *JAMA* 322, no. 19 (2019): 1869–76.

28. World Health Organization (WHO), *WHO Recommendations on Postnatal Care of the Mother and Newborn* (Geneva: WHO, 2013); National Institute for Health and Care Excellence (NICE), *Intrapartum Care for Healthy Women and Babies* (London: NICE, 2014), last updated February 21, 2017, https://www.nice .org.uk/guidance/cg190/chapter/Recommendations#second-stage-of-labour.

29. ACOG Committee on Obstetric Practice, "Committee Opinion No. 684: Delayed Umbilical Cord Clamping after Birth."

30. Chaparro, interview with the author, 2013.

31. Raju, "Timing of Umbilical Cord Clamping after Birth for Optimizing Placental Transfusion," J. S. Mercer and D. A. Erickson-Owens, "Rethinking Placental Transfusion and Cord Clamping Issues," *Journal of Perinatal and Neonatal Nursing* 26, no. 3 (2012): 202–17, doi:10.1097/JPN.0b013e31825d2d9a; S. B. Hooper et al., "The Timing of Umbilical Cord Clamping at Birth: Physiological Considerations," *Maternal Health, Neonatology and Perinatology* 2 (2016):

4, doi:10.1186/s40748-016-0032-y; A. C. Katheria et al., "Placental Transfusion for Asphyxiated Infants," *Frontiers in Pediatrics* 7 (November 2019): 473, doi:10.3389/fped.2019.00473.

32. Tonse Raju, telephone interview with the author, February 11, 2104.

33. M. R. Thomas et al., "Providing Newborn Resuscitation at the Mother's Bedside: Assessing the Safety, Usability and Acceptability of a Mobile Trolley," *BMC Pediatrics* 14, no. 1 (2014): 135, doi:10.1186/1471-2431-14-135; R. Knol et al., "Physiological-Based Cord Clamping in Very Preterm Infants: Randomised Controlled Trial on Effectiveness of Stabilisation," *Resuscitation* 147 (February 2020): 26–33; J. Winter et al., "Ventilation of Preterm Infants during Delayed Cord Clamping (VentFirst): A Pilot Study of Feasibility and Safety," *American Journal of Perinatology* 34, no. 2 (2017): 111–16; L. Duley et al., "Randomised Trial of Cord Clamping and Initial Stabilisation at Very Preterm Birth," *Archives of Disease in Childhood: Fetal & Neonatal Edition* 103 (2018): F6–F14; O. Andersson et al., "Intact Cord Resuscitation versus Early Cord Clamping in the Treatment of Depressed Newborn Infants during the First 10 Minutes of Birth (Nepcord III): A Randomized Clinical Trial," *Maternal Health, Neonatology and Perinatology* 5, no.15 (2019), doi:10.1186/s40748-019-0110-z; D. A. Blank et al., "Baby-Directed Umbilical Cord Clamping: A Feasibility Study," *Resuscitation* 131 (2018): 1–7.

34. R. Sender, S. Fuchs, and R. Milo, "Revised Estimates for the Number of Human and Bacteria Cells in the Body," *PLOS Biology* 14, no. 8 (2016): e1002533.

35. M. C. de Goffau et al., "Human Placenta Has No Microbiome but Can Contain Potential Pathogens," *Nature* 572, no. 7769 (2019): 329–34; E. Yong, "Why the Placental Microbiome Should Be a Cautionary Tale," *Atlantic*, July 31, 2019.

36. Y. Shao et al., "Stunted Microbiota and Opportunistic Pathogen Colonization in Caesarean-section Birth," *Nature* 574, no. 7776 (2019): 117–21; H. Shin et al., "The First Microbial Environment of Infants Born by C-section: The Operating Room Microbes," *Microbiome* 3 (2015): 59, doi:10.1186/s40168-015-0126-1.

37. D. M. Chu et al., "Maturation of the Infant Microbiome Community Structure and Function across Multiple Body Sites and in Relation to Mode of Delivery," *Nature Medicine* 23, no. 3 (2017): 314–26; F. Bäckhed et al., "Dynamics and Stabilization of the Human Gut Microbiome during the First Year of Life," *Cell Host & Microbe* 17, no. 5 (2015): 690–703; F. Fouhy et al., "Perinatal Factors Affect the Gut Microbiota up to Four Years after Birth," *Nature Communications* 10 (2019): 1517, doi: 10.1038/s41467-019-09252-4.

38. C. Yuan et al., "Association between Cesarean Birth and Risk of Obesity in Offspring in Childhood, Adolescence, and Early Adulthood," *JAMA Pediatrics*. 170, no. 11 (2016): e162385; A. Sevelsted et al., "Cesarean Section and Chronic

Immune Disorders," *Pediatrics* 135, no. 1 (2015): e92–e98; A. Sevelsted, J. Stokholm, and H. Bisgaard, "Risk of Asthma from Cesarean Delivery Depends on Membrane Rupture," *Journal of Pediatrics* 171 (2016): 38-42.e4; K. Darmasseelane et al., "Mode of Delivery and Offspring Body Mass Index, Overweight and Obesity in Adult Life: A Systematic Review and Meta-analysis," *PloS One* 9, no. 2 (2014): e87896; S. Y. Huh et al., "Delivery by Caesarean Section and Risk of Obesity in Preschool Age Children: A Prospective Cohort Study," *Archives of Disease in Childhood* 97, no. 7 (2012): 610–16; M. Eggesbø et al., "Is Delivery by Cesarean Section a Risk Factor for Food Allergy?" *Journal of Allergy and Clinical Immunology* 112, no. 2 (2003): 420–26; N. Mitselou et al., "Cesarean Delivery, Preterm Birth, and Risk of Food Allergy: Nationwide Swedish Cohort Study of More Than 1 Million Children, *Journal of Allergy and Clinical Immunology* 142, no. 5 (2018): 1510-1514.e2.

39. S. Tamburini et al., "The Microbiome in Early Life: Implications for Health Outcomes, *Nature Medicine* 22, no. 7 (2016): 713–22.

40. American College of Obstetricians and Gynecologists (ACOG) Committee on Obstetric Practice, "Committee Opinion No. 761: Cesarean Delivery on Maternal Request," *Obstetrics and Gynecology* 133, no. 1 (2019): e73–e77.

41. G. Molina et al., "Relationship between Cesarean Delivery Rate and Maternal and Neonatal Mortality," *JAMA* 314, no. 21 (2015): 2263–70; A. P. Betrán, A. P. et al., "The Increasing Trend in Caesarean Section Rates: Global, Regional and National Estimates: 1990-2014," *PloS One* 11, no. 2 (2016): e0148343.

42. T. Harman and A. Wakeford, *Microbirth* (Brighton, UK: Alto Films, 2014), documentary, 60 min.; J. Gilbert, R. Knight, and S. Blakeslee, *Dirt is Good* (New York: St. Martin's Press, 2017); S. Blakeslee, "Using a Mother's Microbes to Protect Cesarean Babies," *New York Times*, February 1, 2016; J. E. Brody, "The Importance of Infants' Exposure to Micro-Organisms," *New York Times*, February 5, 2018.

43. M. G. Dominguez-Bello et al., "Partial Restoration of the Microbiota of Cesarean-born Infants via Vaginal Microbial Transfer," *Nature Medicine* 22, no. 3 (2016): 250–53.

44. S. Hourigan, "Vaginal Microbiome Seeding and Health Outcomes in Cesarean-delivered Neonates," *ClinicalTrials.gov*, October 2, 2017, https://clinicaltrials.gov/ct2/show/NCT03298334; H. A. Sampson, "Vaginal Microbiome Exposure and Immune Responses in C-section Infants," *ClinicalTrials.gov*, June 26, 2018, https://clinicaltrials.gov/ct2/show/NCT03567707; J. Liu, "Effects of Vaginal Seeding on Infants' Body Mass Index and Allergy Risk for Caesarean-delivered Children," *ClinicalTrials.gov*, January 18, 2019, https://clinicaltrials.gov/ct2/show/NCT03809390.

45. ACOG Committee on Obstetric Practice, "Committee Opinion No. 725: Vaginal Seeding," *Obstetrics and Gynecology* 130, no. 5 (2017): e274–e278;

T. Haahr et al., "Vaginal Seeding or Vaginal Microbial Transfer from the Mother to the Caesarean-born Neonate: A Commentary Regarding Clinical Management," *BJOG: An International Journal of Obstetrics and Gynaecology* 125, no. 5 (2018): 533–36; A. J. Cunnington et al., "'Vaginal Seeding' of Infants Born by Caesarean Section," *BMJ* 352 (2016): i227; L. F. Stinson, M. S. Payne, and J. A. Keelan, "A Critical Review of the Bacterial Baptism Hypothesis and the Impact of Cesarean Delivery on the Infant Microbiome," *Frontiers in Medicine* 5 (May 2018): 135, doi:10.3389/fmed.2018.00135.

46. J. Huynh, P. Palasanthiran, and B. McMullan, "Potential Transmission of Herpes Simplex Virus Via Vaginal Seeding," *Pediatric Infectious Disease Journal* 37, no. 11(2018): e278.

47. Haahr et al., "Vaginal Seeding or Vaginal Microbial Transfer from the Mother to the Caesarean-born Neonate."

48. Brody, "The Importance of Infants' Exposure to Micro-Organisms"; N. T. Mueller et al., "Bacterial Baptism: Scientific, Medical, and Regulatory Issues Raised by Vaginal Seeding of C-Section-Born Babies," *Journal of Law, Medicine & Ethics: A Journal of the American Society of Law, Medicine & Ethics* 47, no. 4 (2019): 568–78.

49. Gilbert, Knight, and Blakeslee, *Dirt is Good.*

50. Blakeslee, "Using a Mother's Microbes to Protect Cesarean Babies."

51. A. U. Lokugamage and S. D. C. Pathberiya, "The Microbiome Seeding Debate: Let's Frame It around Women-Centred Care," *Reproductive Health* 16 (June 2019): 91, doi: 10.1186/s12978-019-0747-0.

52. Stinson, Payne, and Keelan, "A Critical Review of the Bacterial Baptism Hypothesis"; D. M. Chu et al., "The Development of the Human Microbiome: Why Moms Matter," *Gastroenterology Clinics of North America* 48, no. 3 (2019): 357–75.

53. P. Ferretti et al., "Mother-to-Infant Microbial Transmission from Different Body Sites Shapes the Developing Infant Gut Microbiome," *Cell Host & Microbe* 24, no. 1 (2018): 133-45.e5.

54. R. M. Duar, D. Kyle, and R. M. Tribe, "Reintroducing *B. infantis* to the Cesarean-born Neonate: An Ecologically Sound Alternative to "Vaginal Seeding," *FEMS Microbiology Letters* 367, no. 6 (2020): fnaa032, doi: 10.1093/femsle/fnaa032.

55. Ferretti et al., "Mother-to-Infant Microbial Transmission from Different Body Sites"; O. Sakwinska et al., "Does the Maternal Vaginal Microbiota Play a Role in Seeding the Microbiota of Neonatal Gut and Nose?" *Beneficial Microbes* 8, no. 5 (2017): 763–78; L. Wampach et al., "Birth Mode Is Associated with Earliest Strain-Conferred Gut Microbiome Functions and Immunostimulatory Potentia," *Nature Communications* 9 (2018): 5091, doi: 10.1038/s41467-018-07631-x.

56. K. Korpela et al., "Maternal Fecal Microbiota Transplantation in

Cesarean-Born Infants Rapidly Restores Normal Gut Microbial Development: A Proof-of-Concept Study," *Cell* 183, no. 2 (2020): 324-34.e5.

57. C. Lesté-Lasserre, "Eating a Tiny Bit of Mom's Poop Could Give C-section Babies an Immune 'Primer,'" *Science*, October 1, 2020.

58. Stinson, Payne, and Keelan, "A Critical Review of the Bacterial Baptism Hypothesis"; Duar, Kyle, and Tribe, "Reintroducing *B. infantis* to the Cesarean-born Neonate."

59. World Health Organization, *WHO Recommendations on Postnatal Care of the Mother and Newborn*; Association of Women's Health, Obstetric and Neonatal Nurses (AWHONN), *Neonatal Skin Care: Evidence-based Clinical Practice Guidelines*, 4th ed. (Washington, DC: AWHONN, 2018).

60. M. O. Visscher et al., "Newborn Infant Skin: Physiology, Development, and Care," *Clinics in Dermatology* 33, no. 3 (June 2015): 271–80.

61. H. DiCioccio et al., "Initiative to Improve Exclusive Breastfeeding by Delaying the Newborn Bath," *Journal of Obstetric, Gynecologic, and Neonatal Nursing* 48, no. 2 (2019): 189–96; G. Preer et al., "Delaying the Bath and In-Hospital Breastfeeding Rates," *Breastfeeding Medicine* 8, no. 6 (2013): 485–90; S. Warren et al., "Effects of Delayed Newborn Bathing on Breastfeeding, Hypothermia, and Hypoglycemia," *Journal of Obstetric, Gynecologic, and Neonatal Nursing* 49, no. 2 (2020): 181-89, doi:10.1016/j.jogn.2019.12.004.

62. DiCioccio et al., "Initiative to Improve Exclusive Breastfeeding by Delaying the Newborn Bath."

63. J. Brogan and G. Rapkin, "Implementing Evidence-Based Neonatal Skin Care with Parent-Performed, Delayed Immersion Baths," *Nursing for Women's Health* 21, no. 6 (2017): 442–50; C. Suchy et al., "Does Changing Newborn Bath Procedure Alter Newborn Temperatures and Exclusive Breastfeeding?" *Neonatal Network* 37, no. 1 (2018): 4–10; J. Turney et al., "Delayed Newborn First Bath and Exclusive Breastfeeding Rates," *Nursing for Women's Health* 23, no. 1 (2019): 31–37.

64. DiCioccio et al., "Initiative to Improve Exclusive Breastfeeding by Delaying the Newborn Bath"; Warren et al., "Effects of Delayed Newborn Bathing on Breastfeeding, Hypothermia, and Hypoglycemia"; Brogan and Rapkin, "Implementing Evidence-Based Neonatal Skin Care with Parent-Performed, Delayed Immersion Baths"; J. Chamberlain et al., "Impact on Delayed Newborn Bathing on Exclusive Breastfeeding Rates, Glucose and Temperature Stability, and Weight Loss," *Journal of Neonatal Nursing* 25, no. 2 (2019): 74–77.

65. J. Bryanton et al., "Tub Bathing versus Traditional Sponge Bathing for the Newborn," *Journal of Obstetric, Gynecologic, and Neonatal Nursing* 33, no. 6 (2004): 704–12.

66. C. Loring et al., "Tub Bathing Improves Thermoregulation of the Late Preterm Infant," *Journal of Obstetric, Gynecologic, and Neonatal Nursing* 41, no. 2 (2012): 171–79.

67. Bryanton et al., "Tub Bathing versus Traditional Sponge Bathing for the Newborn."

68. J. M. Kuller, "Update on Newborn Bathing," *Newborn Infant Nursing Reviews* 14, no. 4 (2014): 166–70.

3. OF INJECTIONS AND EYE GOOP

1. S. Leavitt, "A Baby Story: Olive Eloise Leavitt," *C'est Si Bon* (blog), January 15, 2014, http://www.cestsibonblog.com/2014/01/a-baby-story-olive-eloiseleavitt.html.

2. S. Leavitt, "The Story of a Miracle: The First 24 Hours," *C'est Si Bon* (blog), February 28, 2014, http://www.cestsibonblog.com/2014/02/the-story-of-miracle-first-24-hours.html.

3. S. Leavitt, "The Story of a Miracle: Getting Out of the Woods," *C'est Si Bon* (blog), March 1, 2014, http://www.cestsibonblog.com/2014/03/the-story-of-miracle-getting-out-of.html.

4. Stefani Leavitt, email to the author, February 23, 2020.

5. J. Loyal et al., "Refusal of Vitamin K by Parents of Newborns: A Survey of the Better Outcomes through Research for Newborns Network," *Academic Pediatrics* 17, no. 4 (2017): 368–73; L. H. Marcewicz et al., "Parental Refusal of Vitamin K and Neonatal Preventive Services: A Need for Surveillance," *Maternal and Child Health Journal* 21, no. 5 (2017) 1079–84; V. Sahni, F. Y. Lai, and S. E. MacDonald, "Neonatal Vitamin K Refusal and Nonimmunization," *Pediatrics* 134, no. 3 (2014): 497–503.

6. Centers for Disease Control and Prevention (CDC), "Notes from the Field: Late Vitamin K Deficiency Bleeding in Infants Whose Parents Declined Vitamin K Prophylaxis—Tennessee, 2013," *Morbidity and Mortality Weekly Report (MMWR)* 62, no. 45 (2013): 901–2; J. Loyal et al., "Refusal of Vitamin K by Parents of Newborns: A Qualitative Study," *Academic Pediatrics* 19, no. 4 (2019): 793–800; J. Loyal and E. D. Shapiro, "Refusal of Intramuscular Vitamin K by Parents of Newborns: A Review," *Hospital Pediatrics* 10, no. 3 (2020): 286-94, doi:10.1542/hpeds.2019-0228.

7. M. J. Shearer, "Vitamin K Deficiency Bleeding (VKDB) in Early Infancy," *Blood Reviews* 23, no. 2 (2009): 49–59, doi:10.1016/j.blre.2008.06.001.

8. J. W. Suttie, "Historical Background," in *Vitamin K in Health and Disease* (Boca Raton, FL: CRC Press, 2009), 1–12.

9. H. Dam, "The Antihaemorrhagic Vitamin of the Chick," *Biochemical Journal* 29, no. 6 (1935): 1273–85.

10. R. Zetterström, "H. C. P. Dam (1895–1976) and E. A. Doisy (1893–1986): The Discovery of Antihaemorrhagic Vitamin and Its Impact on Neonatal Health," *Acta Paediatrica* 95, no. 6 (2006): 642–44, doi:10.1080/08035250600719739.

11. F. R. Greer, "Vitamin K the Basics: What's New?" *Early Human Development* 86, suppl. 1 (2010): 43–47, doi:10.1016/j.earlhumdev.2010.01.015.

12. G. Lippi and M. Franchini, "Vitamin K in Neonates: Facts and Myths," *Blood Transfusion* 9, no. 1 (2011): 4–9, doi:10.2450/2010.0034-10.

13. Shearer, "Vitamin K Deficiency Bleeding (VKDB) in Early Infancy."

14. C. A. Crowther and D. D. Crosby, "Vitamin K prior to Preterm Birth for Preventing Neonatal Periventricular Haemorrhage," *Cochrane Database of Systematic Reviews* 1 (2010): CD000229; L. Mandelbrot et al., "Placental Transfer of Vitamin K₁ and Its Implications in Fetal Hemostasis," *Thrombosis and Haemostasis* 60, no. 1 (1988): 39–43.

15. H. E. Indyk and D. C. Woollard, "Vitamin K in Milk and Infant Formulas: Determination and Distribution of Phylloquinone and Menaquinone-4," *Analyst* 122, no. 5 (1997): 465–69, doi:10.1039/A608221A; S. Kayata et al., "Vitamin K₁ and K₂ in Infant Human Liver," *Journal of Pediatric Gastroenterology and Nutrition* 8, no. 3 (1989): 304–7.

16. J. C. Phillippi et al., "Prevention of Vitamin K Deficiency Bleeding," *Journal of Midwifery & Women's Health* 61, no. 5 (2016): 632–636.

17. Shearer, "Vitamin K Deficiency Bleeding (VKDB) in Early Infancy."

18. American Academy of Pediatrics (AAP), "Policy Statement: Controversies Concerning Vitamin K and the Newborn," *Pediatrics* 112, no. 1 (2003): 191 92.

19. M. J. Sankar et al., "Vitamin K Prophylaxis for Prevention of Vitamin K Deficiency Bleeding: A Systematic Review," *Journal of Perinatology* 36, no. 1 (2016): S29–S35.

20. P. M. Loughnan and P. N. McDougall, "Epidemiology of Late Onset Haemorrhagic Disease: A Pooled Data Analysis," *Journal of Paediatrics and Child Health* 29, no. 3 (1993): 177–81, doi:10.1111/j.1440-1754.1993.tb00480.x.

21. AAP, "Policy Statement: Controversies Concerning Vitamin K and the Newborn."

22. P. Danziger, "Vitamin K for Newborns Is a No-Brainer. Why Are So Many Parents Worried?" *New York Times*, February 19, 2020.

23. Shearer, "Vitamin K Deficiency Bleeding (VKDB) in Early Infancy."

24. Shearer, "Vitamin K Deficiency Bleeding (VKDB) in Early Infancy."

25. S. Leavitt, "Our Alpha-1 Kid," *C'est Si Bon* (blog), March 26, 2014, http://www.cestsibonblog.com/2014/03/our-alpha-1-kid.html.

26. P. M. van Hasselt et al., "Vitamin K Deficiency Bleeding in Cholestatic Infants with Alpha-1-Antitrypsin Deficiency," *Archives of Disease in Childhood: Fetal and Neonatal Edition* 94, no. 6 (2009): F456-60, doi:10.1136/adc.2008.148239; P. M. van Hasselt et al., "Prevention of Vitamin K Deficiency Bleeding in Breastfed Infants: Lessons from the Dutch and Danish Biliary Atresia Registries," *Pediatrics* 121, no. 4 (April 1, 2008): e857-63, doi:10.1542/peds.2007-1788.

27. R. Schulte et al., "Rise in Late Onset Vitamin K Deficiency Bleeding in Young Infants Due to Omission or Refusal of Prophylaxis at Birth," *Pediatric Neurology* 50, no. 6 (2014): 564–68, doi:10.1016/j.pediatrneurol.2014.02.013; R. Decker, "Evidence for the Vitamin K Shot in Newborns," *Evidence Based Birth* (blog), March 18, 2014, http://evidencebasedbirth.com/evidence-for-the-vitamin-k.

28. Schulte et al., "Rise in Late Onset Vitamin K Deficiency Bleeding."

29. Phillippi et al., "Prevention of Vitamin K Deficiency Bleeding."

30. J. Golding et al., "Childhood Cancer, Intramuscular Vitamin K, and Pethidine Given during Labour," *BMJ* 305, no. 6849 (1992): 341–46.

31. Various authors, "Responses to Golding et al. 1992," *BMJ*, August 8, 1992, http://www.bmj.com/content/305/6849/341.

32. G. J. Draper and C. A. Stiller, "Intramuscular Vitamin K and Childhood Cancer," *BMJ* 305, no. 6855 (1992): 709–11; R. W. Miller, "Vitamin K and Childhood Cancer," *BMJ* 305, no. 6860 (1992): 1016.

33. J. A. Ross and S. M. Davies, "Vitamin K Prophylaxis and Childhood Cancer," *Medical and Pediatric Oncology* 34, no. 6 (2000): 434–37, doi:10.1002/(SICI)1096-911X(200006)34:6<434::AID-MPO11>3.0.CO;2-X; E. Roman et al., "Vitamin K and Childhood Cancer: Analysis of Individual Patient Data from Six Case-Control Studies," *British Journal of Cancer* 86, no. 1 (2002): 63–69, doi:10.1038/sj.bjc.6600007; N. T. Fear et al., "Vitamin K and Childhood Cancer: A Report from the United Kingdom Childhood Cancer Study," *British Journal of Cancer* 89, no. 7 (2003): 1228–31, doi:10.1038/sj.bjc.6601278.

34. W. A. Mihatsch et al., "Prevention of Vitamin K Deficiency Bleeding in Newborn Infants: A Position Paper by the ESPGHAN Committee on Nutrition," *Journal of Pediatric Gastroenterology and Nutrition* 63, no. 1 (2016): 123–29.

35. Sankar et al., "Vitamin K Prophylaxis for Prevention of Vitamin K Deficiency Bleeding."

36. Y. N. Löwensteyn et al., "Increasing the Dose of Oral Vitamin K Prophylaxis and Its Effect on Bleeding Risk," *European Journal of Pediatrics* 178, no. 7 (2019): 1033–42.

37. B. Laubscher, O. Bänziger, and G. Schubiger, "Prevention of Vitamin K Deficiency Bleeding with Three Oral Mixed Micellar Phylloquinone Doses: Results of a 6-Year (2005–2011) Surveillance in Switzerland," *European Journal of Pediatrics* 172, no. 3 (2013): 357–60, doi:10.1007/s00431-012-1895-1.

38. Van Hasselt et al., "Prevention of Vitamin K Deficiency Bleeding in Breastfed Infants."

39. Mihatsch et al., "Prevention of Vitamin K Deficiency Bleeding in Newborn Infants"; E. Ng and A. D. Loewy, "Guidelines for Vitamin K Prophylaxis in Newborns," *Paediatrics & Child Health* 23, no. 6 (2018): 394–402; National Institute for Health and Care Excellence (NICE), *Postnatal Care up to 8 Weeks*

after Birth (London: NICE, 2006), last updated February 1, 2015, https://www
.nice.org.uk/guidance/cg37.

40. Phillippi et al., "Prevention of Vitamin K Deficiency Bleeding."

41. M. J. Shearer, X. Fu, and S. L. Booth, "Vitamin K Nutrition, Metabolism, and Requirements: Current Concepts and Future Research," *Advances in Nutrition: An International Review Journal* 3, no. 2 (2012): 182–95, doi:10.3945/an.111.001800.

42. P. M. Loughnan and P. N. McDougall, "Does Intramuscular Vitamin K$_1$ Act as an Unintended Depot Preparation?" *Journal of Paediatrics and Child Health* 32, no. 3 (1996): 251–54.

43. Stanford School of Medicine, "Guidelines for Vitamin K Prophylaxis," Newborn Nursery at Lucile Packard Children's Hospital, accessed April 12, 2014, http://med.stanford.edu/newborns/clinical-guidelines/vitamink.html.

44. "Using Dietary Supplements Wisely," National Center for Complementary and Integrative Health, accessed December 10, 2020, https://www.nccih.nih.gov/health/using-dietary-supplements-wisely.

45. Crowther and Crosby, "Vitamin K prior to Preterm Birth for Preventing Neonatal Periventricular Haemorrhage."

46. B. Pietschnig et al., "Vitamin K in Breast Milk: No Influence of Maternal Dietary Intake," *European Journal of Clinical Nutrition* 47, no. 3 (1993): 209–15.

47. F. R. Greer et al., "Improving the Vitamin K Status of Breastfeeding Infants with Maternal Vitamin K Supplements," *Pediatrics* 99, no. 1 (1997): 88–92, doi:10.1542/peds.99.1.88.

48. US Department of Agriculture (USDA), Agricultural Research Service, FoodData Central, accessed December 10, 2020, fdc.nal.usda.gov.

49. P. S. Shah et al., "Breastfeeding or Breast Milk for Procedural Pain in Neonates," *Cochrane Database of Systematic Reviews*, no. 12 (2012): CD004950; C. Johnston et al., "Skin-to-Skin Care for Procedural Pain in Neonates," *Cochrane Database of Systematic Reviews*, no. 1 (2014): CD008435; AAP, "Prevention and Management of Procedural Pain in the Neonate: An Update," *Pediatrics* 137, no. 2 (2016, reaffirmed July 2020): e20154271.

50. E. Koklu et al., "Anaphylactic Shock due to Vitamin K in a Newborn and Review of Literature," *Journal of Maternal-Fetal and Neonatal Medicine* 27, no. 11 (2014): 1180–81, doi:10.3109/14767058.2013.847425.

51. Frank R. Greer, interview with the author, April 16, 2014.

52. S. J. Fomon, "Infant Feeding and Evolution," in *Nutrition of Normal Infants* (St. Louis, MO: Mosby–Year Book, 1993), 1–5.

53. C. S. F. Credé, "Prevention of Inflammatory Eye Disease in the Newborn," *Archiv Für Gynaekologie* 17 (1881): 50–53.

54. J. D. Oriel, "Eminent Venereologists 5: Carl Credé," *Genitourinary Medicine* 67, no. 1 (1991): 67–69; P. M. Dunn, "Dr Carl Credé (1819–1892) and the

Prevention of Ophthalmia Neonatorum," *Archives of Disease in Childhood: Fetal and Neonatal Edition* 83, no. 2 (2000): F158-59, doi:10.1136/fn.83.2.F158.

55. Credé, "Prevention of Inflammatory Eye Disease in the Newborn."

56. Credé, "Prevention of Inflammatory Eye Disease in the Newborn"; Oriel, "Eminent Venereologists 5: Carl Credé."

57. US Preventive Services Task Force (USPSTF) et al., "Ocular Prophylaxis for Gonococcal Ophthalmia Neonatorum: US Preventive Services Task Force Reaffirmation Recommendation Statement," *JAMA* 321, no. 4 (2019): 394–98.

58. U. C. Schaller and V. Klauss, "Is Credé's Prophylaxis for Ophthalmia Neonatorum Still Valid?" *Bulletin of the World Health Organization* 79, no. 3 (2001): 262–66; E. K. Darling and H. McDonald, "A Meta-analysis of the Efficacy of Ocular Prophylactic Agents Used for the Prevention of Gonococcal and Chlamydial Ophthalmia Neonatorum," *Journal of Midwifery and Women's Health* 55, no. 4 (2010): 319–27, doi:10.1016/j.jmwh.2009.09.003.

59. D. W. Kimberlin et al., eds., "Prevention of Neonatal Ophthalmia," in *Red Book: 2018-2021 Report of the Committee on Infectious Diseases* (Elk Grove Village, IL: American Academy of Pediatrics, 2018), 1046-50.

60. USPSTF et al., "Ocular Prophylaxis for Gonococcal Ophthalmia Neonatorum"; "STDs during Pregnancy: CDC Fact Sheet (Detailed)," Centers for Disease Control and Prevention (CDC), accessed March 4, 2020, https://www.cdc.gov/std/pregnancy/stdfact-pregnancy-detailed.htm.

61. USPSTF et al., "Ocular Prophylaxis for Gonococcal Ophthalmia Neonatorum"; World Health Organization (WHO), *WHO Guidelines for the Treatment of Neisseria gonorrhoeae* (Geneva: WHO, 2016).

62. CDC, *Sexually Transmitted Disease Surveillance 2018* (Atlanta: CDC, 2019), https://www.cdc.gov/std/stats18/default.htm.

63. "Gonorrhea: CDC Fact Sheet (Detailed Version)," CDC, accessed March 4, 2020, last updated November 5, 2019, https://www.cdc.gov/std/gonorrhea/stdfact-gonorrhea-detailed.htm.

64. M. J. K. Osterman and J. A. Martin, "Timing and Adequacy of Prenatal Care in the United States, 2016," *National Vital Statistics Reports* 67, no. 3 (2018): 1–14.

65. "STDs during Pregnancy: CDC Fact Sheet (Detailed)."

66. A. A. Zuppa et al., "Ophthalmia Neonatorum: What Kind of Prophylaxis?" Journal of Maternal-Fetal and Neonatal Medicine 24, no. 6 (2011): 769–73, doi:10.3109/14767058.2010.531326.

67. B. Diener, "Cesarean Section Complicated by Gonococcal Ophthalmia Neonatorum," *Journal of Family Practice* 13, no. 5 (1981): 739, 743–44; C. L. Strand and V. A. Arango, "Gonococcal Ophthalmia Neonatorum after Delivery by Cesarean Section: Report of a Case," *Sexually Transmitted Diseases* 6, no. 2 (1979): 77–78.

68. "2015 STD Treatment Guidelines: Gonococcal Infections," CDC, accessed March 4, 2020, https://www.cdc.gov/std/tg2015/gonorrhea.htm.

69. Kristi Watterberg, interview with the author, April 24, 2014.

70. D. L. Moore et al., "Preventing Ophthalmia Neonatorum," *Canadian Journal of Infectious Diseases and Medical Microbiology* 26, no. 3 (2015): 122–25.

71. European Centre for Disease Prevention and Control (ECDC), *Gonorrhoea: Annual Epidemiological Report for 2018* (Solna, Sweden: ECDC, 2020), https://www.ecdc.europa.eu/en/publications-data/gonorrhoea-annual-epidemiological-report-2018; Public Health Agency of Canada, "Reported Cases from 1991 to 2018 in Canada: Notifiable Diseases On-line," Government of Canada, last updated August 11, 2020, https://diseases.canada.ca/notifiable/charts?c=yl; CDC, *Sexually Transmitted Disease Surveillance 2018*.

72. Margaret R. Hammerschlag, email to the author, April 29, 2014.

73. Douglas Leonard, email to the author, May 1, 2014.

74. P. M. Butterfield, R. N. Emde, and B. B. Platt, "Effects of Silver Nitrate on Initial Visual Behavior," *American Journal of Diseases of Children* 132, no. 4 (1978): 426; P. M. Butterfield, R. N. Emde, and M. J. Svejda, "Does the Early Application of Silver Nitrate Impair Maternal Attachment?" *Pediatrics* 67, no. 5 (1981): 737–38.

75. Kimberlin et al., "Prevention of Neonatal Ophthalmia."

76. K. Hedberg et al., "Outbreak of Erythromycin-Resistant Staphylococcal Conjunctivitis in a Newborn Nursery," *Pediatric Infectious Disease Journal* 9, no. 4 (1990): 268–73.

77. M. G. Dominguez-Bello et al., "Role of the Microbiome in Human Development," *Gut* 68, no. 6 (2019): 1108–14.

78. C. Gray, "Systemic Toxicity with Topical Ophthalmic Medications in Children," *Paediatric and Perinatal Drug Therapy* 7, no. 1 (2006): 23–29.

79. F. Moussa, B. Alaswad, and J. Garcia, "Erythromycin Eye Ointment: Effect on Gastrointestinal Motility," *American Journal of Gastroenterology* 95, no. 3 (2000): 826, doi:10.1111/j.1572-0241.2000.01893.x.

80. S. R. Jadcherla and C. L. Berseth, "Effect of Erythromycin on Gastroduodenal Contractile Activity in Developing Neonates," *Journal of Pediatric Gastroenterology* 34, no. 1 (2002): 16–22.

81. Henry Redel, email to the author, April 24, 2014.

82. A. R. Kemper, "Newborn Screening," *UpToDate*, last updated November 16, 2020, https://www.uptodate.com/contents/newborn-screening.

83. B. R. Vohr, "Screening the Newborn for Hearing Loss," *UpToDate*, last updated July 6, 2020, https://www.uptodate.com/contents/screening-the-newborn-for-hearing-loss.

84. M. Oster, "Newborn Screening for Critical Congenital Heart Disease Using Pulse Oximetry," *UpToDate*, last updated February 11, 2019, https://

www.uptodate.com/contents/newborn-screening-for-critical-congenital-heart-disease-using-pulse-oximetry.

4. GETTING TO KNOW YOU

1. H. M. Dunsworth, "Thank Your Intelligent Mother for Your Big Brain," *Proceedings of the National Academy of Sciences* 113, no. 25 (2016): 6816–18; J. DeSilva and J. Lesnik, "Chimpanzee Neonatal Brain Size: Implications for Brain Growth in *Homō erectus*," *Journal of Human Evolution* 51, no. 2 (2006): 207–12.

2. Leah R., email to the author, June 9, 2013.

3. A.-M. Widström et al., "Newborn Behaviour to Locate the Breast When Skin-to-Skin: A Possible Method for Enabling Early Self-Regulation," *Acta Paediatrica* 100, no. 1 (2011): 79–85, doi:10.1111/j.1651–2227.2010.01983.x.

4. Widström et al., "Newborn Behaviour to Locate the Breast When Skin-to-Skin," 80-81.

5. Kym S., interview with the author, June 4, 2013.

6. Widström et al., "Newborn Behaviour to Locate the Breast When Skin-to-Skin," 84.

7. "Initiation of Breastfeeding by Breast Crawl," *Breast Crawl*, Mother and Child Health Education Trust, accessed June 25, 2020, http://www.breastcrawl.org.

8. K. A. Bard, "Parenting in Nonhuman Primates," in *Handbook of Parenting, Volume 2: Biology and Ecology of Parenting*, ed. M. H. Bornstein (New York, NY: Routledge, 2019), 78-122.

9. M. Shibata et al., "Broad Cortical Activation in Response to Tactile Stimulation in Newborns," *Neuroreport* 23, no. 6 (2012): 373–77, doi:10.1097/WNR.0b013e3283520296.

10. S. Kotagal, "Neurological Examination of the Newborn," *UpToDate*, last updated May 21, 2020, http://www.uptodate.com/contents/neurologic-examination-of-the-newborn.

11. A. A. Anekar and B. Bordoni, "Palmar Grasp Reflex," in *StatPearls* [online] (Treasure Island, FL: StatPearls Publishing, 2020), https://www.ncbi.nlm.nih.gov/books/NBK553133; "Newborn Reflexes," Stanford Children's Health, accessed November 14, 2014, http://www.stanfordchildrens.org/en/topic/default?id=newborn-reflexes-90-P02630.

12. P. Rochat, "Five Levels of Self-Awareness as They Unfold Early in Life," *Consciousness and Cognition* 12, no. 4 (2003): 717–31, doi:10.1016/S1053-8100(03)00081-3.

13. A. Streri, M. Lhote, and S. Dutilleul, "Haptic Perception in Newborns," *Developmental Science* 3, no. 3 (2000): 319–27.

14. L. Marcus et al., "Tactile Sensory Capacity of the Preterm Infant: Manual Perception of Shape from 28 Gestational Weeks," *Pediatrics* 130, no. 1 (2012): e88-94, doi:10.1542/peds.2011-3357.

15. P. Rochat, "Mouthing and Grasping in Neonates: Evidence for the Early Detection of What Hard or Soft Substances Afford for Action," *Infant Behavior and Development* 10, no. 4 (1987): 435–49, doi:10.1016/0163-6383(87)90041-5.

16. L. Gray, L. Watt, and E. M. Blass, "Skin-to-Skin Contact Is Analgesic in Healthy Newborns," *Pediatrics* 105, no. 1 (2000): e14.

17. B. S. Kisilevsky et al., "Effects of Experience on Fetal Voice Recognition," *Psychological Science* 14, no. 3 (2003): 220–24.

18. C. Moon, R. Panneton Cooper, and W. P. Fifer, "Two-Day-Olds Prefer Their Native Language," *Infant Behavior and Development* 16, no. 4 (1993): 495–500, doi:10.1016/0163-6383(93)80007-U; A. J. DeCasper et al., "Fetal Reactions to Recurrent Maternal Speech," *Infant Behavior and Development* 17, no. 2 (1994): 159–64.

19. A. J. DeCasper and W. P. Fifer, "Of Human Bonding: Newborns Prefer Their Mothers' Voices," *Science* 208, no. 4448 (1980): 1174–76.

20. G. Y. Lee and B. S. Kisilevsky, "Fetuses Respond to Father's Voice but Prefer Mother's Voice after Birth," *Developmental Psychobiology* 56, no. 1 (2014): 1–11.

21. H. Kurihara et al., "Behavioral and Adrenocortical Responses to Stress in Neonates and the Stabilizing Effects of Maternal Heartbeat on Them," *Early Human Development* 46, no. 1–2 (1996): 117–27, doi:10.1016/0378-3782(96) 01749-5.

22. P. Glass, "Development of the Visual System and Implications for Early Intervention," *Infants and Young Children* 15, no. 1 (2002): 1–10.

23. D. Y. Teller, "First Glances: The Vision of Infants. The Friedenwald Lecture," *Investigative Ophthalmology and Visual Science* 38, no. 11 (1997): 2183–203.

24. Y. Pan et al., "Visual Acuity Norms in Preschool Children: The Multi-Ethnic Pediatric Eye Disease Study," *Optometry and Vision Science: Official Publication of the American Academy of Optometry* 86, no. 6 (2009): 607–12, doi:10.1097/ OPX.0b013e3181a76e55; R. G. Bosworth and K. R. Dobkins, "Chromatic and Luminance Contrast Sensitivity in Fullterm and Preterm Infants," *Journal of Vision* 9, no. 13 (2009): 15, doi:10.1167/9.13.15.

25. C. C. Goren, M. Sarty, and P. Y. K. Wu, "Visual Following and Pattern Discrimination of Face-Like Stimuli by Newborn Infants," *Pediatrics* 56, no. 4 (1975): 544–49.

26. O. R. Salva et al., "The Evolution of Social Orienting: Evidence from Chicks (*Gallus gallus*) and Human Newborns," *PLoS ONE* 6, no. 4 (2011): e18802, doi:10.1371/journal.pone.0018802; E. Valenza et al., "Face Preference at Birth," *Journal of Experimental Psychology: Human Perception and Performance* 22, no. 4 (1996): 892–903.

27. Glass, "Development of the Visual System; D. Ricci et al., "Application of a Neonatal Assessment of Visual Function in a Population of Low Risk Full-Term Newborn," *Early Human Development* 84, no. 4 (2008): 277–80, doi:10.1016

/j.earlhumdev.2007.10.002; L. M. Dubowitz et al., "Visual Function in the Pre-term and Fullterm Newborn Infant," *Developmental Medicine and Child Neurology* 22, no. 4 (1980): 465–75.

28. A. Batki et al., "Is There an Innate Gaze Module? Evidence from Human Neonates," *Infant Behavior and Development* 23, no. 2 (2000): 223–29, doi:10 .1016/S0163-6383(01)00037-6.

29. T. Farroni et al., "Eye Contact Detection in Humans from Birth," *Proceed-ings of the National Academy of Sciences of the United States of America* 99, no. 14 (2002): 9602–5, doi:10.1073/pnas.152159999.

30. F. Z. Sai, "The Role of the Mother's Voice in Developing Mother's Face Preference: Evidence for Intermodal Perception at Birth," *Infant and Child Devel-opment* 14, no. 1 (2005): 29–50, doi:10.1002/icd.376.

31. H. Varendi, R. H. Porter, and J. Winberg, "Does the Newborn Baby Find the Nipple by Smell?" *Lancet* 344 (1994): 989–90.

32. H. Varendi, R. H. Porter, and J. Winberg, "Natural Odour Preferences of Newborn Infants Change Over Time," *Acta Paediatrica* 86, no. 9 (1997): 985–90.

33. H. Varendi et al., "Soothing Effect of Amniotic Fluid Smell in Newborn Infants," *Early Human Development* 51, no. 1 (1998): 47–55, doi:10.1016/S0378-3782(97)00082-0.

34. H. Varendi, R. H. Porter, and J. Winberg, "Attractiveness of Amniotic Fluid Odor: Evidence of Prenatal Olfactory Learning?" *Acta Paediatrica* 85, no. 10 (1996): 1223–27.

35. Varendi, Porter, and Winberg, "Natural Odour Preferences of Newborn Infants"; R. H. Porter and J. Winberg, "Unique Salience of Maternal Breast Odors for Newborn Infants," *Neuroscience and Biobehavioral Reviews* 23, no. 3 (1999): 439–49; J. M. Cernoch and R. H. Porter, "Recognition of Maternal Axil-lary Odors by Infants," *Child Development* 56 (1985): 1593–98.

36. J. A. Mennella, A. Johnson, and G. K. Beauchamp, "Garlic Ingestion by Pregnant Women Alters the Odor of Amniotic Fluid," *Chemical Senses* 20, no. 2 (1995): 207–9; J. A. Mennella and G. K. Beauchamp, "Maternal Diet Alters the Sensory Qualities of Human Milk and the Nursling's Behavior," *Pediatrics* 88 (1991): 737–44.

37. M. Kaitz and R. Bronner, "Parturient Women Can Recognize Their Infants by Touch," *Developmental Psychology* 28, no. 1 (1992): 35–39.

38. M. Kaitz et al., "Mothers' and Fathers' Recognition of Their Newborns' Photographs during the Postpartum Period," *Developmental and Behavioral Pediatrics* 9, no. 4 (1988): 223–26.

39. J. N. Lundström et al., "Maternal Status Regulates Cortical Responses to the Body Odor of Newborns," *Frontiers in Psychology* 4 (2013), doi:10.3389/ fpsyg.2013.00597.

40. M. Kaitz et al., "Mothers' Recognition of Their Newborns by Olfactory Cues," *Developmental Psychobiology* 20, no. 6 (1987): 587–91.

41. E. Gustafsson et al., "Fathers Are Just as Good as Mothers at Recognizing the Cries of Their Baby," *Nature Communications* 4 (2013): 1698, doi:10.1038/ncomms2713.

42. J. A. Green and G. E. Gustafson, "Individual Recognition of Human Infants on the Basis of Cries Alone," *Developmental Psychobiology* 16, no. 6 (1983) 485–93; A. R. Wiesenfeld, C. Z. Malatesta, and L. L. Deloach, "Differential Parental Response to Familiar and Unfamiliar Infant Distress Signals," *Infant Behavior and Development* 4 (March 1981): 281–95.

43. R. C. White-Traut et al., "Salivary Cortisol and Behavioral State Responses of Healthy Newborn Infants to Tactile-Only and Multisensory Interventions," *Journal of Obstetric, Gynecologic, and Neonatal Nursing* 38, no. 1 (2009): 22–34, doi:10.1111/j.1552-6909.2008.00307.x.

44. C. Blair et al., "Maternal Sensitivity Is Related to Hypothalamic-Pituitary-Adrenal Axis Stress Reactivity and Regulation in Response to Emotion Challenge in 6-Month-Old Infants," *Annals of the New York Academy of Sciences* 1094, no. 1 (2006): 263–67, doi:10.1196/annals.1376.031.

45. E. M. Albers et al., "Maternal Behavior Predicts Infant Cortisol Recovery from a Mild Everyday Stressor," *Journal of Child Psychology and Psychiatry* 49, no. 1 (2008): 97–103, doi:10.1111/j.1469-7610.2007.01818.x.

46. D. Divecha, "Why Attachment Parenting Is Not the Same as Secure Attachment," *Greater Good Magazine*, May 2, 2018, https://greatergood.berkeley.edu/article/item/why_attachment_parenting_is_not_the_same_as_secure_attachment.

47. J. R. Britton, H. L. Britton, and V. Gronwaldt, "Breastfeeding, Sensitivity, and Attachment," *Pediatrics* 118, no. 5 (2006): e1436–43, doi:10.1542/peds.2005-2916; A. Tharner et al., "Breastfeeding and Its Relation to Maternal Sensitivity and Infant Attachment," *Journal of Developmental and Behavioral Pediatrics* 33, no. 5 (2012): 396–404; Douglas M. Teti, interview with the author, February 11, 2014; N. Koren-Karie et al., "Mothers' Insightfulness Regarding Their Infants' Internal Experience: Relations with Maternal Sensitivity and Infant Attachment," *Developmental Psychology* 38, no. 4 (July 2002): 534–42, doi:10.1037/0012-1649.38.4.534; N. L. McElwain and C. Booth-LaForce, "Maternal Sensitivity to Infant Distress and Nondistress as Predictors of Infant-Mother Attachment Security," *Journal of Family Psychology* 20, no. 2 (2006): 247–55, doi:10.1037/0893-3200.20.2.247; E. M. Leerkes, A. Nayena Blankson, and M. O'Brien, "Differential Effects of Maternal Sensitivity to Infant Distress and Nondistress on Social-Emotional Functioning," *Child Development* 80, no. 3 (2009): 762–75; S. H. Landry, K. E. Smith, and P. R. Swank, "Responsive Parenting: Establishing Early Foundations for Social, Communication, and Independent Problem-Solving Skills," *Developmental Psychology* 42, no. 4 (2006): 627–42, doi:10.1037/0012-1649.42.4.627; I. S. Hairston et al., "Mother-Infant Bonding Is Not Associated with Feeding Type: A Community

Study Sample," *BMC Pregnancy Childbirth* 19, no. 1 (2019): 125, doi: 10.1186/s12884-019-2264-0.

5. VACCINES AND YOUR CHILD

1. Margaret Jordan Green, interview with the author, March 1, 2014.

2. W. J. Moss and D. E. Griffin, "Measles," *Lancet* 379, no. 9811 (2012): 153–64, doi:10.1016/S0140-6736(10)62352-5.

3. Moss and Griffin, "Measles."

4. R. Buchanan and D. J. Bonthius, "Measles Virus and Associated Central Nervous System Sequelae," *Seminars in Pediatric Neurology* 19, no. 3 (2012): 107–14, doi:10.1016/j.spen.2012.02.003.

5. Centers for Disease Control and Prevention (CDC), "MMWR Summary of Notifiable Diseases, United States, 1993," October 21, 1994, https://www.cdc.gov/mmwr/preview/mmwrhtml/00035381.htm.

6. A. Allen, "Battling Measles, Remodeling Society," in *Vaccine: The Controversial Story of Medicine's Greatest Lifesaver* (New York: W. W. Norton, 2007), 215–47.

7. National Communicable Disease Center, "Reported Incidence of Notifiable Diseases in the United States, 1966: Measles (Rubeola), 1965-1966," *Morbidity and Mortality Weekly Report* 15, no. 53 (1967): 1-60, http://stacks.cdc.gov/view/cdc/615.

8. C. E. Koop, *Measles Continues to Spread in the US: 1916* (video), Measles Timeline, Vaccine Makers Project, accessed February 5, 2014, http://www.historyofvaccines.org/content/timelines/measles.

9. World Health Organization, "WHO Coronavirus Disease (COVID-19) Dashboard," accessed December 13, 2020, https://covid19.who.int; S. E. Oliver et al., "The Advisory Committee on Immunization Practices' Interim Recommendation for Use of Pfizer-BioNTech COVID-19 Vaccine—United States, December 2020," *Morbidity and Mortality Weekly Report (MMWR)* Early Release 69, no. 50 (2020): 1922-24, doi:10.15585/mmwr.mm6950e2.

10. C. A. Pierce et al., "Immune Responses to SARS-CoV-2 Infection in Hospitalized Pediatric and Adult Patients," *Science Translational Medicine* 12, no. 564 (2020): eabd5487.

11. J. P. Baker, "The First Measles Vaccine," *Pediatrics* 128, no. 3 (2011): 435–37, doi:10.1542/peds.2011-1430.

12. Nobel Media, "John F. Enders—Biographical," Nobelprize.org, accessed February 5, 2014, http://www.nobelprize.org/nobel_prizes/medicine/laureates/1954/enders-bio.html.

13. S. L. Katz, *Thomas Peebles Isolates the Measles Virus: 1954* (video), Measles Timeline, Vaccine Makers Project, accessed June 17, 2014, http://www.historyofvaccines.org/content/timelines/measles.

14. Baker, "The First Measles Vaccine."

15. Baker, "The First Measles Vaccine"; S. L. Katz, "The History of Measles Vaccine and Attempts to Control Measles," in *Microbe Hunters: Then and Now* (Bloomington, IL: Medi-Ed Press, 1996), 69–76.

16. P. A. Offit, "The Destroying Angel," in *Vaccinated: One Man's Quest to Defeat the World's Deadliest Diseases* (New York: Harper Collins, 2007), 44–56.

17. Allen, "Battling Measles, Remodeling Society."

18. CDC, "Measles," chapter 13 in *Epidemiology and Prevention of Vaccine-Preventable Diseases*, ed. J. Hamborsky, A. Kroger, and C. Wolf, 13th ed. (Washington, DC: Public Health Foundation, 2015), 209-30, https://www.cdc.gov/vaccines/pubs/pinkbook/meas.html.

19. CDC, "Measles History," last updated November 5, 2020, https://www.cdc.gov/measles/about/history.html.

20. A. P. Fiebelkorn et al., "Measles in the United States during the Postelimination Era," *Journal of Infectious Diseases* 202, no. 10 (November 15, 2010): 1520–28, doi:10.1086/656914; National Center for Health Statistics, "Health, United States, 2018: Data Finder," CDC, last updated October 30, 2019, https://www.cdc.gov/nchs/hus/contents2018.htm.

21. CDC, "Measles Cases and Outbreaks," last updated November 5, 2020, https://www.cdc.gov/measles/cases-outbreaks.html.

22. N. S. Clemmons et al., "Measles: United States, January 4–April 2, 2015," *Morbidity and Mortality Weekly Report (MMWR)* 64, no. 14 (2015): 373-76, https://www.cdc.gov/mmwr/preview/mmwrhtml/mm6414a1.htm.

23. CDC, "Measles Elimination," last updated November 5, 2020, https://www.cdc.gov/measles/elimination.html.

24. WHO, "European Region Loses Ground in Effort to Eliminate Measles," press release, August 29, 2019, http://www.euro.who.int/en/media-centre/sections/press-releases/2019/european-region-loses-ground-in-effort-to-eliminate-measles.

25. M. K. Patel et al., "Progress Toward Regional Measles Elimination: Worldwide, 2000–2018," *Morbidity and Mortality Weekly Report (MMWR)* 68, no. 48 (2019): 1105-1111; WHO, "More Than 140,000 Die from Measles as Cases Surge Worldwide," joint news release, December 5, 2019, https://www.who.int/news-room/detail/05-12-2019-more-than-140-000-die-from-measles-as-cases-surge-worldwide.

26. CDC, "Table 1: Recommended Child and Adolescent Immunization Schedule for Ages 18 Years or Younger, United States, 2020" last updated February 3, 2020, https://www.cdc.gov/vaccines/schedules/hcp/imz/child-adolescent.html.

27. S. W. Roush, T. V. Murphy, and Vaccine-Preventable Disease Table Working Group, "Historical Comparisons of Morbidity and Mortality for Vaccine-Preventable Diseases in the United States," *JAMA* 298, no. 18 (2007): 2155–63, doi:10.1001/jama.298.18.2155.

28. F. Zhou et al., "Economic Evaluation of the Routine Childhood Immuni-

zation Program in the United States, 2009," *Pediatrics* 133, no. 4 (2014): 577–85, doi:10.1542/peds.2013-0698.

29. CDC, "*Haemophilus influenzae*," chapter 8 in *Epidemiology and Prevention of Vaccine-Preventable Diseases*, ed. J. Hamborsky, A. Kroger, and C. Wolf (Washington, DC: Public Health Foundation, 2015), 119–33, https://www.cdc.gov/vaccines/pubs/pinkbook/hib.html.

30. CDC, "Pneumococcal Disease," chapter 17 in *Epidemiology and Prevention of Vaccine-Preventable Diseases*, ed. J. Hamborsky, A. Kroger, and C. Wolf (Washington, DC: Public Health Foundation, 2015), 279–95, https://www.cdc.gov/vaccines/pubs/pinkbook/pneumo.html; CDC, "Trends by Serotype Group," Active Bacterial Core Surveillance (ABCs), last updated July 17, 2018, https://www.cdc.gov/abcs/reports-findings/survreports/spneu-types.html.

31. X. Zhou et al., "National Impact of 13-valent Pneumococcal Conjugate Vaccine on Ambulatory Care Visits for Otitis Media in Children under 5 Years in the United States," *International Journal of Pediatric Otorhinolaryngology* 119 (2019): 96–102.

32. R. I. Glass et al., "Rotavirus Vaccines: Successes and Challenges," *Journal of Infection* 68, suppl. 1 (2014): S9-18, doi:10.1016/j.jinf.2013.09.010.

33. CDC, "Rotavirus," chapter 19 in *Epidemiology and Prevention of Vaccine-Preventable Diseases*, ed. J. Hamborsky, A. Kroger, and C. Wolf (Washington, DC: Public Health Foundation, 2015), 311–23, https://www.cdc.gov/vaccines/pubs/pinkbook/rota.html.

34. C. A. Panozzo et al., "Direct, Indirect, Total, and Overall Effectiveness of the Rotavirus Vaccines for the Prevention of Gastroenteritis Hospitalizations in Privately Insured US Children, 2007–2010," *American Journal of Epidemiology* 179, no. 7 (2014): 895–909, doi:10.1093/aje/kwu001.

35. D. R. Feikin et al., "Individual and Community Risks of Measles and Pertussis Associated with Personal Exemptions to Immunization," *JAMA* 284, no. 24 (2000): 3145–50, doi:10.1001/jama.284.24.3145; J. M. Glanz et al., "Parental Refusal of Pertussis Vaccination Is Associated with an Increased Risk of Pertussis Infection in Children," *Pediatrics* 123, no. 6 (2009): 1446–51, doi:10.1542/peds.2008-2150; J. E. Atwell et al., "Nonmedical Vaccine Exemptions and Pertussis in California, 2010," *Pediatrics* 132, no. 4 (2013): 624–30, doi:10.1542/peds.2013-0878; S. B. Omer et al., "Nonmedical Exemptions to School Immunization Requirements: Secular Trends and Association of State Policies with Pertussis Incidence," *JAMA* 296, no. 14 (2006): 1757–63, doi:10.1001/jama.296.14.1757; S. B. Omer et al., "Geographic Clustering of Nonmedical Exemptions to School Immunization Requirements and Associations with Geographic Clustering of Pertussis," *American Journal of Epidemiology* 168, no. 12 (2008): 1389–96, doi:10.1093/aje/kwn263; J. M. Glanz et al., "Parental Decline of Pneumococcal Vaccination and Risk of Pneumococcal Related Disease in Children," *Vaccine* 29, no. 5 (2011): 994–99, doi:10.1016/j.vaccine.2010.11.085.

36. R. S. Barlow et al., "Vaccinated Children and Adolescents with Pertussis Infections Have Decreased Illness Severity and Duration, Oregon 2010–2012," *Clinical Infectious Diseases* 58, no. 11 (2014): 1523–29, doi:10.1093/cid/ciu156; P. Mitchell et al., "Previous Vaccination Modifies Both the Clinical Disease and Immunological Features in Children with Measles," *Journal of Primary Health Care* 5, no. 2 (2013): 93–98.

37. P. Fine, K. Eames, and D. L. Heymann, "'Herd Immunity': A Rough Guide," *Clinical Infectious Diseases* 52, no. 7 (2011): 911–16, doi:10.1093/cid/cir007; H. Rashid, G. Khandaker, and R. Booy, "Vaccination and Herd Immunity: What More Do We Know?" *Current Opinion in Infectious Diseases* 25, no. 3 (2012): 243–49, doi:10.1097/QCO.0b013e328352f727.

38. P. G. Smith, "Concepts of Herd Protection and Immunity," *Procedia in Vaccinology* 2, no. 2 (2010): 134–39, doi:10.1016/j.provac.2010.07.005; S. Funk et al., "Combining Serological and Contact Data to Derive Target Immunity Levels for Achieving and Maintaining Measles Elimination," *BMC Medicine* 17 (2019): 180, doi: 10.1186/s12916-019-1413-7.

39. D. E. Sugerman et al., "Measles Outbreak in a Highly Vaccinated Population, San Diego, 2008: Role of the Intentionally Undervaccinated," *Pediatrics* 125, no. 4 (2010): 747–55.

40. Sugerman et al., "Measles Outbreak in a Highly Vaccinated Population."

41. W. A. Orenstein, "The Role of Measles Elimination in Development of a National Immunization Program," *Pediatric Infectious Disease Journal* 25, no. 12 (2006): 1093–1101, doi:10.1097/01.inf.0000246840.13477.28.

42. Patel et al., "Progress Toward Regional Measles Elimination"; R. McDonald, "Notes from the Field: Measles Outbreaks from Imported Cases in Orthodox Jewish Communities, New York and New Jersey, 2018–2019," *Morbidity and Mortality Weekly Report (MMWR)* 68, no. 19 (2019): 444-45.

43. S. Sarkar et al. "Measles Resurgence in the USA: How International Travel Compounds Vaccine Resistance," *Lancet Infectious Diseases* 19, no. 7 (2019): 684–86.

44. S. S. Chaves et al., "Varicella in Infants after Implementation of the US Varicella Vaccination Program," *Pediatrics* 128, no. 6 (2011): 1071–77, doi:10.1542/peds.2011-0017.

45. M. M. Patel et al., "Fulfilling the Promise of Rotavirus Vaccines: How Far Have We Come since Licensure?" *Lancet Infectious Diseases* 12, no. 7 (2012): 561–70, doi:10.1016/S1473-3099(12)70029-4; P. A. Gastañaduy et al., "Gastroenteritis Hospitalizations in Older Children and Adults in the United States before and after Implementation of Infant Rotavirus Vaccination," *JAMA* 310, no. 8 (2013): 851–53, doi:10.1001/jama.2013.170800.

46. Rashid, Khandaker, and Booy, "Vaccination and Herd Immunity."

47. Feikin et al., "Individual and Community Risks of Measles and Pertussis."

48. V. Demicheli et al., "Vaccines for Measles, Mumps and Rubella in Chil-

dren," *Cochrane Database of Systematic Reviews* 2 (2012): CD004407, doi:10. 1002/14651858.CD004407.pub3.

49. F. Kowalzik, J. Faber, and M. Knuf, "MMR and MMRV Vaccines," *Vaccine* 36, no. 36 (2018): 5402–7; CDC, "Measles," in *Epidemiology and Prevention of Vaccine-Preventable Diseases*.

50. N. Principi and S. Esposito, "Vaccines and Febrile Seizures," *Expert Review of Vaccines* 12, no. 8 (2013): 885–92, doi:10.1586/14760584.2013.814781.

51. CDC, "Measles," in *Epidemiology and Prevention of Vaccine-Preventable Diseases*.

52. K. Bohlke et al., "Risk of Anaphylaxis after Vaccination of Children and Adolescents," *Pediatrics* 112, no. 4 (2003): 815–20, doi:10.1542/peds.112.4.815.

53. Institute of Medicine (IOM), *Childhood Immunization Schedule and Safety: Stakeholder Concerns, Scientific Evidence, and Future Studies* (Washington, DC: National Academies Press, 2013), https://www.nap.edu/catalog/13563/the -childhood-immunization-schedule-and-safety-stakeholder-concerns-scientific -evidence.

54. J. L. Schwartz, "The First Rotavirus Vaccine and the Politics of Acceptable Risk," *Milbank Quarterly* 90, no. 2 (2012): 278–310, doi:10.1111/j.1468-0009 .2012.00664.x.

55. US Food and Drug Administration (FDA), "Vaccine Development — 101," last updated December 14, 2020, https://www.fda.gov/vaccines-blood -biologics/development-approval-process-cber/vaccine-development-101.

56. J. C. Smith, D. E. Snider, and L. K. Pickering, "Immunization Policy Development in the United States: The Role of the Advisory Committee on Immunization Practices," *Annals of Internal Medicine* 150, no. 1 (January 2009): 45–49, doi:10.7326/0003-4819-150-1-200901060-00009.

57. CDC, "Rotavirus Vaccine for the Prevention of Rotavirus Gastroenteritis among Children: Recommendations of the Advisory Committee on Immunization Practices (ACIP)," *MMWR Recommendations and Reports* 48, no. RR-2 (1999), http://www.cdc.gov/mmwr/preview/mmwrhtml/00056669.htm.

58. CDC, "Vaccine Adverse Event Reporting System (VAERS)," 2013, http:// www.cdc.gov/vaccinesafety/Activities/vaers.html; F. Varricchio et al., "Understanding Vaccine Safety Information from the Vaccine Adverse Event Reporting System," *Pediatric Infectious Disease Journal* 23, no. 4 (2004): 287–94.

59. Schwartz, "The First Rotavirus Vaccine and the Politics of Acceptable Risk"; CDC, "Withdrawal of Rotavirus Vaccine Recommendation," *MMWR Recommendations and Reports* 48, no. 43 (1999), http://www.cdc.gov/mmwr /preview/mmwrhtml/mm4843a5.htm.

60. A. Allen, "No Good Deed Goes Unpunished," in *Vaccine: The Controversial Story of Medicine's Greatest Lifesaver* (New York: W. W. Norton, 2007), 294–326.

61. J. Baggs et al., "The Vaccine Safety Datalink: A Model for Monitoring

Immunization Safety," *Pediatrics* 127, suppl. (2011): S45-53, doi:10.1542/peds.2010-1722H; CDC, "Vaccine Safety Datalink (VSD)," last updated August 24, 2020, http://www.cdc.gov/vaccinesafety/Activities/vsd.html.

62. W. K. Yih et al., "Intussusception Risk after Rotavirus Vaccination in US Infants," *New England Journal of Medicine* 370, no. 6 (2014): 503–12, doi:10.1056/NEJMoa1303164.

63. K. Soares-Weiser et al., "Vaccines for Preventing Rotavirus Diarrhoea: Vaccines in Use," *Cochrane Database Systematic Reviews*, no. 3 (2019): CD008521.

64. R. Desai et al., "Potential Intussusception Risk versus Benefits of Rotavirus Vaccination in the United States," *Pediatric Infectious Disease Journal* 32, no. 1 (2013): 1–7, doi:10.1097/INF.0b013e318270362c.

65. Janie Oyakawa, email to the author, March 12, 2014.

66. J. Oyakawa, "A Crunchy Mom's Reversal on Vaccinations," *The Mom of OZ* (blog), November 10, 2013, http://rubyslippersx3.blogspot.co.uk/2013/11/a-crunchy-moms-reversal-on-vaccinations.html.

67. A. Kennedy et al., "Confidence about Vaccines in the United States: Understanding Parents' Perceptions," *Health Affairs (Millwood)* 30, no. 6 (2011): 1151–59, doi:10.1377/hlthaff.2011.0396; M. Mason McCauley et al., "Exploring the Choice to Refuse or Delay Vaccines: A National Survey of Parents of 6- through 23-Month-Olds," *Academic Pediatrics* 12, no. 5 (2012): 375–83, doi:10.1016/j.acap.2012.06.007.

68. Paul Slovic, interview with the author, February 18, 2014.

69. D. Kahneman, "Of Two Minds: How Fast and Slow Thinking Shape Perception and Choice," *Scientific American*, June 15, 2012, http://www.scientificamerican.com/article/kahneman-excerpt-thinking-fast-and-slow; P. Slovic et al., "Risk as Analysis and Risk as Feelings: Some Thoughts about Affect, Reason, Risk, and Rationality," *Risk Analysis* 24, no. 2 (2004): 311–22, doi:10.1111/j.0272-4332.2004.00433.x.

70. P. Slovic, "Perception of Risk," *Science* 236, no. 4799 (1987): 280–85; L. K. Ball, G. Evans, and A. Bostrom, "Risky Business: Challenges in Vaccine Risk Communication," *Pediatrics* 101, no. 3 (1998): 453–58; M. Siddiqui, D. A. Salmon, and S. B. Omer, "Epidemiology of Vaccine Hesitancy in the United States," *Human Vaccines and Immunotherapeutics* 9, no. 12 (2013): 2643–48, doi:10.4161/hv.27243.

71. Slovic, interview, 2014.

72. Slovic, "Perception of Risk"; D. M. Kahan et al., "Who Fears the HPV Vaccine, Who Doesn't, and Why? An Experimental Study of the Mechanisms of Cultural Cognition," *Law and Human Behavior* 34, no. 6 (2010): 501–16, doi:10.1007/s10979-009-9201-0.

73. Oyakawa, "A Crunchy Mom's Reversal on Vaccinations."

6. SLEEP SAFELY, SLEEP SWEETLY

1. Esmee McKee, email to the author, August 21, 2012.

2. G. A. Morelli et al., "Cultural Variation in Infants' Sleeping Arrangements: Questions of Independence," *Developmental Psychology* 28 (1992): 604–13.

3. S. Latz, A. W. Wolf, and B. Lozoff, "Cosleeping in Context: Sleep Practices and Problems in Young Children in Japan and the United States," *Archives of Pediatrics and Adolescent Medicine* 153 (1999): 339–46.

4. Shimizu, M., Park, H. & Greenfield, P. M. "Infant Sleeping Arrangements and Cultural Values among Contemporary Japanese Mothers," *Frontiers in Psychology* 5 (2014): 718, 10.3389/fpsyg.2014.00718.

5. B. Lozoff, G. L. Askew, and A. W. Wolf, "Cosleeping and Early Childhood Sleep Problems: Effects of Ethnicity and Socioeconomic Status," *Journal of Developmental Behavioral Pediatrics* 17 (1996): 9–15.

6. E. R. Colson et al., "Trends and Factors Associated with Infant Bed Sharing, 1993-2010: The National Infant Sleep Position Study," *JAMA Pediatrics* 167, no. 11 (2013): 1032–37; J. M. Bombard, "Vital Signs: Trends and Disparities in Infant Safe Sleep Practices: United States, 2009–2015," *Morbidity and Mortality Weekly Report (MMWR)* 67, no. 1 (2018): 39-46; H. L. Ball et al., "Bed-Sharing by Breastfeeding Mothers: Who Bed-Shares and What Is the Relationship with Breastfeeding Duration?" *Acta Paediatrica* 105, no. 6 (2016): 628–34; P. S. Blair, "The Prevalence and Characteristics Associated with Parent-Infant Bed-Sharing in England," *Archives of Disease in Childhood* 89, no. 12 (2004): 1106–10, doi:10.1136/adc.2003.038067; J. Young, and R. Shipstone, "Shared Sleeping Surfaces and Dangerous Sleeping Environments," in *SIDS, Sudden Infant and Early Childhood Death: The Past, the Present and the Future*, ed. J. R. Duncan and R. W. Byard (South Australia: University of Adelaide Press, 2018), 187-215.

7. S. L. Blunden, K. R. Thompson, and D. Dawson, "Behavioural Sleep Treatments and Night Time Crying in Infants: Challenging the Status Quo," *Sleep Medicine Reviews* 15 (2011): 327–34, doi:10.1016/j.smrv.2010.11.002; J. J. McKenna, H. L. Ball, and L. T. Gettler, "Mother-Infant Cosleeping, Breastfeeding and Sudden Infant Death Syndrome: What Biological Anthropology Has Discovered about Normal Infant Sleep and Pediatric Sleep Medicine," *American Journal of Physical Anthropology* 134, suppl. 45 (2007): 133–61, doi:10.1002/ajpa.20736; M. Small, *Our Babies, Ourselves: How Biology and Culture Shape the Way We Parent* (New York: Anchor Books, 1999).

8. American Academy of Pediatrics (AAP) Task Force on Sudden Infant Death Syndrome, "SIDS and Other Sleep-Related Infant Deaths: Updated 2016 Recommendations for a Safe Infant Sleeping Environment," *Pediatrics* 138, no. 5 (2016): e20162938.

9. Ask Dr. Sears, "Scientific Benefits of Co-Sleeping," accessed November 7, 2014, http://www.askdrsears.com/topics/sleep-problems/scientific-benefits -co-sleeping.

10. J. McKenna, "Frequently Asked Questions on Infant Sleep, SIDS Risks, Cosleeping, and Breastfeeding," Mother-Baby Behavioral Sleep Laboratory, accessed November 7, 2014, http://cosleeping.nd.edu/frequently-asked -questions/#40.

11. C. K. Shapiro-Mendoza et al., "The Epidemiology of Sudden Infant Death Syndrome and Sudden Unexpected Infant Deaths: Diagnostic Shift and other Temporal Changes," in *SIDS Sudden Infant and Early Childhood Death: The Past, the Present and the Future*, ed. J. R. Duncan and R. W. Byard (South Australia: University of Adelaide Press, 2018), 257-82.

12. B. J. Taylor et al., "International Comparison of Sudden Unexpected Death in Infancy Rates Using a Newly Proposed Set of Cause-of-Death Codes," *Archives of Disease in Childhood* 100, no. 11 (2015): 1018–23.

13. Centers for Disease Control and Prevention (CDC), "SUID and SIDS: Data and Statistics," last updated November 10, 2020, https://www.cdc.gov/sids /data.htm.

14. N. Matoba and J. W. Collins, "Racial Disparity in Infant Mortality," *Seminars in Perinatology* 41, no. 6 (2017): 354-359.

15. C. K. Shapiro-Mendoza et al., "Variations in Cause-of-Death Determination for Sudden Unexpected Infant Deaths," *Pediatrics* 140, no. 5 (2017): e1293-e1300.

16. Shapiro-Mendoza et al., "Epidemiology of Sudden Infant Death Syndrome and Sudden Unexpected Infant Deaths."

17. L. R. Rechtman et al., "Sofas and Infant Mortality," *Pediatrics* 134, no. 5 (2014): e1293–e1300.

18. A. B. Erck Lambert et al., "Sleep-Related Infant Suffocation Deaths Attributable to Soft Bedding, Overlay, and Wedging," *Pediatrics* 143, no. 5 (2019): e20183408.

19. N. J. Scheers, D. W. Woodard, and B. T. Thach, "Crib Bumpers Continue to Cause Infant Deaths: A Need for a New Preventive Approach," *Journal of Pediatrics* 169 (2016): 93-97.e1.

20. P. Liaw et al., "Infant Deaths in Sitting Devices," *Pediatrics* 144, no. 1 (2019): e20182576.

21. R. R. Peachman, "While They Were Sleeping," *Consumer Reports*, December 30, 2019, https://www.consumerreports.org/child-safety/while-they-were -sleeping.

22. E. M. Mannen et al., "Biomechanical Analysis of Inclined Sleep Products: Final Report 09.18.2019," in *Supplemental Notice of Proposed Rulemaking for Infant Sleep Products* (Bethesda, MD: United States Consumer Product Safety Commission, 2019), 31-107, https://www.cpsc.gov/s3fs-public/Supplemental NoticeofProposedRulemakingforInfantSleepProducts_10_16_2019.pdf.

23. S. R. Orenstein, P. F. Whitington, and D. M. Orenstein, "The Infant Seat as Treatment for Gastroesophageal Reflux," *New England Journal of Medicine* 309 (1983): 760–63.

24. P. G. Schnitzer, T. M. Covington, and H. K. Dykstra, "Sudden Unexpected Infant Deaths: Sleep Environment and Circumstances," *American Journal of Public Health* 102 (2012): 1204–12, doi:10.2105/AJPH.2011.300613.

25. Erck Lambert et al., "Sleep-Related Infant Suffocation Deaths."

26. F. R. Hauck et al., "Sleep Environment and the Risk of Sudden Infant Death Syndrome in an Urban Population: The Chicago Infant Mortality Study," *Pediatrics* 111, suppl. 1 (2003): 1207–14.

27. H. C. Kinney et al., "The Brainstem and Serotonin in the Sudden Infant Death Syndrome," *Annual Review of Pathology: Mechanisms of Disease* 4, no. 1 (2009): 517–50, doi:10.1146/annurev.pathol.4.110807.092322.

28. R. F. Carlin and R. Y. Moon, "Risk Factors, Protective Factors, and Current Recommendations to Reduce Sudden Infant Death Syndrome: A Review," *JAMA Pediatrics* 171, no. 2 (2017): 175–80.

29. Carlin and Moon, "Risk Factors, Protective Factors, and Current Recommendations"; J. Spinelli, "Evolution and Significance of the Triple Risk Model in Sudden Infant Death Syndrome," *Journal of Paediatrics and Child Health* 53, no. 2 (2017): 112–15.

30. R. Gilbert, "Infant Sleeping Position and the Sudden Infant Death Syndrome: Systematic Review of Observational Studies and Historical Review of Recommendations from 1940 to 2002," *International Journal of Epidemiology* 34, no. 4 (2005): 874–87.

31. Gilbert, "Infant Sleeping Position."

32. A. Kahn et al., "Prone or Supine Body Position and Sleep Characteristics in Infants," *Pediatrics* 91, no. 6 (1993): 1112–15.

33. P. Franco et al., "Arousal from Sleep Mechanisms in Infants," *Sleep Medicine* 11, no. 7 (2010): 603–14.

34. E. Pace, "Benjamin Spock, World's Pediatrician, Dies at 94," *New York Times*, March 17, 1998.

35. Gilbert, "Infant Sleeping Position."

36. R. Carpenter et al., "Bed Sharing When Parents Do Not Smoke: Is There a Risk of SIDS? An Individual Level Analysis of Five Major Case-Control Studies," *BMJ Open* 3, no. 5 (2013), doi:10.1136/bmjopen-2012-002299.

37. P. S. Blair et al., "Bed-Sharing in the Absence of Hazardous Circumstances: Is There a Risk of Sudden Infant Death Syndrome? An Analysis from Two Case-Control Studies Conducted in the UK," *PLoS ONE* 9, no. 9 (September 19, 2014): e107799, doi:10.1371/journal.pone.0107799.

38. Blair et al., "Bed-Sharing in the Absence of Hazardous Circumstances."

39. Carpenter et al., "Bed Sharing When Parents Do Not Smoke," 10.

40. Blair et al., "Bed-Sharing in the Absence of Hazardous Circumstances."

41. R. Y. Moon and AAP Task Force on Sudden Infant Death Syndrome, "SIDS and Other Sleep-Related Infant Deaths: Evidence Base for 2016 Updated

Recommendations for a Safe Infant Sleeping Environment," *Pediatrics* 138, no. 5 (2016): e20162940, doi:10.1542/peds.2016-2940.

42. AAP Task Force on Sudden Infant Death Syndrome, "SIDS and Other Sleep-Related Infant Deaths: Updated 2016 Recommendations for a Safe Infant Sleeping Environment," *Pediatrics* 138, no. 5 (2016): e20162938, doi:10.1542/peds.2016-2938; Public Health Agency (PHA) of Canada, *Joint Statement on Safe Sleep: Preventing Sudden Infant Deaths in Canada* (Ontario: PHA of Canada, 2011), https://www.canada.ca/en/public-health/services/health-promotion/childhood-adolescence/stages-childhood/infancy-birth-two-years/safe-sleep/joint-statement-on-safe-sleep.html.

43. Blair et al., "Bed-Sharing in the Absence of Hazardous Circumstances."

44. AAP Task Force on Sudden Infant Death Syndrome, "SIDS and Other Sleep-Related Infant Deaths."

45. UNICEF UK, Baby Friendly Initiative, *Caring for Your Baby at Night: A Guide for Parents* (London: UNICEF, 2019), https://www.unicef.org.uk/babyfriendly/wp-content/uploads/sites/2/2018/08/Caring-for-your-baby-at-night-web.pdf; Red Nose, National Scientific Advisory Group (NSAG), *Sleeping with a Baby* (Melbourne: National SIDS Council of Australia, 2019), https://rednose.org.au/downloads/InfoStatement_SharingSleepSurfacewithBaby_Dec2019.pdf; National Institute for Health and Care Excellence (NICE), *Postnatal Care up to 8 Weeks after Birth* (London: NICE, 2006), last updated February 1, 2015, https://www.nice.org.uk/guidance/cg37; P. S. Blair et al., "Bedsharing and Breastfeeding: The Academy of Breastfeeding Medicine Protocol #6, Revision 2019," *Breastfeeding Medicine* 15, no. 1 (2020): 5–16.

46. S. A. Baddock et al., "The Influence of Bed-Sharing on Infant Physiology, Breastfeeding and Behaviour: A Systematic Review," *Sleep Medicine Reviews* 43 (February 2019): 106–17.

47. S. A. Baddock et al., "Hypoxic and Hypercapnic Events in Young Infants during Bed-Sharing," *Pediatrics*, July 16, 2012, doi:10.1542/peds.2011-3390.

48. H. Ball, "Airway Covering during Bed-Sharing," *Child: Care, Health, and Development* 35, no. 5 (September 2009): 728–37, doi:10.1111/j.1365-2214.2009.00979.x.

49. D. P. Davies, "Cot Death in Hong Kong: A Rare Problem?" *Lancet* 2, no. 8468 (1985): 1346–49; N. N. Lee et al., "Sudden Infant Death Syndrome in Hong Kong: Confirmation of Low Incidence," *BMJ* 298, no. 6675 (1989): 721.

50. Davies, "Cot Death in Hong Kong," 1347.

51. E. A. Nelson et al., "International Child Care Practices Study: Infant Sleeping Environment," *Early Human Development* 62, no. 1 (2001): 43–55.

52. P. G. Tuohy, A. M. Counsell, and D. C. Geddis, "Sociodemographic Factors Associated with Sleeping Position and Location," *Archives of Disease in Childhood* 69, no. 6 (1993): 664–66; S. Farooqi, I. J. Perry, and D. G. Beevers, "Ethnic Differences in Infant-Rearing Practices and Their Possible Relationship to the

Incidence of Sudden Infant Death Syndrome (SIDS)," *Paediatric and Perinatal Epidemiology* 7, no. 3 (1993): 245–52; M. Gantley, D. P. Davies, and A. Murcott, "Sudden Infant Death Syndrome: Links with Infant Care Practices," *BMJ* 306, no. 6869 (1993): 16–20.

53. Rachel Y. Moon, interview with the author, April 15, 2013.

54. Shapiro-Mendoza et al., "Epidemiology of Sudden Infant Death Syndrome and Sudden Unexpected Infant Deaths."

55. Taylor et al., "International Comparison of Sudden Unexpected Death in Infancy Rates."

56. R. G. Carpenter et al., "Sudden Unexplained Infant Death in 20 Regions in Europe: Case Control Study," *Lancet* 363, no. 9404 (2004): 185–91.

57. D. Tappin, R. Ecob, and H. Brooke, "Bedsharing, Roomsharing, and Sudden Infant Death Syndrome in Scotland: A Case-Control Study," *Journal of Pediatrics* 147, no. 1 (2005): 32–37, doi:10.1016/j.jpeds.2005.01.035; P. S. Blair et al., "Hazardous Cosleeping Environments and Risk Factors Amenable to Change: Case-Control Study of SIDS in South West England," *BMJ* 339 (2009): b3666, doi:10.1136/bmj.b3666.

58. AAP Task Force on Sudden Infant Death Syndrome, "SIDS and Other Sleep-Related Infant Deaths."

59. PHA of Canada, *Joint Statement on Safe Sleep*; New Zealand Ministry of Health, "Keeping Baby Safe in Bed: The First 6 Weeks," last updated January 8, 2020, https://www.health.govt.nz/your-health/pregnancy-and-kids /first-year/first-6-weeks/keeping-baby-safe-bed-first-6-weeks; The Lullaby Trust, *Safer Sleep: Saving Babies Lives, A Guide for Professionals* (London: Public Health England, n.d.), https://www.lullabytrust.org.uk/product/a-guide-for -professionals-safer-sleep-saving-babies-lives; R. Y. Moon and F. R. Hauck, "Are There Long-Term Consequences of Room-Sharing During Infancy?" *Pediatrics* 140, no. 1 (2017): e20171323.

60. R. Y. Moon and AAP Task Force on Sudden Infant Death Syndrome, "SIDS and Other Sleep-Related Infant Deaths: Evidence Base for 2016 Updated Recommendations for a Safe Infant Sleeping Environment."

61. Small, *Our Babies, Ourselves*.

62. J. J. McKenna, S. S. Mosko, and C. A. Richard, "Bedsharing Promotes Breastfeeding," *Pediatrics* 100 (1997): 214–19; S. S. Mosko et al., "Infant Sleep Architecture during Bedsharing and Possible Implications for SIDS," *Sleep* 19, no. 9 (1996): 677–84; S. S. Mosko, C. A. Richard, and J. J. McKenna, "Infant Arousals during Mother-Infant Bed Sharing: Implications for Infant Sleep and Sudden Infant Death Syndrome Research," Pediatrics 100, no. 5 (1997): 841–49, doi:10.1542/peds.100.5.841; S. S. Mosko, C. A. Richard, and J. J. McKenna, "Maternal Sleep and Arousals during Bedsharing with Infants," *Sleep* 20 (1997): 142–50.

63. J. J. McKenna and T. McDade, "Why Babies Should Never Sleep Alone:

A Review of the Co-Sleeping Controversy in Relation to SID S, Bedsharing and Breast Feeding," *Paediatric Respiratory Reviews* 6 (2005): 134–52, doi:10.1016 /j.prrv.2005.03.006.

64. Blair et al., "Bed-Sharing in the Absence of Hazardous Circumstances."

65. K. Hinde and L. A. Milligan, "Primate Milk: Proximate Mechanisms and Ultimate Perspectives," *Evolutionary Anthropology: Issues, News, and Reviews* 20, no. 1 (2011): 9–23, doi:10.1002/evan.20289.

66. Ball et al., "Bed-Sharing by Breastfeeding Mothers"; H. L. Ball, "Breast-feeding, Bed-Sharing, and Infant Sleep," *Birth* 30, no. 3 (2003): 181–88; M. L. Bovbjerg et al., "Women Who Bedshare More Frequently at 14 Weeks Postpartum Subsequently Report Longer Durations of Breastfeeding," *Journal of Midwifery & Women's Health* 63, no. 4 (2018): 418–24; Y. Huang et al., "Influence of Bedsharing Activity on Breastfeeding Duration among US Mothers," *JAMA Pediatrics* 167, no. 11 (2013): 1038–44, doi:10.1001/jamapediatrics.2013. 2632.

67. P. S. Blair, J. Heron, and P. J. Fleming, "Relationship between Bed Sharing and Breastfeeding: Longitudinal, Population-Based Analysis," *Pediatrics* 126, no. 5 (2010): e1119-26, doi:10.1542/peds.2010-1277.

68. L. A. Smith et al., "Infant Sleep Location and Breastfeeding Practices in the United States, 2011-2014," *Academic Pediatrics* 16, no. 6 (2016): 540–49.

69. Baddock et al., "The Influence of Bed-Sharing on Infant Physiology, Breastfeeding and Behaviour"

70. K. Kendall-Tackett, Z. Cong, and T. W. Hale, "Mother-Infant Sleep Locations and Nighttime Feeding Behavior," *Clinical Lactation* 1, no. 1 (2010): 27–30.

71. C. McGarvey et al., "Factors Relating to the Infant's Last Sleep Environment in Sudden Infant Death Syndrome in the Republic of Ireland," *Archives of Disease in Childhood* 88, no. 12 (2003): 1058–64; P. J. Fleming et al., "Environment of Infants during Sleep and Risk of the Sudden Infant Death Syndrome: Results of 1993–5 Case-Control Study for Confidential Inquiry into Stillbirths and Deaths in Infancy," *BMJ* 313, no. 7051 (1996): 191–95, doi:10.1136/bmj. 313.7051.191.

72. Moon and AAP Task Force on Sudden Infant Death Syndrome, "SIDS and Other Sleep-Related Infant Deaths"; F. R. Hauck et al., "Breastfeeding and Reduced Risk of Sudden Infant Death Syndrome: A Meta-analysis," *Pediatrics* 128, no. 1 (2011): 103–10, doi:10.1542/peds.2010-3000; J. M. D. Thompson et al., "Duration of Breastfeeding and Risk of SIDS: An Individual Participant Data Meta-analysis," *Pediatrics* 140, no. 5 (2017): e20171324.

73. Hauck et al., "Breastfeeding and Reduced Risk"; R. S. C. Horne et al., "Comparison of Evoked Arousability in Breast and Formula Fed Infants," *Archives of Disease in Childhood* 89, no. 1 (2004): 22–25.

74. Moon, interview, 2013.

7. IN SEARCH OF A GOOD NIGHT'S SLEEP

1. S.-S. Yoo, et al. "The Human Emotional Brain without Sleep: A Prefrontal Amygdala Disconnect," *Current Biology* 17, no. 20 (2007): R877–78; S.-S. Yoo, et al., "A Deficit in the Ability to Form New Human Memories without Sleep," *Nature Neuroscience* 10, no. 3 (2007): 385–92; H. P. A. Van Dongen et al., "The Cumulative Cost of Additional Wakefulness: Dose-Response Effects on Neurobehavioral Functions and Sleep Physiology from Chronic Sleep Restriction and Total Sleep Deprivation," *Sleep* 26, no. 2 (2003): 117–26; G. N. Pires et al., "Effects of Acute Sleep Deprivation on State Anxiety Levels: A Systematic Review and Meta-analysis," *Sleep Medicine* 24 (August 2016): 109–18.

2. Centers for Disease Control and Prevention (CDC), "Drowsy Driving: 19 States and the District of Columbia, 2009–2010," *Morbidity and Mortality Weekly Report (MMWR)* 61, no. 51 (2013): 1033-37, https://www.cdc.gov /mmwr/preview/mmwrhtml/mm6151a1.htm; S. R. Patel et al., "Association between Reduced Sleep and Weight Gain in Women," *American Journal of Epidemiology* 164, no. 10 (2006): 947–54; A. A. Prather et al., "Behaviorally Assessed Sleep and Susceptibility to the Common Cold," *Sleep* 38, no. 9 (2015): 1353–59.

3. F. Cook et al., "Depression and Anger in Fathers of Unsettled Infants: A Community Cohort Study," *Journal of Paediatrics and Child Health* 53, no. 2 (2017): 131–35; A. M. Medina, C. L. Lederhos, and T. A. Lillis, "Sleep Disruption and Decline in Marital Satisfaction across the Transition to Parenthood," *Families, Systems, and Health* 27, no. 2 (2009): 153–60, doi:10.1037/a0015762; M. L. Okun, "Disturbed Sleep and Postpartum Depression," *Current Psychiatry Reports* 18, no. 7 (2016): 66, 10.1007/s11920-016-0705-2.

4. L. E. Philbrook and D. M. Teti, "Bidirectional Associations between Bedtime Parenting and Infant Sleep: Parenting Quality, Parenting Practices, and Their Interaction," *Journal of Family Psychology* 30, no. 4 (2016): 431–41.

5. M. Kahn et al., "Effects of One Night of Induced Night-Wakings versus Sleep Restriction on Sustained Attention and Mood: A Pilot Study," *Sleep Medicine* 15, no. 7 (2014): 825–32.

6. L. Tikotzky, A. Sadeh, and T. Glickman-Gavrieli, "Infant Sleep and Paternal Involvement in Infant Caregiving During the First 6 Months of Life," *Journal of Pediatric Psychology* 36, no. 1 (2011): 36–46; L. Tikotzky, "Infant Sleep Development from 3 to 6 Months Postpartum: Links with Maternal Sleep and Paternal Involvement," *Monographs for the Society for Research in Child Development* 80, no. 1 (2015): 107–24.

7. I. Iglowstein et al., "Sleep Duration from Infancy to Adolescence: Reference Values and Generational Trends," *Pediatrics* 111, no. 2 (2003): 302–7.

8. B. Cavell, "Gastric Emptying in Infants Fed Human Milk or Infant Formula," *Acta Paediatrica Scandinavica* 70 (1981): 639–41; E. Sievers et al., "Feeding

Patterns in Breast-Fed and Formula-Fed Infants," *Annals of Nutrition and Metabolism* 46, no. 6 (2002): 243–48, doi:10.1159/000066498.

9. M. De Carvalho, S. Robertson, and A. Friedman, "Effect of Frequent Breast-Feeding on Early Milk Production and Infant Weight Gain," *Pediatrics* 72, no. 3 (1983): 307–11.

10. A. W. de Weerd and R. A. van den Bossche, "The Development of Sleep during the First Months of Life," *Sleep Medicine Reviews* 7, no. 2 (2003): 179–91, doi:10.1053/smrv.2002.0198.

11. de Weerd and van den Bossche, "The Development of Sleep"; T. F. Anders, "Organization and Development of Sleep in Early Life," in *Encyclopedia on Early Childhood Development*, ed. R. E. Tremblay, M. Boivin, and R. Peters (Montreal: Centre of Excellence for Early Childhood Development and Strategic Knowledge Cluster on Early Child Development, 2010), 1–8, http://child-encyclopedia.com/pages/PDF/sleeping_behaviour/according-experts/organization-and-development-sleep-early-life.

12. de Weerd and van den Bossche, "The Development of Sleep"; Anders, "Organization and Development of Sleep"; S. Coons and C. Guilleminault, "Development of Sleep-Wake Patterns and Non-Rapid Eye Movement Sleep Stages during the First Six Months of Life in Normal Infants," *Pediatrics* 69, no. 6 (1982): 793–98.

13. Sievers et al., "Feeding Patterns in Breast-Fed and Formula-Fed Infants."

14. R. Y. Moore, "Suprachiasmatic Nucleus in Sleep-Wake Regulation," *Sleep Medicine* 8 (2007): 27–33, doi:10.1016/j.sleep.2007.10.003.

15. K. McGraw et al., "The Development of Circadian Rhythms in a Human Infant," *Sleep* 22, no. 3 (1999): 303–10.

16. McGraw et al., "The Development of Circadian Rhythms."

17. J. Ardura et al., "Emergence and Evolution of the Circadian Rhythm of Melatonin in Children," *Hormone Research* 59, no. 2 (2003): 66–72, doi:10.1159/000068571; M. Mirmiran, Y. G. Maas, and R. L. Ariagno, "Development of Fetal and Neonatal Sleep and Circadian Rhythms," *Sleep Medicine Reviews* 7, no. 4 (2003): 321–34, doi:10.1053/smrv.2002.0243; R. J. Custodio et al., "The Emergence of the Cortisol Circadian Rhythm in Monozygotic and Dizygotic Twin Infants: The Twin-Pair Synchrony," *Clinical Endocrinology* 66, no. 2 (2007): 192–97, doi:10.1111/j.1365-2265.2006.02706.x.

18. A. Cohen Engler et al., "Breastfeeding May Improve Nocturnal Sleep and Reduce Infantile Colic: Potential Role of Breast Milk Melatonin," *European Journal of Pediatrics* 171, no. 4 (2011): 729–32, doi:10.1007/s00431-011-1659-3; J. Cubero et al., "The Circadian Rhythm of Tryptophan in Breast Milk Affects the Rhythms of 6-Sulfatoxymelatonin and Sleep in Newborn," *Neuroendocrinology Letters* 26, no. 6 (2005): 657–61; H. Illnerov., M. Buresov., and J. Presl, "Melatonin Rhythm in Human Milk," *Journal of Clinical Endocrinology and Metabolism* 77, no. 3 (1993): 838–41.

19. Y. Harrison, "The Relationship between Daytime Exposure to Light and Night-Time Sleep in 6–12-Week-Old Infants," *Journal of Sleep Research* 13 (2004): 345–52, doi:10.1111/j.1365-2869.2004.00435.x.

20. I. C. McMillen et al., "Development of Circadian Sleep-Wake Rhythms in Preterm and Full-Term Infants," *Pediatric Research* 29, no. 4 (1991): 381–84.

21. McGraw et al., "The Development of Circadian Rhythms."

22. Coons and Guilleminault, "Development of Sleep-Wake Patterns."

23. T. Field et al., "Mothers Massaging Their Newborns with Lotion versus No Lotion Enhances Mothers' and Newborns' Sleep," *Infant Behavior and Development* 45, Part A (2016): 31–37.

24. J. A. Mindell and A. A. Williamson, "Benefits of a Bedtime Routine in Young Children: Sleep, Development, and Beyond," *Sleep Medicine Reviews* 40 (2018): 93–108.

25. J. A. Mindell et al., "A Nightly Bedtime Routine: Impact on Sleep in Young Children and Maternal Mood," *Sleep* 32, no. 5 (2009): 599–606.

26. H. L. Ball, "Breastfeeding, Bed-Sharing, and Infant Sleep," *Birth* 30, no. 3 (2003): 181–88; J. M. T. Henderson et al., "Sleeping through the Night: The Consolidation of Self-Regulated Sleep across the First Year of Life," *Pediatrics* 126, no. 5 (2010): e1081-87, doi:10.1542/peds.2010-0976; J. M. T. Henderson, K. G. France, and N. M. Blampied, "The Consolidation of Infants' Nocturnal Sleep across the First Year of Life," *Sleep Medicine Reviews* 15, no. 4 (2011): 211–20; J. A. Mindell et al., "Development of Infant and Toddler Sleep Patterns: Real-World Data from a Mobile Application," *Journal of Sleep Research* 25, no. 5 (2016): 508–16; B. C. Galland et al., "Normal Sleep Patterns in Infants and Children: A Systematic Review of Observational Studies," *Sleep Medicine Reviews* 16, no. 3 (2012): 213–22.

27. E. Touchette et al., "Genetic and Environmental Influences on Daytime and Nighttime Sleep Duration in Early Childhood," *Pediatrics* 131, no. 6 (2013): e1874-80, doi:10.1542/peds.2012-2284.

28. T. F. Anders and M. Keener, "Developmental Course of Nighttime Sleep-Wake Patterns in Full-Term and Premature Infants during the First Year of Life. I," *Sleep* 8, no. 3 (1985): 173–92; J. Eaton-Evans and A. E. Dugdale, "Sleep Patterns of Infants in the First Year of Life," *Archives of Disease in Childhood* 63, no. 6 (1988): 647–49; C. W. DeLeon and K. H. Karraker, "Intrinsic and Extrinsic Factors Associated with Night Waking in 9-Month-Old Infants," *Infant Behavior and Development* 30 (December 2007): 596–605, doi:10.1016/j.infbeh.2007. 03.009; A. Scher, R. Epstein, and E. Tirosh, "Stability and Changes in Sleep Regulation: A Longitudinal Study from 3 Months to 3 Years," *International Journal of Behavioral Development* 28, no. 3 (2004): 268–74, doi:10.1080/01650 250344000505.

29. A. Scher and D. V. Cohen, "Sleep as a Mirror of Developmental Transitions in Infancy: The Case of Crawling," *Monographs of the Society for Research in Child Development* 80, no.1 (2015): 70–88.

30. K. So, T. M. Adamson, and R. S. Horne, "The Use of Actigraphy for Assessment of the Development of Sleep/Wake Patterns in Infants during the First 12 Months of Life," *Journal of Sleep Research* 16, no. 2 (2007): 181–87.

31. National Sleep Foundation, *2004 Children and Sleep*, accessed July 7, 2013, http://www.sleepfoundation.org/professionals/sleep-america-polls/2004-children-and-sleep.

32. Ball, "Breastfeeding, Bed-Sharing, and Infant Sleep."

33. Mindell et al., "Development of Infant and Toddler Sleep Patterns."

34. Mindell et al., "Development of Infant and Toddler Sleep Patterns"; Galland et al., "Normal Sleep Patterns in Infants and Children."

35. J. J. McKenna and L. E. Volpe, "Sleeping with Baby: An Internet-Based Sampling of Parental Experiences, Choices, Perceptions, and Interpretations in a Western Industrialized Context," *Infant and Child Development* 16, no. 4 (2007): 359–85, doi:10.1002/icd.525.

36. S. A. Baddock et al., "The Influence of Bed-Sharing on Infant Physiology, Breastfeeding and Behaviour: A Systematic Review," *Sleep Medicine Reviews* 43 (February 2019): 106–17.

37. McKenna and Volpe, "Sleeping with Baby"; F. R. Hauck et al., "Infant Sleeping Arrangements and Practices during the First Year of Life," *Pediatrics* 122, suppl. 2 (2008): S113-20, doi:10.1542/peds.2008-1315o; M. F. Elias et al., "Sleep/Wake Patterns of Breast-Fed Infants in the First 2 Years of Life," *Pediatrics* 77, no. 3 (1986): 322–29.

38. Hauck et al., "Infant Sleeping Arrangements and Practices during the First Year of Life."

39. Elias et al., "Sleep/Wake Patterns of Breast-Fed Infants."

40. Elias et al., "Sleep/Wake Patterns of Breast-Fed Infants."

41. J. A. Mindell et al., "Cross-Cultural Differences in Infant and Toddler Sleep," *Sleep Medicine* 11, no. 3 (2010): 274–80, doi:10.1016/j.sleep.2009.04.012.

42. A. N. Crittenden et al., "Infant Co-sleeping Patterns and Maternal Sleep Quality among Hadza Hunter-Gatherers," *Sleep Health* 4, no. 6 (2018): 527–34.

43. Mindell et al., "Development of Infant and Toddler Sleep Patterns."

44. I. M. Paul et al., "Mother-Infant Room-Sharing and Sleep Outcomes in the INSIGHT Study," *Pediatrics* 140, no. 1 (2017): e20170122, doi:10.1542/peds.2017-0122.

45. Mindell et al., "Development of Infant and Toddler Sleep Patterns"; Paul et al., "Mother-Infant Room-Sharing."

46. E. Volkovich et al., "Mother-Infant Sleep Patterns and Parental Functioning of Room-Sharing and Solitary-Sleeping Families: A Longitudinal Study from 3 to 18 Months," *Sleep* 41, no. 2 (2018): 1-14, doi:10.1093/sleep/zsx207.

47. D. M. Teti et al., "Sleep Arrangements, Parent-Infant Sleep during the First Year, and Family Functioning," *Developmental Psychology* 52, no. 8 (2016): 1169–81.

48. T. Pinilla and L. L. Birch, "Help Me Make It through the Night: Behav-

ioral Entrainment of Breast-Fed Infants' Sleep Patterns," *Pediatrics* 91, no. 2 (February 1993): 436–44.

49. V. R. Mileva-Seitz et al., "Association between Infant Nighttime-Sleep Location and Attachment Security: No Easy Verdict," *Infant Mental Health Journal* 37, no. 1 (2016): 5–16.

50. Douglas M. Teti, interview with the author, February 11, 2014; D. M. Teti et al., "Maternal Emotional Availability at Bedtime Predicts Infant Sleep Quality," *Journal of Family Psychology* 24, no. 3 (2010): 307–15, doi:10.1037/a0019306.

51. Leita Dzubay, interview with the author, August 23, 2012.

52. Thomas F. Anders, interview with the author, April 26, 2013.

53. Anders, interview, 2013.

54. T. F. Anders, "Home-Recorded Sleep in 2- and 9-Month-Old Infants," *Journal of the American Academy of Child Psychiatry* 17, no. 3 (1978): 421–32.

55. T. F. Anders, "Night-Waking in Infants during the First Year of Life," *Pediatrics* 63, no. 6 (1979): 860–64.

56. Anders and Keener, "Developmental Course of Nighttime Sleep-Wake Patterns."

57. Anders, interview, 2013.

58. T. F. Anders, L. F. Halpern, and J. Hua, "Sleeping through the Night: A Developmental Perspective," *Pediatrics* 90, no. 4 (1992): 554–60.

59. Anders, Halpern, and Hua, "Sleeping through the Night"; W. Anuntaseree et al., "Night Waking in Thai Infants at 3 Months of Age: Association between Parental Practices and Infant Sleep," *Sleep Medicine* 9, no. 5 (2008): 564–71, doi:10.1016/j.sleep.2007.07.009; M. M. Burnham et al., "Nighttime Sleep-Wake Patterns and Self-Soothing from Birth to One Year of Age: A Longitudinal Intervention Study," *Journal of Child Psychology and Psychiatry* 43, no. 6 (2002): 713–25; É. Touchette et al., "Factors Associated with Fragmented Sleep at Night across Early Childhood," *Archives of Pediatrics and Adolescent Medicine* 159, no. 3 (2005): 242; J. A. Mindell et al., "Parental Behaviors and Sleep Outcomes in Infants and Toddlers: A Cross-Cultural Comparison," *Sleep Medicine* 11, no. 4 (2010): 393–99, doi:10.1016/j.sleep.2009.11.011.

60. Anders, interview, 2013.

61. Burnham et al., "Nighttime Sleep-Wake Patterns."

62. M. A. Keener, C. H. Zeanah, and T. F. Anders, "Infant Temperament, Sleep Organization, and Nighttime Parental Interventions," *Pediatrics* 81, no. 6 (1988): 762–71.

63. I. St James-Roberts et al., "Video Evidence that Parenting Methods Predict which Infants Develop Long Night-Time Sleep Periods by Three Months of Age," *Primary Health Care Research & Development* 18, no. 3 (2017): 212–26.

64. Pinilla and Birch, "Help Me Make It through the Night"; A. Wolfson, P. Lacks, and A. Futterman, "Effects of Parent Training on Infant Sleeping Pat-

terns, Parents' Stress, and Perceived Parental Competence," *Journal of Consulting and Clinical Psychology* 60, no. 1 (1992): 41–48.

65. W. Sears et al., *The Baby Book, Revised Edition: Everything You Need to Know About Your Baby from Birth to Age Two* (New York: Little, Brown, 2013), 334.

66. M. B. Ramamurthy et al., "Effect of Current Breastfeeding on Sleep Patterns in Infants from Asia-Pacific Region," *Journal of Paediatrics and Child Health* 48, no. 8 (2012): 669–74, doi:10.1111/j.1440-1754.2012.02453.x.

67. S. Latz, A. W. Wolf, and B. Lozoff, "Cosleeping in Context: Sleep Practices and Problems in Young Children in Japan and the United States," *Archives of Pediatrics and Adolescent Medicine* 153, no. 4 (1999): 339–46.

68. L. Tikotzky and A. Sadeh, "Maternal Sleep-Related Cognitions and Infant Sleep: A Longitudinal Study from Pregnancy through the 1st Year," *Child Development* 80, no. 3 (2009): 860–74.

69. Tikotzky and Sadeh, "Maternal Sleep-Related Cognitions and Infant Sleep."

70. L. Tikotzky and L. Shaashua, "Infant Sleep and Early Parental Sleep-Related Cognitions Predict Sleep in Pre-School Children," *Sleep Medicine* 13, no. 2 (2012): 185–92, doi:10.1016/j.sleep.2011.07.013.

71. Tikotzky and Sadeh, "Maternal Sleep-Related Cognitions and Infant Sleep," 871.

72. Anders, Halpern, and Hua, "Sleeping through the Night."

73. Touchette et al., "Genetic and Environmental Influences."

74. A. Callahan, "How I Helped My Baby Learn to Sleep," *Janet Lansbury, Elevating Child Care*, February 19, 2016, https://www.janetlansbury.com/2016/02/how-i-helped-my-baby-learn-to-sleep-guest-post-by-alice-callahan-phd.

75. A. Reuter et al., "A Systematic Review of Prevention and Treatment of Infant Behavioural Sleep Problems," *Acta Paediatrica* 109, no. 9 (2020): 1717-32, doi:10.1111/apa.15182; L. J. Meltzer and J. A. Mindell, "Systematic Review and Meta-Analysis of Behavioral Interventions for Pediatric Insomnia," *Journal of Pediatric Psychology* 39, no. 8 (2014): 932–48; M. Gradisar et al., "Behavioral Interventions for Infant Sleep Problems: A Randomized Controlled Trial," *Pediatrics* 137, no. 6 (2016): e20151486, 10.1542/peds.2015-1486; W. A. Hall et al., "A Randomized Controlled Trial of an Intervention for Infants' Behavioral Sleep Problems," *BMC Pediatrics* 15 (2015): 181, doi:10.1186/s12887-015-0492-7.

76. Jodi A. Mindell, email to the author, May 6, 2013.

77. D. Narvaez, "Dangers of 'Crying It Out,'" *Moral Landscapes* (blog), *Psychology Today*, December 11, 2011, http://www.psychologytoday.com/blog/moral-landscapes/201112/dangers-crying-it-out.

78. J. P. Shonkoff and A. S. Garner, "The Lifelong Effects of Early Childhood Adversity and Toxic Stress," *Pediatrics* 129, no. 1 (2012): e232-46, doi:10.1542/peds.2011-2663.

79. H. Hiscock et al., "Long-term Mother and Child Mental Health Effects of a Population-based Infant Sleep Intervention: Cluster-Randomized, Controlled Trial," *Pediatrics* 122, no. 3 (2008): e621-27; A. M. Price et al., "Five-Year Follow-up of Harms and Benefits of Behavioral Infant Sleep Intervention: Randomized Trial," *Pediatrics* 130, no. 4 (2012): 643-51, doi:10.1542/peds.2011-3467.

80. Gradisar et al., "Behavioral Interventions for Infant Sleep Problems."

81. W. Middlemiss et al., "Asynchrony of Mother-Infant Hypothalamic-Pituitary-Adrenal Axis Activity Following Extinction of Infant Crying Responses Induced during the Transition to Sleep," *Early Human Development* 88, no. 4 (2011): 227–32.

82. Anders, interview, 2013.

8. MILK AND MOTHERHOOD

1. Jordan P. Green, interview with the author, May 25, 2014; Cheryl R. L. Green, interview with the author, May 25, 2014.

2. J. P. Green, interview, 2014.

3. C. R. L. Green, interview, 2014.

4. S. J. Fomon, "History," in *Nutrition of Normal Infants* 6–14 (St. Louis, MO: Mosby–Year Book, 1993), 6-14; S. J. Fomon, "Infant Feeding in the 20th Century: Formula and Beikost," *Journal of Nutrition* 131, no. 2 (2001): 409-20S; D. Thulier, "Breastfeeding in America: A History of Influencing Factors," *Journal of Human Lactation* 25, no. 1 (2009): 85–94, doi:10.1177/0890334408324452.

5. Thulier, "Breastfeeding in America"; M. Obladen, "Pap, Gruel, and Panada: Early Approaches to Artificial Infant Feeding," *Neonatology* 105, no. 4 (2014): 267–74.

6. Fomon, "History"; Obladen, "Pap, Gruel, and Panada."

7. B. Lozoff, "Birth and 'Bonding' in Non-Industrial Societies," *Developmental Medicine and Child Neurology* 25, no. 5 (1983): 595–600.

8. Fomon, "History."

9. Fomon, "History."

10. Fomon, "History."

11. Thulier, "Breastfeeding in America"; E. E. Stevens, T. E. Patrick, and R. Pickler, "A History of Infant Feeding," *Journal of Perinatal Education* 18, no. 2 (2009): 32–39.

12. T. Cassidy, "The Hut, the Home, and the Hospital," in *Birth: The Surprising History of How We Are Born* (New York, Atlantic Monthly Press, 2006), 54-63; E. Temkin, "Rooming-In: Redesigning Hospitals and Motherhood in Cold War America," *Bulletin of the History of Medicine* 76, no. 2 (2002): 271–98, doi:10.1353/bhm.2002.0101.

13. Fomon, "Infant Feeding in the 20th Century"; D. Thulier, "Breastfeeding in America."

14. M. Van Den Driessche, "Gastric Emptying in Formula-Fed and Breast-Fed

Infants Measured with the 13C-Octanoic Acid Breath Test," *Journal of Pediatric Gastroenterology* 29, no. 1 (1999): 46–51.

15. H. Lee et al., "Compositional Dynamics of the Milk Fat Globule and Its Role in Infant Development," *Frontiers in Pediatrics* 6 (October 2018): 313, doi: 10.3389/fped.2018.00313.

16. B. Lönnerdal, "Bioactive Proteins in Breast Milk," *Journal of Paediatrics and Child Health* 49, suppl. 1 (2013): 1–7, doi:10.1111/jpc.12104; O. Ballard and A. L. Morrow, "Human Milk Composition," *Pediatric Clinics of North America* 60, no. 1 (2013): 49–74, doi:10.1016/j.pcl.2012.10.002; L. Bode et al., "Understanding the Mother-Breastmilk-Infant 'Triad,'" *Science* 367, no. 6482 (2020): 1070–72.

17. L. Fernández et al., "The Microbiota of the Human Mammary Ecosystem," *Frontiers in Cellular and Infection Microbiology* 10 (2020): 586667, https://doi.org/10.3389/fcimb.2020.586667; V. Triantis, L. Bode, and R. J. J.van Neerven, "Immunological Effects of Human Milk Oligosaccharides," *Frontiers in Pediatrics* 6 (2018): 190, doi: 10.3389/fped.2018.00190.

18. L. R. Mitoulas et al., "Variation in Fat, Lactose and Protein in Human Milk over 24h and throughout the First Year of Lactation," *British Journal of Nutrition* 88, no. 1 (2002): 29–37; D. Katzer et al., "Melatonin Concentrations and Antioxidative Capacity of Human Breast Milk According to Gestational Age and the Time of Day," *Journal of Human Lactation* 32, no. 4 (2016): NP105–10; S. Pundir et al., "Variation of Human Milk Glucocorticoids over 24 Hour Period," *Journal of Mammary Gland Biology and Neoplasia* 22, no. 1 (2017): 85–92.

19. M. S. Kramer et al., "Promotion of Breastfeeding Intervention Trial (PROBIT): A Randomized Trial in the Republic of Belarus," *JAMA* 285, no. 4 (January 24, 2001): 413–20, doi:10.1001/jama.285.4.413.

20. G. Der, G. D. Batty, and I. J. Deary, "Effect of Breast Feeding on Intelligence in Children: Prospective Study, Sibling Pairs Analysis, and Meta-analysis," *BMJ* 333, no. 7575 (2006): 945, doi:10.1136/bmj.38978.699583.55.

21. Der, Batty, and Deary, "Effect of Breast Feeding on Intelligence."

22. M. S. Kramer, "Methodological Challenges in Studying Long-Term Effects of Breast-Feeding," in *Breast-Feeding: Early Influences on Later Health*, ed. G. Goldberg et al., Advances in Experimental Medicine and Biology 639 (Dordrecht: Springer Netherlands, 2009), 121–33.

23. Kramer et al., "Promotion of Breastfeeding Intervention Trial (PROBIT)."

24. L. Duijts, M. K. Ramadhani, and H. A. Moll, "Breastfeeding Protects against Infectious Diseases during Infancy in Industrialized Countries: A Systematic Review," *Maternal and Child Nutrition* 5, no. 3 (2009): 199–210, doi:10.1111/j.1740-8709.2008.00176.x; L. Duijts et al., "Prolonged and Exclusive Breastfeeding Reduces the Risk of Infectious Diseases in Infancy," *Pediatrics* 126, no. 1 (2010): e18–25, doi:10.1542/peds.2008-3256; M. A. Quigley et al., "Exclusive Breastfeeding Duration and Infant Infection," *European Journal*

of Clinical Nutrition 70, no. 12 (2016): 1420–27; S. Ip et al., "A Summary of the Agency for Healthcare Research and Quality's Evidence Report on Breastfeeding in Developed Countries," *Breastfeeding Medicine* 4, suppl. 1 (2009): S17–30.

25. N. M. Frank et al., "The Relationship between Breastfeeding and Reported Respiratory and Gastrointestinal Infection Rates in Young Children," *BMC Pediatrics* 19, no. 1 (2019): 339.

26. Duijts, Ramadhani, and Moll, "Breastfeeding Protects against Infectious Diseases"; Duijts et al., "Prolonged and Exclusive Breastfeeding"; Quigley et al., "Exclusive Breastfeeding"; Ip et al., "A Summary"; Frank et al., "The Relationship between Breastfeeding and Reported Respiratory and Gastrointestinal Infection Rates"; A. Kørvel-Hanquist et al., "Risk Factors of Early Otitis Media in the Danish National Birth Cohort," *PLoS ONE* 11, no. 11 (2016): e0171901, doi: 10.1371/journal.pone.0166465; G. Bowatte et al., "Breastfeeding and Childhood Acute Otitis Media: A Systematic Review and Meta-analysis," *Acta Paediatrica* 104, no. 467 (2015): 85–95.

27. Frank et al., "The Relationship between Breastfeeding and Reported Respiratory and Gastrointestinal Infection Rates"; Bowatte et al., "Breastfeeding and Childhood Acute Otitis Media"; C. M. Fisk et al., "Breastfeeding and Reported Morbidity during Infancy: Findings from the Southampton Women's Survey," *Maternal and Child Nutrition* 7, no. 1 (2011): 61–70, doi:10.1111/j.1740-8709.2010.00241.x; M. A. Quigley, Y. J. Kelly, and A. Sacker, "Breastfeeding and Hospitalization for Diarrheal and Respiratory Infection in the United Kingdom Millennium Cohort Study," *Pediatrics* 119, no. 4 (2007): e837–42, doi:10.1542/peds.2006-2256; M. Tarrant et al., "Breast-Feeding and Childhood Hospitalizations for Infections," *Epidemiology* 21, no. 6 (2010): 847–54, doi:10.1097/EDE.0b013e3181f55803.

28. A. A. Breakey et al., "Illness in Breastfeeding Infants Relates to Concentration of Lactoferrin and Secretory Immunoglobulin A in Mother's Milk," *Evolution, Medicine, and Public Health* 2015, no. 1 (2015): 21–31; F. Hassiotou et al., "Maternal and Infant Infections Stimulate a Rapid Leukocyte Response in Breastmilk," *Clinical & Translational Immunology* 2, no. 4 (2013): e3, doi: 10.1038/cti.2013.1.

29. Bode et al., "Understanding the Mother-Breastmilk-Infant 'Triad,'"; Triantis, Bode, and van Neerven, "Immunological Effects of Human Milk Oligosaccharides."

30. Bode et al., "Understanding the Mother-Breastmilk-Infant 'Triad,'"; M. L. Power and J. Schulkin, "Milk Protects," in *Milk: The Biology of Lactation* (Baltimore: Johns Hopkins University Press, 2016): 159–74.

31. Bowatte et al., "Breastfeeding and Childhood Acute Otitis Media"; S. W. Abrahams and M. H. Labbok, "Breastfeeding and Otitis Media: A Review of Recent Evidence," *Current Allergy and Asthma Reports* 11, no. 6 (2011): 508–12, doi:10.1007/s11882-011-0218-3; S. B. Tully, Y. Bar-Haim, and R. L. Bradley,

"Abnormal Tympanography after Supine Bottle Feeding," *Journal of Pediatrics* 126, no. 6 (1995): S105–11; K. M. Boone, S. R. Geraghty, and S. A. Keim, "Feeding at the Breast and Expressed Milk Feeding: Associations with Otitis Media and Diarrhea in Infants," *Journal of Pediatrics* 174 (July 2016): 118–25.

32. T. R. Coker et al., "Diagnosis, Microbial Epidemiology, and Antibiotic Treatment of Acute Otitis Media in Children: A Systematic Review," *JAMA* 304, no. 19 (2010): 2161–69.

33. Centers for Disease Control and Prevention (CDC), "Antibiotic Resistance Questions and Answers," last updated January 31, 2020, https://www.cdc.gov /antibiotic-use/community/about/antibiotic-resistance-faqs.html.

34. N. Shehab et al., "US Emergency Department Visits for Outpatient Adverse Drug Events, 2013–2014," *JAMA* 316, no. 20 (2016): 2115–25.

35. J. M. D. Thompson et al., "Duration of Breastfeeding and Risk of SIDS: An Individual Participant Data Meta-analysis," *Pediatrics* 140, no. 5 (2017): e20171324.

36. M. Quigley, N. D. Embleton, and W. McGuire, "Formula versus Donor Breast Milk for Feeding Preterm or Low Birth Weight Infants," *Cochrane Database of Systematic Reviews*, no. 6 (2018): CD002971, doi: 10.1002/14651858. CD002971.pub4.

37. C. G. Colen and D. M. Ramey, "Is Breast Truly Best? Estimating the Effects of Breastfeeding on Long-term Child Health and Wellbeing in the United States Using Sibling Comparisons," *Social Science and Medicine* 109 (May 2014): 55–65, doi:10.1016/j.socscimed.2014.01.027.

38. L. G. Smithers, M. S. Kramer, and J. W. Lynch, "Effects of Breastfeeding on Obesity and Intelligence: Causal Insights from Different Study Designs," *JAMA Pediatrics* 169, no. 8 (2015): 707–8.

39. J. Grose, "New Study Confirms It: Breastfeeding Benefits Have Been Drastically Overstated," *Slate*, February 27, 2014, http://www.slate.com/blogs /xx_factor/2014/02/27/breast_feeding_study_benefits_of_breast_over_bottle _have_been_exaggerated.html.

40. E. Innes, "Breast Milk Is No Better for a Baby Than Bottled Milk, Expert Claims," *Mail Online*, February 26, 2014, http://www.dailymail.co.uk/health /article-2568426/Breast-milk-no-better-baby-bottled-milk-INCREASES-risk-asthma-expert-claims.html.

41. T. Cassels, "'Is Breast Really Best?' The Debate Doesn't End Here," *Evolutionary Parenting*, February 28, 2014, http://evolutionaryparenting.com/is -breast-really-best-the-debate-doesnt-end-here; M. Beyer, "New 'Breast Isn't Best' Study Has the Potential to Derail Nursing," *SheKnows Parenting*, February 28, 2014, http://www.sheknows.com/parenting/articles/1031627/new-breast -isnt-best-study-has-the-potential-to-derail-nursing.

42. American Academy of Pediatrics (AAP) Section on Breastfeeding,

"Breastfeeding and the Use of Human Milk," *Pediatrics* 129, no. 3 (2012): e827–41, doi:10.1542/peds.2011-3552.

43. Let's Move!, "For Health Care Providers," accessed July 8, 2020, https://letsmove.obamawhitehouse.archives.gov/health-care-providers.

44. M. S. Kramer, "'Breast Is Best': The Evidence," *Early Human Development* 86, no. 11 (2010): 729–32, doi:10.1016/j.earlhumdev.2010.08.005; M. S. Kramer et al., "Effects of Prolonged and Exclusive Breastfeeding on Child Behavior and Maternal Adjustment: Evidence From a Large, Randomized Trial," *Pediatrics* 121, no. 3 (2008): e435–40; M. S. Kramer et al., "Effect of Prolonged and Exclusive Breast Feeding on Risk of Allergy and Asthma: Cluster Randomised Trial," *BMJ* 335, no. 7624 (2007): 815, doi:10.1136/bmj.39304.464016.AE; M. S. Kramer et al., "A Randomized Breast-feeding Promotion Intervention Did Not Reduce Child Obesity in Belarus," *Journal of Nutrition* 139, no. 2 (2009): 417–21S, doi:10.3945/jn.108.097675.

45. R. M. Martin et al., "Effects of Promoting Longer-Term and Exclusive Breastfeeding on Cardiometabolic Risk Factors at Age 11.5 Years A Cluster-Randomized, Controlled Trial," *Circulation* 129, no. 3 (2014): 321–29; R. M. Martin et al., "Effects of Promoting Longer-Term and Exclusive Breast-feeding on Adiposity and Insulin-like Growth Factor-I at Age 11.5 Years: A Randomized Trial," *JAMA* 309, no. 10 (2013): 1005–13, doi:10.1001/jama.2013.167.

46. M. S. Kramer et al., "Breastfeeding and Child Cognitive Development: New Evidence from a Large Randomized Trial," *Archives of General Psychiatry* 65, no. 5 (2008): 578–84, doi:10.1001/archpsyc.65.5.578; S. Yang et al., "Breast-feeding during Infancy and Neurocognitive Function in Adolescence: 16-Year Follow-Up of the PROBIT Cluster-Randomized Trial," *PLoS Medicine* 15, no. 4 (2018): e1002554, doi: 10.1371/journal.pmed.1002554.

47. B. L. Horta, C. Loret de Mola, and C. G. Victora, "Breastfeeding and Intelligence: A Systematic Review and Meta-analysis," *Acta Paediatrica* 104, no. 467 (2015): 14–19.

48. M. J. Brion et al., "What Are the Causal Effects of Breastfeeding on IQ, Obesity and Blood Pressure? Evidence from Comparing High-Income with Middle-Income Cohorts," *International Journal of Epidemiology* 40, no. 3 (2011): 670–80, doi:10.1093/ije/dyr020.

49. Der, Batty, and Deary, "Effect of Breast Feeding on Intelligence"; Grose, "New Study Confirms It"; E. Evenhouse and S. Reilly, "Improved Estimates of the Benefits of Breastfeeding Using Sibling Comparisons to Reduce Selection Bias," *Health Services Research* 40, no. 6, pt. 1 (2005): 1781–802, doi:10.1111/j.1475-6773.2005.00453.x.

50. Smithers, Kramer, and Lynch, "Effects of Breastfeeding on Obesity and Intelligence."

51. S. M. Innis, "Impact of Maternal Diet on Human Milk Composition and Neurological Development of Infants," *American Journal of Clinical Nutrition* 99, no. 3 (2014): 734–41S, doi:10.3945/ajcn.113.072595.

52. N. Timby et al., "Neurodevelopment, Nutrition, and Growth until 12 mo of Age in Infants Fed a Low-Energy, Low-Protein Formula Supplemented with Bovine Milk Fat Globule Membranes: A Randomized Controlled Trial," *American Journal of Clinical Nutrition* 99, no. 4 (2014): 860–68.

53. K. F. Michaelsen, L. Lauritzen, and E. L. Mortensen, "Effects of Breast-Feeding on Cognitive Function," in Goldberg et al., *Breast-Feeding*, 199–215.

54. Kramer et al., "Promotion of Breastfeeding Intervention Trial (PROBIT)"; Martin et al., "Effects of Promoting Longer-Term and Exclusive Breastfeeding on Cardiometabolic Risk Factors"; Martin et al., "Effects of Promoting Longer-Term and Exclusive Breastfeeding on Adiposity and Insulin-like Growth Factor-I."

55. S. S. Hawkins et al., "Examining Associations between Perinatal and Postnatal Risk Factors for Childhood Obesity Using Sibling Comparisons," *Childhood Obesity* 15, no. 4 (2019): 254–61.

56. Brion et al., "What Are the Causal Effects of Breastfeeding on IQ, Obesity and Blood Pressure?"; C. H. Fall et al., "Infant-Feeding Patterns and Cardiovascular Risk Factors in Young Adulthood: Data from Five Cohorts in Low- and Middle-Income Countries," *International Journal of Epidemiology* 40, no. 1 (2011): 47–62, doi:10.1093/ije/dyq155;

57. Horta, Loret de Mola, and Victora, "Breastfeeding and Intelligence"; J. A. Woo Baidal et al., "Risk Factors for Childhood Obesity in the First 1,000 Days: A Systematic Review," *American Journal of Preventive Medicine* 50, no. 6 (2016): 761–79; J. Qiao et al., "A Meta-analysis of the Association between Breastfeeding and Early Childhood Obesity," *Journal of Pediatric Nursing* 53 (July–August 2020): 57–66; B. Patro-Gołąb et al., "Nutritional Interventions or Exposures in Infants and Children Aged up to 3 Years and Their Effects on Subsequent Risk of Overweight, Obesity and Body Fat: A Systematic Review of Systematic Reviews," *Obesity Reviews* 17, no. 12 (2016): 1245–57.

58. A. Mazzocchi et al., "Hormones in Breast Milk and Effect on Infants' Growth: A Systematic Review," *Nutrients* 11, no. 8 (2019): 1845, doi: 10.3390/nu11081845.

59. Kramer et al., "Promotion of Breastfeeding Intervention Trial (PROBIT)"; C. Flohr et al., "Effect of an Intervention to Promote Breastfeeding on Asthma, Lung Function, and Atopic Eczema at Age 16 Years: Follow-Up of the PROBIT Randomized Trial," *JAMA Pediatrics* 172, no. 1 (2018): e174064.

60. D. Güngör et al., "Infant Milk-Feeding Practices and Food Allergies, Allergic Rhinitis, Atopic Dermatitis, and Asthma throughout the Life Span: A Systematic Review," *American Journal of Clinical Nutrition* 109, suppl. 7 (2019): 772S–99S.

61. Güngör et al., "Infant Milk-Feeding Practices"; C. J. Lodge et al., "Breast-feeding and Asthma and Allergies: A Systematic Review and Meta-analysis," *Acta Paediatrica* 104, no. S467 (2015): 38–53; C. M. Dogaru et al., "Breastfeeding and Childhood Asthma: Systematic Review and Meta-Analysis," *American Journal of Epidemiology* 179, no. 10 (2014): 1153–67, doi:10.1093/aje/kwu072.

62. A. K. Lossius et al., "Prospective Cohort Study of Breastfeeding and the Risk of Childhood Asthma," *Journal of Pediatrics* 195 (April 2018): 182-89.e2.

63. Lodge et al., "Breastfeeding and Asthma and Allergies"; M. S. Kramer et al., "Effect of Prolonged and Exclusive Breast Feeding on Risk of Allergy and Asthma: Cluster Randomised Trial," *BMJ* 335, no. 7624 (2007): 815, doi:10.1136/bmj.39304.464016.AE; D. de Silva et al., "Preventing Food Allergy in Infancy and Childhood: Systematic Review of Randomised Controlled Trials," *Pediatric Allergy and Immunology* 31, no. 7 (2020): 813–26 doi:10.1111/pai.13273.

64. D. Güngör et al., "Infant Milk-Feeding Practices and Childhood Leukemia: A Systematic Review," *American Journal of Clinical Nutrition* 109, suppl. 7 (2019): 757S–71S; D. Güngör et al., "Infant Milk-Feeding Practices and Diabetes Outcomes in Offspring: A Systematic Review," *American Journal of Clinical Nutrition* 109, suppl. 1 (2019): 817S–37S.

65. Eunice Kennedy Shriver National Institute of Child Health and Human Development, "When Breastfeeding, How Many Calories Should Moms and Babies Consume?" last updated January 31, 2017, https://www.nichd.nih.gov /health/topics/breastfeeding/conditioninfo/calories.

66. C. Feltner et al., *Breastfeeding Programs and Policies, Breastfeeding Uptake, and Maternal Health Outcomes in Developed Countries*, Comparative Effectiveness Review No. 210 prepared by the RTI International–University of North Carolina at Chapel Hill Evidence-based Practice Center under Contract No. 290-2015-00011-I, AHRQ Publication No. 18-EHC014-EF (Rockville, MD: Agency for Healthcare Research and Quality, July 2018), https://doi.org/10.23970 /AHRQEPCCER210; E. Bonifacino et al., "Effect of Lactation on Maternal Hypertension: A Systematic Review," *Breastfeeding Medicine* 13, no. 9 (2018): 578–88; R. Chowdhury et al., "Breastfeeding and Maternal Health Outcomes: A Systematic Review and Meta-analysis," *Acta Paediatrica* 104, no. 467 (2015): 96–113.

67. R. M. Rameez et al., "Association of Maternal Lactation with Diabetes and Hypertension: A Systematic Review and Meta-analysis," *JAMA Network Open* 2, no. 10 (2019): e1913401.

68. Chowdhury et al., "Breastfeeding and Maternal Health Outcomes."

69. Feltner et al., *Breastfeeding Programs and Policies*; Chowdhury et al., "Breastfeeding and Maternal Health Outcomes."

70. AAP Section on Breastfeeding, "Breastfeeding and the Use of Human Milk"; World Health Organization (WHO), "Breastfeeding," Health Topics, accessed July 30, 2020, http://www.who.int/topics/breastfeeding/en.

71. UNICEF, "Infant and Young Child Feeding," UNICEF Data, October 2019, https://data.unicef.org/topic/nutrition/infant-and-young-child-feeding.

72. CDC, "2020 Breastfeeding Report Card," last updated September 17, 2020, https://www.cdc.gov/breastfeeding/data/reportcard.htm.

73. Y. Chzhen, A. Gromada, and G. Rees, *Are the World's Richest Countries Family Friendly? Policy in the OECD and EU* (Florence: UNICEF Office of Research, 2019).

74. Patient Protection and Affordable Care Act of 2010, H.R. 3590, 111th Cong. (2010).

75. WHO, *Marketing of Breast-milk Substitutes: National Implementation of the International Code, Status Report 2020* (Geneva: WHO, 2020).

76. Organisation for Economic Co-operation and Development (OECD), "Public Policies for Families with Children," OECD Family Database, accessed August 1, 2020, http://www.oecd.org/social/family/database.htm.

77. C. G. Victora et al., "Breastfeeding in the 21st century: Epidemiology, Mechanisms, and Lifelong Effect," *Lancet* 387, no. 10017 (2016): 475–90.

78. C. J. Chantry et al., "Excess Weight Loss in First-Born Breastfed Newborns Relates to Maternal Intrapartum Fluid Balance," *Pediatrics* 127, no. 1 (2011): e171–79, doi:10.1542/peds.2009-2663.

79. L. Feldman-Winter et al., "Evidence-Based Updates on the First Week of Exclusive Breastfeeding Among Infants ≥35 Weeks," *Pediatrics* 145, no. 4 (2020): e20183696, doi: 10.1542/peds.2018-3696.

80. A. M. Stuebe et al., "Prevalence and Risk Factors for Early, Undesired Weaning Attributed to Lactation Dysfunction," *Journal of Women's Health* 23, no. 5 (2014): 404–12, doi:10.1089/jwh.2013.4506.

81. Feldman-Winter et al., "Evidence-Based Updates on the First Week of Exclusive Breastfeeding"; M. Neifert and M. Bunik, "Overcoming Clinical Barriers to Exclusive Breastfeeding," *Pediatric Clinics of North America* 60, no. 1 (2013): 115–45, doi:10.1016/j.pcl.2012.10.001; R. Grajeda and R. Pérez-Escamilla, "Stress during Labor and Delivery Is Associated with Delayed Onset of Lactation among Urban Guatemalan Women," *Journal of Nutrition* 132, no. 10 (2002): 3055–60; P. Zhu et al., "New Insight into Onset of Lactation: Mediating the Negative Effect of Multiple Perinatal Biopsychosocial Stress on Breastfeeding Duration," *Breastfeeding Medicine* 8 (2013): 151–58, doi:10.1089/bfm.2012.0010.

82. S. L. Matias et al., "Risk Factors for Early Lactation Problems among Peruvian Primiparous Mothers," *Maternal and Child Nutrition* 6, no. 2 (2010): 120–33, doi:10.1111/j.1740-8709.2009.00195.x; G. E. Otoo et al., "HIV-Negative Status Is Associated with Very Early Onset of Lactation among Ghanaian Women," *Journal of Human Lactation* 26, no. 2 (2010): 107–17, doi:10.1177/0890334409348214.

83. B. S. Hewlett and S. Winn, "Allomaternal Nursing in Humans," *Current Anthropology* 55, no. 2 (2014): 200–29.

84. D. W. Sellen, "Comparison of Infant Feeding Patterns Reported for Nonindustrial Populations with Current Recommendations," *Journal of Nutrition* 131, no. 10 (2001): 2707–15.

85. Lozoff, "Birth and 'Bonding' in Non-Industrial Societies," 598.

86. A. Viguera, "Postpartum Unipolar Major Depression: Epidemiology, Clinical Features, Assessment, and Diagnosis," *UpToDate*, last updated October 13,

2020, https://www.uptodate.com/contents/postpartum-unipolar-major
-depression-epidemiology-clinical-features-assessment-and-diagnosis.

87. A. M. Stuebe, K. Grewen, and S. Meltzer Brody, "Association between Maternal Mood and Oxytocin Response to Breastfeeding," *Journal of Women's Health* 22, no. 4 (2013): 352–61, doi:10.1089/jwh.2012.3768; E. Sibolboro Mezzacappa and E. S. Katkin, "Breast-Feeding Is Associated with Reduced Perceived Stress and Negative Mood in Mothers," *Health Psychology* 21, no. 2 (2002): 187–93, doi:10.1037/0278-6133.21.2.187.

88. Stuebe et al., "Prevalence and Risk Factors for Early, Undesired Weaning"; A. M. Stuebe et al., "Failed Lactation and Perinatal Depression: Common Problems with Shared Neuroendocrine Mechanisms?" *Journal of Women's Health* 21, no. 3 (2012): 264–72, doi:10.1089/jwh.2011.3083; C.-L. Dennis and K. McQueen, "The Relationship between Infant-Feeding Outcomes and Postpartum Depression: A Qualitative Systematic Review," *Pediatrics* 123, no. 4 (2009): e736–51, doi:10.1542/peds.2008-1629; S. Watkins et al., "Early Breastfeeding Experiences and Postpartum Depression," *Obstetrics and Gynecology* 118, no. 2 (2011): 214–21, doi:10.1097/AOG.0b013e3182260a2d; I. M. Paul et al., "Postpartum Anxiety and Maternal-Infant Health Outcomes," *Pediatrics* 131, no. 4 (2013): e1218–24, doi:10.1542/peds.2012-2147; E. M. Taveras et al., "Clinician Support and Psychosocial Risk Factors Associated With Breastfeeding Discontinuation," *Pediatrics* 112, no. 1 (2003): 108–15.

89. A. M. Stuebe, "Is Breastfeeding Promotion Bad for Mothers?" *Breastfeeding Medicine* (blog), February 21, 2011, http://bfmed.wordpress.com/2011/02/21/is-breastfeeding-promotion-bad-for-mothers.

90. M. Sapp and A. Vandeven, "Update on Childhood Sexual Abuse," *Current Opinion in Pediatrics* 17, no. 2 (2005): 258–64.

91. J. Coles, "Qualitative Study of Breastfeeding after Childhood Sexual Assault," *Journal of Human Lactation* 25, no. 3 (2009): 317–24, doi:10.1177/0890334409334926; C. T. Beck, "An Adult Survivor of Child Sexual Abuse and Her Breastfeeding Experience: A Case Study," *American Journal of Maternal/Child Nursing* 34, no. 2 (2009): 91–97, doi:10.1097/01.NMC.0000347302.85455; S. K. Klingelhafer, "Sexual Abuse and Breastfeeding," *Journal of Human Lactation* 23, no. 2 (2007): 194–97, doi:10.1177/0890334407300387; C. Elfgen et al., "Breastfeeding in Women Having Experienced Childhood Sexual Abuse," *Journal of Human Lactation* 33, no. 1 (2017): 119–27, doi:10.1177/0890334416680789.

92. H. Stapleton, A. Fielder, and M. Kirkham, "Breast or Bottle? Eating Disordered Childbearing Women and Infant-Feeding Decisions," *Maternal and Child Nutrition* 4, no. 2 (2008): 106–20, doi:10.1111/j.1740-8709.2007.00121.x; E. Astrachan-Fletcher et al., "The Reciprocal Effects of Eating Disorders and the Postpartum Period: A Review of the Literature and Recommendations for Clinical Care," *Journal of Women's Health* 17, no. 2 (2008): 227–39; E. Waugh and

C. M. Bulik, "Offspring of Women with Eating Disorders," *International Journal of Eating Disorders* 25, no. 2 (1999): 123–33; S. Barston, "Of Human Bonding," in *Bottled Up: How the Way We Feed Babies Has Come to Define Motherhood, and Why It Shouldn't* (Berkeley: University of California Press, 2012): 70–95.

93. E. Burns et al., "A Meta-Ethnographic Synthesis of Women's Experience of Breastfeeding," *Maternal and Child Nutrition* 6, no. 3 (2010): 201–19, doi:10.1111/j.1740-8709.2009.00209.x; V. Schmied and D. Lupton, "Blurring the Boundaries: Breastfeeding and Maternal Subjectivity," *Sociology of Health and Illness* 23, no. 2 (2001): 234–50, doi:10.1111/1467-9566.00249; A. Sheehan, V. Schmied, and L. Barclay, "Women's Experiences of Infant Feeding Support in the First 6 Weeks Post-Birth," *Maternal and Child Nutrition* 5, no. 2 (2009): 138–50, doi:10.1111/j.1740-8709.2008.00163.x; P. Hoddinott et al., "A Serial Qualitative Interview Study of Infant Feeding Experiences: Idealism Meets Realism," *BMJ Open* 2, no. 2 (2012): e000504, doi:10.1136/bmjopen-2011-000504.

94. L. J. Henrickson, "Breastfeeding: It's So Easy," *KellyMom.com*, last updated January 14, 2018, https://kellymom.com/pregnancy/bf-prep/cache-bfeasy/ (2011).

95. New York State Department of Health, "Breastfeed: Give the Gift of a Lifetime to Your Baby," accessed June 6, 2014, http://www.health.ny.gov/publi cations/3998.

96. D. Hegney, T. Fallon, and M. L. O'Brien, "Against All Odds: A Retrospective Case-Controlled Study of Women Who Experienced Extraordinary Breastfeeding Problems," *Journal of Clinical Nursing* 17, no. 9 (2008): 1182–92, doi:10.1111/j.1365-2702.2008.02300.x.

97. E. Satter, "Understanding Your Newborn," in *Child of Mine: Feeding with Love and Good Sense* (Boulder, CO: Bull Publishing, 2000): 111–35.

98. J. P. Green, interview, 2014.

9. GETTING STARTED WITH SOLID FOODS

1. S. J. Fomon, "Infant Feeding in the 20th Century: Formula and Beikost," *Journal of Nutrition* 131, no. 2 (2001): 409–20S.

2. K. G. Dewey and C. M. Chaparro, "Session 4: Mineral Metabolism and Body Composition Iron Status of Breast-Fed Infants," *Proceedings of the Nutrition Society* 66 (August 2007): 412–22, doi:10.1017/S002966510700568X.

3. C. J. Chantry, C. R. Howard, and P. Auinger, "Full Breastfeeding Duration and Risk for Iron Deficiency in US Infants," *Breastfeeding Medicine* 2, no. 2 (2007): 63–73, doi:10.1089/bfm.2007.0002; E. B. Calvo, A. C. Galindo, and N. B. Aspres, "Iron Status in Exclusively Breast-Fed Infants," *Pediatrics* 90, no. 3 (1992): 375; D. Hopkins et al., "Infant Feeding in the Second 6 Months of Life Related to Iron Status: An Observational Study," *Archives of Disease in Childhood* 92 (2007): 850–54; J. L. Maguire et al., "Association between Total Duration of Breastfeeding and Iron Deficiency," *Pediatrics* 131, no. 5 (2013): e1530–37.

4. N. F. Krebs et al., "Zinc Supplementation during Lactation: Effects on Maternal Status and Milk Zinc Concentrations," *American Journal of Clinical Nutrition* 61, no. 5 (May 1, 1995): 1030–36.

5. "Krebs et al., "Zinc Supplementation during Lactation"; M. A. Siimes, L. Salmenper., and J. Perheentupa, "Exclusive Breast-Feeding for 9 Months: Risk of Iron Deficiency," *Journal of Pediatrics* 104, no. 2 (1984): 196–99.

6. N. F. Krebs et al., "Meat as a First Complementary Food for Breastfed Infants: Feasibility and Impact on Zinc Intake and Status," *Journal of Pediatric Gastroenterology and Nutrition* 42, no. 2 (2006): 207–14; L. Persson et al., "Are Weaning Foods Causing Impaired Iron and Zinc Status in 1-Year-Old Swedish Infants? A Cohort Study," *Acta Paediatrica* 87, no. 6 (1998): 618–22, doi:10.1111/j.1651-2227.1998.tb01518.x; R. G. Sezer et al., "Effect of Breast-feeding on Serum Zinc Levels and Growth in Healthy Infants," *Breastfeeding Medicine* 8, no. 2 (2013): 159–63, doi:10.1089/bfm.2012.0014.

7. Pan American Health Organization (PAHO) and World Health Organization (WHO), *Guiding Principles for Complementary Feeding of the Breastfed Child* (Washington, DC: PAHO, 2003), http://www.who.int/maternal_child _adolescent/documents/a85622/en.

8. K. G. Dewey, "The Challenge of Meeting Nutrient Needs of Infants and Young Children during the Period of Complementary Feeding: An Evolutionary Perspective," *Journal of Nutrition* 143, no. 12 (2013): 2050–54, doi:10.3945/jn.113.182527.

9. World Health Organization (WHO), "Breastfeeding," Health Topics, accessed July 30, 2020, http://www.who.int/topics/breastfeeding/en.

10. Sezer et al., "Effect of Breastfeeding on Serum Zinc"; R. D. Baker and F. R. Greer, "Diagnosis and Prevention of Iron Deficiency and Iron-Deficiency Anemia in Infants and Young Children (0–3 Years of Age)," *Pediatrics* 126, no. 5 (2010): 1040–50, doi:10.1542/peds.2010-2576.

11. WHO, "Breastfeeding."

12. Health Canada, Canadian Paediatric Society, Dietitians of Canada, and Breastfeeding Committee for Canada, "Nutrition for Healthy Term Infants: Recommendations from Birth to Six Months," last updated August 18, 2015, https://www.canada.ca/en/health-canada/services/canada-food-guide/resources /infant-feeding/nutrition-healthy-term-infants-recommendations-birth-six -months.html; American Academy of Pediatrics (AAP) Section on Breastfeeding, "Breastfeeding and the Use of Human Milk," *Pediatrics* 129, no. 3 (2012): e827–41, doi:10.1542/peds.2011-3552.

13. M. Fewtrell et al., "Complementary Feeding: A Position Paper by the European Society for Paediatric Gastroenterology, Hepatology, and Nutrition (ESPGHAN) Committee on Nutrition," *Journal of Pediatric Gastroenterology and Nutrition* 64, no. 1 (2017): 119–32.

14. W. Samady et al., "Recommendations on Complementary Food Intro-

duction among Pediatric Practitioners," *JAMA Network Open* 3, no. 8 (2020): e2013070.

15. Valerie Wheat, email to the author, November 23, 2013.

16. M. Fewtrell et al., "Six Months of Exclusive Breast Feeding: How Good Is the Evidence?" *BMJ* 342 (2011): 209–12, doi:10.1136/bmj.c5955.

17. M. R. Perkin et al., "Randomized Trial of Introduction of Allergenic Foods in Breast-Fed Infants," *New England Journal of Medicine* 374, no. 18 (2016): 1733–43; M. R. Perkin et al., "Enquiring About Tolerance (EAT) Study: Feasibility of an Early Allergenic Food Introduction Regimen," *Journal of Allergy Clinical Immunology* 137, no. 5 (2016): 1477–86.e8.

18. O. H. Jonsdottir et al., "Timing of the Introduction of Complementary Foods in Infancy: A Randomized Controlled Trial," *Pediatrics* 130, no. 6 (2012): 1038–45; O. H. Jonsdottir et al., "Exclusive Breastfeeding for 4 versus 6 Months and Growth in Early Childhood," *Acta Paediatrica* 103, no. 1 (2013): 105–11, doi:10.1111/apa.12433.

19. R. J. Cohen et al., "Effects of Age of Introduction of Complementary Foods on Infant Breast Milk Intake, Total Energy Intake, and Growth: A Randomised Intervention Study in Honduras," *Lancet* 344, no. 8918 (1994): 288–93, doi:10.1016/S0140-6736(94)91337-4; K. G. Dewey et al., "Age of Introduction of Complementary Foods and Growth of Term, Low-Birth-Weight, Breast-Fed Infants: A Randomized Intervention Study in Honduras," *American Journal of Clinical Nutrition* 69, no. 4 (1999): 679–86.

20. M. S. Kramer and R. Kakuma, "Optimal Duration of Exclusive Breastfeeding," *Cochrane Database of Systematic Reviews*, no. 8 (2012): CD003517, doi:10.1002/14651858.CD003517.pub2.

21. B. M. Popkin et al., "Breast-Feeding and Diarrheal Morbidity," *Pediatrics* 86, no. 6 (1990): 874–82.

22. Perkin et al., "Randomized Trial of Introduction of Allergenic Foods."

23. Cohen et al., "Effects of Age of Introduction of Complementary Foods"; Dewey et al., "Age of Introduction of Complementary Foods."

24. M. A. Quigley, Y. J. Kelly, and A. Sacker, "Infant Feeding, Solid Foods and Hospitalisation in the First 8 Months after Birth," *Archives of Disease in Childhood* 94, no. 2 (February 1, 2009): 148–50, doi:10.1136/adc.2008.146126.

25. K. Størdal et al., "Breast-feeding and Infant Hospitalization for Infections: Large Cohort and Sibling Analysis," *Journal of Pediatric Gastroenterology and Nutrition* 65, no. 2 (2017): 225–31.

26. M. R. Perkin et al., "Association of Early Introduction of Solids with Infant Sleep: A Secondary Analysis of a Randomized Clinical Trial," *JAMA Pediatrics* 172, no. 8 (2018): e180739.

27. M. L. Macknin, S. V. Medendorp, and M. C. Maier, "Infant Sleep and Bedtime Cereal," *American Journal of Diseases of Children* 143, no. 9 (1989): 1066–68; M. J. Heinig et al., "Intake and Growth of Breast-Fed and Formula-Fed

Infants in Relation to the Timing of Introduction of Complementary Foods: The DARLING Study," *Acta Paediatrica* 82, no. 12 (1993): 999–1006.

28. AAP Committee on Nutrition, "Hypoallergenic Infant Formulas," *Pediatrics* 106, no. 2 (2000): 346–49; Department of Health Committee on Toxicity of Chemicals in Food, Consumer Products, and the Environment, *Peanut Allergy* (London: Crown, 1998), https://cot.food.gov.uk/sites/default/files/cot/cot peanutall.pdf.

29. S. H. Sicherer et al., "US Prevalence of Self-Reported Peanut, Tree Nut, and Sesame Allergy: 11-year Follow-up," *Journal of Allergy and Clinical Immunology* 125, no. 6 (2010): 1322–26; K. D. Jackson, L. D. Howie, and L. J. Akinbami, *Trends in Allergic Conditions among Children: United States, 1997–2011*, NCHS Data Brief, no. 121 (Hyattsville, MD: National Center for Health Statistics, 2013).

30. E. M. Abrams and E. S. Chan, "It's Not Mom's Fault: Prenatal and Early Life Exposures that Do and Do Not Contribute to Food Allergy Development," *Immunology and Allergy Clinics of North America* 39, no. 4 (2019): 447–57.

31. J. A. Poole et al., "Timing of Initial Exposure to Cereal Grains and the Risk of Wheat Allergy," *Pediatrics* 117, no. 6 (2006): 2175–82, doi:10.1542/peds.2005-1803.

32. J. J. Koplin et al., "Can Early Introduction of Egg Prevent Egg Allergy in Infants? A Population-Based Study," *Journal of Allergy and Clinical Immunology* 126, no. 4 (2010): 807–13, doi:10.1016/j.jaci.2010.07.028.

33. G. Du Toit et al., "Early Consumption of Peanuts in Infancy Is Associated with a Low Prevalence of Peanut Allergy," *Journal of Allergy and Clinical Immunology* 122, no. 5 (2008): 984–91, doi:10.1016/j.jaci.2008.08.039.

34. F. R. Greer, S. H. Sicherer, and A. W. Burks, "Effects of Early Nutritional Interventions on the Development of Atopic Disease in Infants and Children: The Role of Maternal Dietary Restriction, Breastfeeding, Timing of Introduction of Complementary Foods, and Hydrolyzed Formulas," *Pediatrics* 121, no. 1 (2008): 183–91.

35. C. Agostoni et al., "Complementary Feeding: A Commentary by the ESPGHAN Committee on Nutrition," *Journal of Pediatric Gastroenterology and Nutrition* 46, no. 1 (2008): 99–110; E. S. Chan, C. Cummings, and Canadian Paediatric Society, Community Paediatrics Committee, Allergy Section, "Dietary Exposures and Allergy Prevention in High-Risk Infants," *Paediatrics and Child Health* 18, no. 10 (2013): 545–49; S. L. Prescott and M. L. K. Tang, "The Australasian Society of Clinical Immunology and Allergy Position Statement: Summary of Allergy Prevention in Children," *Medical Journal of Australia* 182, no. 9 (2005): 464–67.

36. G. Du Toit et al., "Randomized Trial of Peanut Consumption in Infants at Risk for Peanut Allergy," *New England Journal of Medicine* 372, no. 9 (2015): 803–13.

37. G. Du Toit et al., "Effect of Avoidance on Peanut Allergy after Early Peanut Consumption," *New England Journal of Medicine* 374, no. 15 (2016): 1435–43.

38. D. M. Fleischer et al., "Consensus Communication on Early Peanut Introduction and the Prevention of Peanut Allergy in High-Risk Infants," *Annals of Allergy, Asthma & Immunology* 115, no. 2 (2015): 87–90.

39. Perkin et al., "Randomized Trial of Introduction of Allergenic Foods."

40. J. A. Burgess et al., "Age at Introduction to Complementary Solid Food and Food Allergy and Sensitization: A Systematic Review and Meta-analysis," *Clinical and Experimental Allergy* 49, no. 6 (2019): 754–69; D. Ierodiakonou et al., "Timing of Allergenic Food Introduction to the Infant Diet and Risk of Allergic or Autoimmune Disease: A Systematic Review and Meta-analysis," *JAMA* 316, no. 11 (2016): 1181–92; K. Logan et al., "Pediatric Allergic Diseases, Food Allergy, and Oral Tolerance," *Annual Review of Cell and Developmental Biology* 36 (2020): 511–28, doi:10.1146/annurev-cellbio-100818-125346.

41. E. M. Abrams et al., "Timing of Introduction of Allergenic Solids for Infants at High Risk," *Paediatrics & Child Health* 24, no. 1 (2019): 56–57; A. Togias et al., "Addendum Guidelines for the Prevention of Peanut Allergy in the United States: Report of the National Institute of Allergy and Infectious Diseases, Sponsored Expert Panel," *World Allergy Organization Journal* 10 (2017): 1, doi:10.1186/s40413-016-0137-9; British Dietetic Association (BDA) and British Society for Allergy and Clinical Immunology (BSACI), *Preventing Food Allergy in Higher Risk Infants: Guidance for Healthcare Professionals* (London: BSACI, 2018), https://www.bsaci.org/wp-content/uploads/2020/02/pdf_Early-feeding-guidance-for-HCPs-2.pdf.

42. P. A. Joshi et al., "The Australasian Society of Clinical Immunology and Allergy Infant Feeding for Allergy Prevention Guidelines," *Medical Journal of Australia* 210, no. 2 (2019): 89–93.

43. Togias et al., "Addendum Guidelines for the Prevention of Peanut Allergy in the United States: Report of the National Institute of Allergy and Infectious Diseases, Sponsored Expert Panel."

44. Logan et al., "Pediatric Allergic Diseases, Food Allergy, and Oral Tolerance."

45. R. S. Gupta et al., "Assessment of Pediatrician Awareness and Implementation of the Addendum Guidelines for the Prevention of Peanut Allergy in the United States," *JAMA Network Open* 3, no. 7 (2020): e2010511; Togias et al., "Addendum Guidelines for the Prevention of Peanut Allergy in the United States: Report of the National Institute of Allergy and Infectious Diseases, Sponsored Expert Panel."

46. M. Greenhawt and M. Shaker, "Determining Levers of Cost-Effectiveness for Screening Infants at High Risk for Peanut Sensitization before Early Peanut Introduction," *JAMA Network Open* 2, no. 12 (2019): e1918041; M. Shaker et al., "'To Screen or Not to Screen': Comparing the Health and Economic Benefits

of Early Peanut Introduction Strategies in Five Countries," *Allergy* 73, no. 8 (2018): 1707–14; M. Shaker, E. M. Abrams, and M. Greenhawt, "Clinician Adoption of US Peanut Introduction Guidelines—A Case for Conditional Recommendations and Contextual Considerations to Empower Shared Decision-Making," *JAMA Network Open* 3, no. 7 (2020): e2011535–e2011535, https://doi.org/10.1001/jamanetworkopen.2020.11535.

47. BDA and BSACI, *Preventing Food Allergy in Higher Risk Infants*; Shaker, Abrams, and Greenhawt, "Clinician Adoption of US Peanut Introduction Guidelines."

48. M. P. W. Platt, "Demand Weaning: Infants' Answer to Professionals' Dilemmas," *Archives of Disease in Childhood* 94, no. 2 (2009): 79–80, doi:10.1136/adc.2008.150011.

49. J. Castenmiller et al., "Appropriate Age Range for Introduction of Complementary Feeding into an Infant's Diet," *European Food Safety Authority Journal* 17, no. 9 (2019): e05780

50. E. Satter, "Feeding Your Older Baby: Oral-Motor Development," in *Child of Mine: Feeding with Love and Good Sense* (Boulder, Colorado: Bull Publishing, 2000), 267–69.

51. B. R. Carruth and J. D. Skinner, "Feeding Behaviors and Other Motor Development in Healthy Children (2–24 Months)," *Journal of the American College of Nutrition* 21, no. 2 (2002): 88–96, doi:10.1080/07315724.2002.10719199.

52. Carruth and Skinner, "Feeding Behaviors and Other Motor Development"; B. R. Carruth et al., "Developmental Milestones and Self-Feeding Behaviors in Infants and Toddlers," *Journal of the American Dietetic Association* 104, suppl. 1 (2004): 51–56, doi:10.1016/j.jada.2003.10.019.

53. E. G. Gisel, "Effect of Food Texture on the Development of Chewing of Children between Six Months and Two Years of Age," *Developmental Medicine and Child Neurology* 33, no. 1 (1991): 69–79, doi:10.1111/j.1469-8749.1991.tb14786.x.

54. Carruth et al., "Developmental Milestones and Self-Feeding Behaviors."

55. K. Northstone et al., "The Effect of Age of Introduction to Lumpy Solids on Foods Eaten and Reported Feeding Difficulties at 6 and 15 Months," *Journal of Human Nutrition and Dietetics* 14, no. 1 (2001): 43–54, doi:10.1046/j.1365-277x.2001.00264.x; H. Coulthard, G. Harris, and P. Emmett, "Delayed Introduction of Lumpy Foods to Children during the Complementary Feeding Period Affects Child's Food Acceptance and Feeding at 7 Years of Age," *Maternal and Child Nutrition* 5, no. 1 (2009): 75–85, doi:10.1111/j.1740-8709.2008.00153.x.

56. P. Voorheis et al., "Challenges Experienced with Early Introduction and Sustained Consumption of Allergenic Foods in the Enquiring About Tolerance (EAT) Study: A Qualitative Analysis," *Journal of Allergy and Clinical Immunology* 144, no. 6 (2019): 1615–23, https://doi.org/10.1016/j.jaci.2019.09.004.

57. A. Callahan, "The New Rules of Food Allergy Prevention, Testing and Diagnosis," *New York Times*, August 9, 2019.

58. M. M. Black and F. E. Aboud, "Responsive Feeding Is Embedded in a Theoretical Framework of Responsive Parenting," *Journal of Nutrition* 141, no. 3 (2011): 490–94, doi:10.3945/jn.110.129973; M. K. Fox et al., "Relationship between Portion Size and Energy Intake among Infants and Toddlers: Evidence of Self-Regulation," *Journal of the American Dietetic Association* 106, no. 1, suppl. (January 2006): 77–83, doi:10.1016/j.jada.2005.09.039.

59. C. Schwartz et al., "Development of Healthy Eating Habits Early in Life: Review of Recent Evidence and Selected Guidelines," *Appetite* 57, no. 3 (2011): 796–807, doi:10.1016/j.appet.2011.05.316; A. K. Ventura and L. L. Birch, "Does Parenting Affect Children's Eating and Weight Status?" *International Journal of Behavioral Nutrition and Physical Activity* 5 (2008): 15, doi:10.1186/1479-5868-5-15.

60. C. Farrow and J. Blissett, "Does Maternal Control during Feeding Moderate Early Infant Weight Gain?" *Pediatrics* 118, no. 2 (2006): e293–98; C. V. Farrow and J. Blissett, "Controlling Feeding Practices: Cause or Consequence of Early Child Weight?" *Pediatrics* 121, no. 1 (2008): e164–69.

61. Black and Aboud, "Responsive Feeding Is Embedded in a Theoretical Framework."

62. G. Rapley, "Baby-Led Weaning Pamphlet," accessed December 29, 2013, http://www.rapleyweaning.com; S. Cameron, A.-L. Heath, and R. Taylor, "How Feasible Is Baby-Led Weaning as an Approach to Infant Feeding? A Review of the Evidence," *Nutrients* 4, no. 12 (2012): 1575–1609.

63. E. D'Auria et al., "Baby-Led Weaning: What a Systematic Review of the Literature Adds On," *Italian Journal of Pediatrics* 44, no. 1 (2018): 49, doi:10.1186/s13052-018-0487-8.

64. D'Auria et al., "Baby-Led Weaning"; S. Komninou, J. C. G. Halford, and J. A. Harrold, "Differences in Parental Feeding Styles and Practices and Toddler Eating Behaviour across Complementary Feeding Methods: Managing Expectations through Consideration of Effect Size," *Appetite* 137 (June 1, 2019): 198–206; A. Brown and M. Lee, "Maternal Control of Child Feeding during the Weaning Period: Differences between Mothers Following a Baby-Led or Standard Weaning Approach," *Maternal and Child Health Journal* 15, no. 8 (November 2011): 1265–71, doi:10.1007/s10995-010-0678-4.

65. E. Dogan et al., "Baby-Led Complementary Feeding: Randomized Controlled Study," *Pediatrics International: Official Journal of the Japan Pediatric Society* 60, no. 12 (2018): 1073–80; L. J. Fangupo et al., "A Baby-Led Approach to Eating Solids and Risk of Choking," *Pediatrics* 138, no. 4 (2016): e20160772.

66. L. Daniels et al., "Impact of a Modified Version of Baby-Led Weaning on Iron Intake and Status: A Randomised Controlled Trial," *BMJ Open* 8, no. 6

(June 27, 2018): e019036, doi:10.1136/bmjopen-2017-019036; Dogan et al., "Baby-Led Complementary Feeding."

67. A. Brown, "No Difference in Self-Reported Frequency of Choking between Infants Introduced to Solid Foods Using a Baby-Led Weaning or Traditional Spoon-Feeding Approach," *Journal of Human Nutrition and Dietetics: The Official Journal of the British Dietetic Association* 31, no. 4 (August 2018): 496–504, https://doi.org/10.1111/jhn.12528.

68. Fangupo et al., "A Baby-Led Approach to Eating Solids and Risk of Choking."

69. Dogan et al., "Baby-Led Complementary Feeding"; R. W. Taylor et al., "Effect of a Baby-Led Approach to Complementary Feeding on Infant Growth and Overweight: A Randomized Clinical Trial," *JAMA Pediatrics* 171, no. 9 (2017): 838–46.

70. Taylor et al., "Effect of a Baby-Led Approach to Complementary Feeding on Infant Growth and Overweight."

71. B. J. Morison et al., "Impact of a Modified Version of Baby-Led Weaning on Dietary Variety and Food Preferences in Infants," *Nutrients* 10, no. 8 (2018): 1092, doi:10.3390/nu10081092; L. Williams Erickson et al., "Impact of a Modified Version of Baby-Led Weaning on Infant Food and Nutrient Intakes: The BLISS Randomized Controlled Trial," *Nutrients* 10, no. 6 (2018): 740, doi:10.3390/nu10060740.

10. EAT, GROW, AND LEARN

1. Eve F., post on *Natural Mother Magazine* Facebook page asking for advice about how to start solid foods, accessed October 20, 2013, https://www.face book.com/NaturalMotherMagazine.

2. S. J. Fomon, "Infant Feeding in the 20th Century: Formula and Beikost," *Journal of Nutrition* 131, no. 2 (2001): 409–20S.

3. E. W. Duffy et al., "Trends in Food Consumption Patterns of US Infants and Toddlers from Feeding Infants and Toddlers Studies (FITS) in 2002, 2008, 2016," *Nutrients* 11, no. 11 (2019): 2807, doi: 10.3390/nu11112807.

4. B. S. Vitta and K. G. Dewey, *Identifying Micronutrient Gaps in the Diets of Breastfed 6–11-Mo-Old Infants in Bangladesh, Ethiopia, and Vietnam Using Linear Programming* (Washington, DC: Alive and Thrive, 2012).

5. K. G. Dewey, "The Challenge of Meeting Nutrient Needs of Infants and Young Children during the Period of Complementary Feeding: An Evolutionary Perspective," *Journal of Nutrition* 143, no. 12 (2013): 2050–54, doi:10.3945/jn.113.182527.

6. Pan American Health Organization (PAHO) and World Health Organization (WHO), *Guiding Principles for Complementary Feeding of the Breastfed Child* (Washington, DC: PAHO, 2003), 25, http://www.who.int/maternal_child_adolescent/documents/a85622/en.

7. R. Yip et al., "Declining Prevalence of Anemia among Low-Income Children in the United States," *JAMA* 258, no. 12 (1987): 1619–23.

8. Dewey, "The Challenge of Meeting Nutrient Needs."

9. G. H. Pelto, Y. Zhang, and J. Habicht, "Premastication: The Second Arm of Infant and Young Child Feeding for Health and Survival?" *Maternal and Child Nutrition* 6, no. 1 (2010): 4–18, doi:10.1111/j.1740-8709.2009.00200.x.

10. L. Cordain et al., "Fatty Acid Analysis of Wild Ruminant Tissues: Evolutionary Implications or Reducing Diet-Related Chronic Disease," *European Journal of Clinical Nutrition* 56, no. 3 (2002): 181–91.

11. E. E. Birch et al., "The DIAMOND (DHA Intake And Measurement Of Neural Development) Study: A Double-Masked, Randomized Controlled Clinical Trial of the Maturation of Infant Visual Acuity as a Function of the Dietary Level of Docosahexaenoic Acid," *American Journal of Clinical Nutrition* 91, no. 4 (2010): 848–59, doi:10.3945/ajcn.2009.28557; S. E. Carlson and J. Colombo, "Docosahexaenoic Acid and Arachidonic Acid Nutrition in Early Development," *Advances in Pediatrics* 63, no. 1 (2016): 453–71.

12. C. Campoy et al., "Omega 3 Fatty Acids on Child Growth, Visual Acuity and Neurodevelopment," *British Journal of Nutrition* 107, suppl. 2 (2012): S85–106, doi:10.1017/S0007114512001493.

13. G. A. Olaya, M. Lawson, and M. S. Fewtrell, "Efficacy and Safety of New Complementary Feeding Guidelines with an Emphasis on Red Meat Consumption: A Randomized Trial in Bogota, Colombia," *American Journal of Clinical Nutrition* 98, no. 4 (October 2013): 983–93, doi:10.3945/ajcn.112.053595; N. F. Krebs et al., "Comparison of Complementary Feeding Strategies to Meet Zinc Requirements of Older Breastfed Infants," *American Journal of Clinical Nutrition* 96, no. 1 (2012): 30–35, doi:10.3945/ajcn.112.036046.

14. K. M. Hambidge et al., "Evaluation of Meat as a First Complementary Food for Breastfed Infants: Impact on Iron Intake," *Nutrition Reviews* 69, suppl. 1 (2011): S57–63.

15. L. Davidsson et al., "Iron Bioavailability in Infants from an Infant Cereal Fortified with Ferric Pyrophosphate or Ferrous Fumarate," *American Journal of Clinical Nutrition* 71, no. 6 (2000): 1597–1602; Joint FAO/WHO Expert Consultation on Human Vitamin and Mineral Requirements and WHO Department of Nutrition for Health and Development, *Vitamin and Mineral Requirements in Human Nutrition*, 2nd ed. (Geneva: World Health Organization, 2005).

16. J. D. Cook and E. R. Monsen, "Food Iron Absorption in Human Subjects: III. Comparison of the Effect of Animal Proteins on Nonheme Iron Absorption," *American Journal of Clinical Nutrition* 29, no. 8 (1976): 859–67.

17. A. A. Roess et al., "Food Consumption Patterns of Infants and Toddlers: Findings from the Feeding Infants and Toddlers Study (FITS) 2016," *Journal of Nutrition* 148, suppl. 3 (2018): 1525S–35S.

18. Duffy et al., "Trends in Food Consumption Patterns"; American Academy

of Pediatrics (AAP), "Starting Solid Foods," HealthyChildren.org, accessed September 28, 2020, https://www.healthychildren.org/English/ages-stages/baby/feeding-nutrition/Pages
/Starting-Solid-Foods.aspx.

19. Hambidge et al., "Evaluation of Meat as a First Complementary Food."

20. I. Kull et al., "Fish Consumption during the First Year of Life and Development of Allergic Diseases during Childhood," *Allergy* 61, no. 8 (2006): 1009–15.

21. AAP, "Metals in Baby Food," HealthyChildren.org, accessed September 29, 2020, https://www.healthychildren.org/English/ages-stages/baby/feeding -nutrition/Pages/Metals-in-Baby-Food.aspx; US Food and Drug Administration, "Advice About Eating Fish: For Women Who Are or Might Become Pregnant, Breastfeeding Mothers, and Young Children," accessed September 29, 2020, https://www.fda.gov/food/consumers/advice-about-eating-fish.

22. A. S. Bernstein et al., "Fish, Shellfish, and Children's Health: An Assessment of Benefits, Risks, and Sustainability," *Pediatrics* 143, no. 6 (2019): e20190999, doi: 10.1542/peds.2019-0999.

23. L. Hallberg and L. Hulthén, "Prediction of Dietary Iron Absorption: An Algorithm for Calculating Absorption and Bioavailability of Dietary Iron," *American Journal of Clinical Nutrition* 71, no. 5 (2000): 1147–60; R. F. Hurrell et al., "Iron Absorption in Humans: Bovine Serum Albumin Compared with Beef Muscle and Egg White," *American Journal of Clinical Nutrition* 47, no. 1 (1988): 102–7.

24. M. Makrides et al., "Nutritional Effect of Including Egg Yolk in the Weaning Diet of Breast-Fed and Formula-Fed Infants: A Randomized Controlled Trial," *American Journal of Clinical Nutrition* 75, no. 6 (2002): 1084–92.

25. Makrides et al., "Nutritional Effect of Including Egg Yolk."

26. I. Fraeye et al., "Dietary Enrichment of Eggs with Omega-3 Fatty Acids: A Review," *Food Research International* 48, no. 2 (2012): 961–69, doi:10.1016/ j.foodres.2012.03.014.

27. D. R. Hoffman et al., "Maturation of Visual Acuity Is Accelerated in Breast-Fed Term Infants Fed Baby Food Containing DHA-Enriched Egg Yolk, *Journal of Nutrition* 134, no. 9 (2004): 2307–13.

28. A. P. Simopoulos and N. Salem, "Egg Yolk as a Source of Long-Chain Polyunsaturated Fatty Acids in Infant Feeding," *American Journal of Clinical Nutrition* 55, no. 2 (1992): 411–14; H. D. Karsten et al., "Vitamins A, E and Fatty Acid Composition of the Eggs of Caged Hens and Pastured Hens," *Renewable Agriculture and Food Systems* 25, special issue 1 (2010): 45–54, doi:10.1017/ S1742170509990214.

29. USDA Food Safety and Inspection Service, "Meat and Poultry Labeling Terms," accessed September 29, 2020, http://www.fsis.usda.gov/wps/portal

/fsis/topics/food-safety-education/get-answers/food-safety-fact-sheets/food
-labeling/meat-and-poultry labeling terms/meat-and-poultry-labeling-terms.

30. Makrides et al., "Nutritional Effect of Including Egg Yolk."

31. S. H. Zeisel and K. A. da Costa, "Choline: An Essential Nutrient for Public
Health," *Nutrition Reviews* 67, no. 11 (2009): 615–23.

32. E. E. Ziegler, "Consumption of Cow's Milk as a Cause of Iron Deficiency
in Infants and Toddlers," *Nutrition Reviews* 69, suppl. 1 (2011): S37–42, doi:10.
1111/j.1753-4887.2011.00431.x.

33. M. Lott et al., *Healthy Beverage Consumption in Early Childhood: Recommendations from Key National Health and Nutrition Organizations*, Technical Scientific Report (Durham, NC: Healthy Eating Research, 2019), https://healthy
eatingresearch.org/research/technical-scientific-report-healthy-beverage
-consumption-in-early-childhood-recommendations-from-key-national-health
-and-nutrition-organizations.

34. AAP Committee on Nutrition, "Complementary Feeding," in *Pediatric
Nutrition*, ed. R. E. Kleinman and F. R. Gree, 7th ed. (Elk Grove Village, IL:
American Academy of Pediatrics, 2014), 123–39; Lott et al., *Healthy Beverage
Consumption in Early Childhood*.

35. World Resources Institute, "Protein Scorecard," April 2016, https://www
.wri.org/resources/data-visualizations/protein-scorecard.

36. S. M. Innis, "Dietary Omega 3 Fatty Acids and the Developing
Brain," *Brain Research* 1237 (October 27, 2008): 35–43, doi:10.1016/j.brain-
res.2008.08.078; C. A. Daley et al., "A Review of Fatty Acid Profiles and Antiox-
idant Content in Grass-Fed and Grain-Fed Beef," *Nutrition Journal* 9 (2010): 10,
doi:10.1186/1475-2891-9-10.

37. AAP Committee on Nutrition, "Complementary Feeding."

38. PAHO and WHO, *Guiding Principles for Complementary Feeding*, 22.

39. P. C. Dagnelie and W. A. van Staveren, "Macrobiotic Nutrition and Child
Health: Results of a Population-Based, Mixed-Longitudinal Cohort Study in
the Netherlands," *American Journal of Clinical Nutrition* 59, no. 5 (May 1994):
1187S–96S. 40. M. Van Winckel et al., "Vegetarian Infant and Child Nutrition," *European Journal of Pediatrics* 170, no. 12 (December 1, 2011): 1489–94,
doi:10.1007/s00431-011-1547-x.

41. J. E. Obbagy et al., "Complementary Feeding and Micronutrient Status:
A Systematic Review," *American Journal of Clinical Nutrition* 109, suppl. 1
(2019): 852S–71S. 42. E. E. Ziegler, S. E. Nelson, and J. M. Jeter, "Iron Status of
Breastfed Infants Is Improved Equally by Medicinal Iron and Iron-Fortified Cereal," *American Journal of Clinical Nutrition* 90 (July 2009): 76–87, doi:10.3945/
ajcn.2008.27350.

43. J. Mennella and G. Beauchamp, "Mothers' Milk Enhances the Acceptance
of Cereal during Weaning," *Pediatric Research* 41, no. 2 (1997): 188–92.

44. Joint FAO/WHO, *Vitamin and Mineral Requirements in Human Nutrition*.

45. M. B. Zimmermann and R. F. Hurrell, "Nutritional Iron Deficiency," *Lancet* 370, no. 9586 (2007): 511–20, doi:10.1016/S0140-6736(07)61235-5.

46. J. D. Cook et al., "The Influence of Different Cereal Grains on Iron Absorption from Infant Cereal Foods," *American Journal of Clinical Nutrition* 65, no. 4 (1997): 964–69.

47. N. Roos et al., "Screening for Anti-Nutritional Compounds in Complementary Foods and Food Aid Products for Infants and Young Children: Anti-Nutritional Compounds in Complementary Foods and Products," *Maternal and Child Nutrition* 9, suppl. 1 (2013): 47–71, doi:10.1111/j.1740-8709.2012.00449.x.

48. N. F. Krebs et al., "Effects of Different Complementary Feeding Regimens on Iron Status and Enteric Microbiota in Breastfed Infants," *Journal of Pediatrics* 163, no. 2 (2013): 416–23, doi:10.1016/j.jpeds.2013.01.024.

49. L. A. Perlas and R. S. Gibson, "Household Dietary Strategies to Enhance the Content and Bioavailability of Iron, Zinc and Calcium of Selected Rice- and Maize-Based Philippine Complementary Foods," *Maternal and Child Nutrition* 1, no. 4 (October 2005): 263–73, doi:10.1111/j.1740-8709.2005.00037.x.

50. R. S. Gibson et al., "A Review of Phytate, Iron, Zinc, and Calcium Concentrations in Plant-Based Complementary Foods Used in Low-Income Countries and Implications for Bioavailability," *Food and Nutrition Bulletin* 31, no. 2 (2010): 134–46.

51. B. Hadorn et al., "Quantitative Assessment of Exocrine Pancreatic Function in Infants and Children," *Journal of Pediatrics* 73, no. 1 (1968): 39–50, doi:10.1016/S0022-3476(68)80037-X; G. Zoppi et al., "Exocrine Pancreas Function in Premature and Full Term Neonates," *Pediatric Research* 6, no. 12 (1972): 880–86. https://doi.org/10.1203/00006450-197212000-00005.

52. B. De Vizia et al., "Digestibility of Starches in Infants and Children," *Journal of Pediatrics* 86, no. 1 (1975): 50–55, doi:10.1016/S0022-3476(75)80703-7.

53. Fomon, "Infant Feeding in the 20th Century."

54. G. H. Pelto, E. Levitt, and L. Thairu, "Improving Feeding Practices: Current Patterns, Common Constraints, and the Design of Interventions," *Food and Nutrition Bulletin* 24, no. 1 (2003): 45–82.

55. M. A. Rossiter et al., "Amylase Content of Mixed Saliva in Children," *Acta Paediatrica* 63, no. 3 (1974): 389–92, doi:10.1111/j.1651-2227.1974.tb04815.x; G. P. Sevenhuysen, C. Holodinsky, and C. Dawes, "Development of Salivary Alpha-Amylase in Infants from Birth to 5 Months," *American Journal of Clinical Nutrition* 39, no. 4 (1984): 584–88.

56. R. D. Murray et al., "The Contribution of Salivary Amylase to Glucose Polymer Hydrolysis in Premature Infants," *Pediatric Research* 20, no. 2 (1986): 186–91, doi:10.1203/00006450-198602000-00019; J. L. Rosenblum, C. L. Irwin, and D. H. Alpers, "Starch and Glucose Oligosaccharides Protect Salivary-

378

Type Amylase Activity at Acid pH," *American Journal of Physiology* 254, no. 5 (1988): G775—80.

57. K. M. Shahani, A. J. Kwan, and B. A. Friend, "Role and Significance of Enzymes in Human Milk," *American Journal of Clinical Nutrition* 33, no. 8 (August 1, 1980): 1861–68.

58. J. B. Jones, N. R. Mehta, and M. Hamosh, "Alpha-Amylase in Preterm Human Milk," *Journal of Pediatric Gastroenterology and Nutrition* 1, no. 1 (1982): 43–48.

59. T. Lindberg and G. Skude, "Amylase in Human Milk," *Pediatrics* 70, no. 2 (1982): 235–38; L. A. Heitlinger et al., "Mammary Amylase: A Possible Alternate Pathway of Carbohydrate Digestion in Infancy," *Pediatric Research* 17, no. 1 (1983): 15–18, doi:10.1203/00006450-198301000-00003.

60. Jones, Mehta, and Hamosh, "Alpha-Amylase in Preterm Human Milk."

61. P. C. Lee et al., "Glucoamylase Activity in Infants and Children: Normal Values and Relationship to Symptoms and Histological Findings," *Journal of Pediatric Gastroenterology and Nutrition* 39, no. 2 (2004): 161–65; E. Lebenthal and P. C. Lee, "Glucoamylase and Disaccharidase Activities in Normal Subjects and in Patients with Mucosal Injury of the Small Intestine," *Journal of Pediatrics* 97, no. 3 (1980): 389–93, doi:10.1016/S0022-3476(80)80187-9.

62. R. J. Shulman et al., "Utilization of Dietary Cereal by Young Infants," *Journal of Pediatrics* 103, no. 1 (1983): 23–28, doi:10.1016/S0022-3476(83)80769-0; M. T. Christian et al., "Modeling 13C Breath Curves to Determine Site and Extent of Starch Digestion and Fermentation in Infants," *Journal of Pediatric Gastroenterology* 34, no. 2 (2002): 158–64.

63. J. M. W. Wong et al., "Colonic Health: Fermentation and Short Chain Fatty Acids," *Journal of Clinical Gastroenterology* 40, no. 3 (2006): 235–43.

64. J. Scheiwiller et al., "Human Faecal Microbiota Develops the Ability to Degrade Type 3 Resistant Starch during Weaning," *Journal of Pediatric Gastroenterology and Nutrition* 43, no. 5 (2006): 584–91.

65. Joint FAO/WHO, *Vitamin and Mineral Requirements in Human Nutrition.*

66. C. Schwartz et al., "Development of Healthy Eating Habits Early in Life: Review of Recent Evidence and Selected Guidelines," *Appetite* 57, no. 3 (2011): 796–807, doi:10.1016/j.appet.2011.05.316.

67. G. Harris and S. Mason, "Are There Sensitive Periods for Food Acceptance in Infancy?" *Current Nutrition Reports* 6, no. 2 (2017): 190–96.

68. C. Barends et al., "A Systematic Review of Practices to Promote Vegetable Acceptance in the First Three Years of Life," *Appetite* 137 (June 2019): 174–97; J. A. Mennella, A. R. Reiter, and L. M. Daniels, "Vegetable and Fruit Acceptance during Infancy: Impact of Ontogeny, Genetics, and Early Experiences," *Advances in Nutrition* 7, no. 1 (2016): 211S–19S; A. Maier-Nöth et al., "The Lasting Influences of Early Food-Related Variety Experience: A Longitudinal Study of

Vegetable Acceptance from 5 Months to 6 Years in Two Populations," *PLoS ONE* 11, no. 3 (2016): e0151356.

69. M. K. Spill et al., "Repeated Exposure to Food and Food Acceptability in Infants and Toddlers: A Systematic Review," *American Journal of Clinical Nutrition* 109, suppl. 7 (2019): 978S–89S.

70. R. Pérez-Escamilla, S. Segura-Perez, and M. Lott, *Feeding Guidelines for Infants and Young Toddlers: A Responsive Parenting Approach* (Durham, NC: Healthy Eating Research, 2017), http://healthy eatingresearch.org/research/feeding-guidelines-for-infants-and-young -toddlers-a-responsive-parenting-approach.

71. L. Chambers et al., "Reaching Consensus on a 'Vegetables First' Approach to Complementary Feeding," *Nutrition Bulletin* 41, no. 3 (2016): 270–76.

72. A. Fildes et al., "An Exploratory Trial of Parental Advice for Increasing Vegetable Acceptance in Infancy," *British Journal of Nutrition* 114, no. 2 (2015): 328–36; C. Barends et al., "Effects of Starting Weaning Exclusively with Vegetables on Vegetable Intake at the Age of 12 and 23 Months," *Appetite* 81 (October 2014): 193–99; C. Barends et al., "Effects of Repeated Exposure to Either Vegetables or Fruits on Infant's Vegetable and Fruit Acceptance at the Beginning of Weaning," *Food Quality and Preference* 29, no. 2 (2013): 157–65.

73. Barends et al., "A Systematic Review of Practices to Promote Vegetable Acceptance."

74. A. Fildes et al., "Nature and Nurture in Children's Food Preferences," *American Journal of Clinical Nutrition* 99, no. 4 (2014): 911–17.

75. C. Venter et al., "Different Measures of Diet Diversity During Infancy and the Association with Childhood Food Allergy in a UK Birth Cohort Study," *Journal of Allergy and Clinical Immunology in Practice* 8, no. 6 (2020): 2017–26.

76. C. Roduit et al., "Increased Food Diversity in the First Year of Life Is Inversely Associated with Allergic Diseases," *Journal of Allergy and Clinical Immunology* 133, no. 4 (2014): 1056–64.e7; B. I. Nwaru et al., "Introduction of Complementary Foods in Infancy and Atopic Sensitization at the Age of 5 Years: Timing and Food Diversity in a Finnish Birth Cohort," *Allergy* 68, no. 4 (2013): 507–16.

77. C. Venter et al., "EAACI Position Paper on Diet Diversity in Pregnancy, Infancy and Childhood: Novel Concepts and Implications for Studies in Allergy and Asthma," *Allergy* 75, no. 3 (2020): 497–523.

78. F. R. Greer et al., "The Effects of Early Nutritional Interventions on the Development of Atopic Disease in Infants and Children: The Role of Maternal Dietary Restriction, Breastfeeding, Hydrolyzed Formulas, and Timing of Introduction of Allergenic Complementary Foods," *Pediatrics* 143, no. 4 (2019): e20190281; P. A. Joshi et al., "The Australasian Society of Clinical Immunology and Allergy Infant Feeding for Allergy Prevention Guidelines," *Medical Journal of Australia* 210, no. 2 (2019): 89–93; Allergy UK, *Weaning Your Food Allergic*

Baby (Kent, UK: Allergy UK, 2020), https://www.allergyuk.org/weaning /supportpack.

79. W. Samady et al., "Recommendations on Complementary Food Introduction among Pediatric Practitioners," *JAMA Network Open* 3, no. 8 (2020): e2013070.

80. A. Togias et al., "Addendum Guidelines for the Prevention of Peanut Allergy in the United States: Report of the National Institute of Allergy and Infectious Diseases, Sponsored Expert Panel," *World Allergy Organization Journal* 10 (2017): 1, doi:10.1186/s40413-016-0137-9.

81. W. Samady et al., "Food-induced Anaphylaxis in Infants and Children," *Annals of Allergy, Asthma & Immunology* 121, no. 3 (2018): 360–65.

82. A. Callahan, "The New Rules of Food Allergy Prevention, Testing and Diagnosis," *New York Times*, August 9, 2019.

83. M. R. Perkin et al., "Randomized Trial of Introduction of Allergenic Foods in Breast-Fed Infants," *New England Journal of Medicine* 374, no. 18 (2016): 1733–43.

84. Joshi et al., "The Australasian Society of Clinical Immunology and Allergy Infant Feeding for Allergy Prevention Guidelines"; Allergy UK, *Weaning Your Food Allergic Baby*; Togias et al., "Addendum Guidelines for the Prevention of Peanut Allergy in the United States."

85. Roess et al., "Food Consumption Patterns of Infants and Toddlers."

86. Pérez-Escamilla, Segura-Perez, and Lott, *Feeding Guidelines for Infants and Young Toddlers*.

87. L. L. Birch, "Development of Food Preferences," *Annual Review of Nutrition* 19, no. 1 (1999): 41–62, doi:10.1146/annurev.nutr.19.1.41.

88. Lott et al., *Healthy Beverage Consumption in Early Childhood*; AAP Committee on Nutrition, "Complementary Feeding."

89. AAP, "Infant Constipation," HealthyChildren.org, accessed October 2, 2020, https://www.healthychildren.org/English/ages-stages/baby/diapers -clothing/Pages/Infant-Constipation.aspx.

90. M. G. Tanzi and M. P. Gabay, "Association between Honey Consumption and Infant Botulism," *Pharmacotherapy: Journal of Human Pharmacology and Drug Therapy* 22, no. 11 (2002): 1479–83, doi:10.1592/phco.22.16.1479.33696.

91. J. M. Geleijnse and D. E. Grobbee, "High Salt Intake Early in Life: Does It Increase the Risk of Hypertension?" *Journal of Hypertension* 20, no. 4 (2002): 2121–24.

APPENDIX A. INGREDIENTS IN THE
NEWBORN VITAMIN K SHOT

1. Centers for Disease Control and Prevention (CDC), "Notes from the Field: Late Vitamin K Deficiency Bleeding in Infants Whose Parents Declined Vita-

min K Prophylaxis—Tennessee, 2013," *Morbidity and Mortality Weekly Report (MMWR)* 62, no. 45 (2013): 901–2.

2. Merck Manuals, "Drug Absorption," Merck Manual for Healthcare Professionals, 2014, http://www.merckmanuals.com/professional/clinical_pharmacology/pharmacokinetics/drug_absorption.html.

3. US National Library of Medicine, "Phytonadione Injection, Emulsion," *DailyMed*, last updated April 26, 2019, https://dailymed.nlm.nih.gov/dailymed/drugInfo.cfm?setid=e0b0c8f1-75be-4f25-898a-7b97b608c615.

4. N. Shehab et al., "Exposure to the Pharmaceutical Excipients Benzyl Alcohol and Propylene Glycol among Critically Ill Neonates," *Pediatric Critical Care Medicine* 10, no. 2 (2009): 256–59, doi:10.1097/PCC.0b013e31819a383c; S. P. Nordt and L. E. Vivero, "Pharmaceutical Additives," in *Goldfrank's Toxicologic Emergencies*, ed. L. S. Nelson et al., 9th ed. (New York: McGraw-Hill, 2011), 803-16.

5. H. D. Goff, "Colloidal Aspects of Ice Cream: A Review," *International Dairy Journal* 7, no. 6–7 (1997): 363–73, doi:10.1016/S0958-6946(97)00040-X.

6. V. Lorch et al., "Unusual Syndrome among Premature Infants: Association with a New Intravenous Vitamin E Product," *Pediatrics* 75, no. 3 (1985): 598; S. C. Smolinske, *CRC Handbook of Food, Drug, and Cosmetic Excipients* (Boca Raton, FL: CRC Press, 1992).

7. US National Library of Medicine, "Sodium Acetate Injection, Solution, Concentrate," *DailyMed*, last updated December 31, 2019, https://dailymed.nlm.nih.gov/dailymed/drugInfo.cfm?setid=d7fabf08-d4e0-4bb5-8416-2e8ffe27c04b; R. J. Mitkus et al., "Updated Aluminum Pharmacokinetics Following Infant Exposures through Diet and Vaccination," *Vaccine* 29, no. 51 (2011): 9538–43, doi:10.1016/j.vaccine.2011.09.124.

8. National Center for Biotechnology Information, "Acetic Acid," *PubChem*, accessed April 9, 2014, https://pubchem.ncbi.nlm.nih.gov/compound/176.

9. US National Library of Medicine, "VITAMIN K1 - Phytonadione Injection, Emulsion," *DailyMed*, last updated December 6, 2019, https://dailymed.nlm.nih.gov/dailymed/drugInfo.cfm?setid=e8808230-2c44-44c6-8cab-8f29b6b34051.

10. Shehab et al., "Exposure to the Pharmaceutical Excipients Benzyl Alcohol and Propylene Glycol"; Nordt and Vivero, "Pharmaceutical Additives"; American Academy of Pediatrics (AAP), "'Inactive' Ingredients in Pharmaceutical Products: Update (Subject Review)," *Pediatrics* 99, no. 2 (1997): 268–78, doi:10.1542/peds.99.2.268.

11. D. L. Riegert-Johnson and G. W. Volcheck, "The Incidence of Anaphylaxis Following Intravenous Phytonadione (Vitamin K1): A 5-Year Retrospective Review," *Annals of Allergy, Asthma, and Immunology* 89, no. 4 (2002): 400–406, doi:10.1016/S1081-1206(10)62042-X. 12. US National Library of Medicine, "Dextrose (Dextrose Monohydrate), Injection, Solution," *DailyMed*, accessed

April 8, 2014, https://dailymed.nlm.nih.gov/dailymed/drugInfo .cfm?setid=3a9d9c4a-5e4e-4bb6-b2a9-55e1b0b98f02.

13. Datapharm, "Konakion MM Paediatric 2 mg/0.2 ml: Summary of Product Characteristics (SmPC)," *Electronic Medicines Compendium (emc)*, last updated November 17, 2020, https://www.medicines.org.uk/emc/product/9754/smpc; F. R. Greer et al., "A New Mixed Micellar Preparation for Oral Vitamin K Prophylaxis: Randomised Controlled Comparison with an Intramuscular Formulation in Breast Fed Infants," *Archives of Disease in Childhood* 79, no. 4 (1998): 300–305, doi:10.1136/adc.79.4.300; G. Schubiger et al., "Prevention of Vitamin K Deficiency Bleeding with Oral Mixed Micellar Phylloquinone: Results of a 6-Year Surveillance in Switzerland," *European Journal of Pediatrics* 162, no. 12 (December 2003): 885–88, doi:10.1007/s00431-003-1327-3.

14. E. Hey, "Vitamin K: What, Why, and When," *Archives of Disease in Childhood: Fetal and Neonatal Edition* 88, no. 2 (2003): F80–83, doi:10.1136/fn.88.2.F80.

APPENDIX B. WHY THE HEPATITIS B VACCINE IS RECOMMENDED AT BIRTH

1. World Health Organization (WHO), "Hepatitis B," accessed October 10, 2020, http://www.who.int/immunization/diseases/hepatitisB/en.

2. S. Schillie et al., "Prevention of Hepatitis B Virus Infection in the United States: Recommendations of the Advisory Committee on Immunization Practices," *Morbidity and Mortality Weekly Report (MMWR)* 67, no. 1 (2018): 1–31.

3. C. W. Shepard et al., "Epidemiology of Hepatitis B and Hepatitis B Virus Infection in United States Children," *Pediatric Infectious Disease Journal* 24, no. 9 (2005): 755–60, doi:10.1097/01.inf.0000177279.72993.d5; G. L. Armstrong et al., "Childhood Hepatitis B Virus Infections in the United States Before Hepatitis B Immunization," *Pediatrics* 108, no. 5 (2001): 1123–28, doi:10.1542/peds.108.5.1123.

4. Schillie et al., "Prevention of Hepatitis B Virus Infection in the United States."

5. Shepard et al., "Epidemiology of Hepatitis B and Hepatitis B Virus Infection in United States Children."

6. J. Hayashi et al., "Hepatitis B Virus Transmission in Nursery Schools," *American Journal of Epidemiology* 125, no. 3 (1987): 492–98; E. D. Mcintosh et al., "Horizontal Transmission of Hepatitis B in a Children's Day-Care Centre: A Preventable Event," *Australian and New Zealand Journal of Public Health* 21, no. 7 (1997): 791–92, doi:10.1111/j.1467-842X.1997.tb01797.x.

7. S. F. Schillie and T. V. Murphy, "Seroprotection after Recombinant Hepatitis B Vaccination among Newborn Infants: A Review," *Vaccine* 31, no. 21 (2013): 2506–16, doi:10.1016/j.vaccine.2012.12.012.

8. Armstrong et al., "Childhood Hepatitis B Virus Infections in the United States."

9. Centers for Disease Control and Prevention (CDC), "A Comprehensive Immunization Strategy to Eliminate Transmission of Hepatitis B Virus in the United States," *MMWR Recommendations and Reports* 54, no. RR–16 (2005): 1–33.

10. Shepard et al., "Epidemiology of Hepatitis B and Hepatitis B Virus Infection in United States Children."

11. Schillie et al., "Prevention of Hepatitis B Virus Infection in the United States."

APPENDIX C. NOT TOO MANY VACCINES TOO SOON

1. Centers for Disease Control and Prevention (CDC), "Table 1: Recommended Child and Adolescent Immunization Schedule for Ages 18 Years or Younger, United States, 2020," last updated February 3, 2020, https://www.cdc.gov/vaccines/schedules/hcp/imz/child-adolescent.html.

2. P. A. Offit et al., "Addressing Parents' Concerns: Do Multiple Vaccines Overwhelm or Weaken the Infant's Immune System?" *Pediatrics* 109, no. 1 (2002): 124–29.

3. S. Otto et al., "General Non-Specific Morbidity Is Reduced after Vaccination within the Third Month of Life: The Greifswald Study," *Journal of Infection* 41, no. 2 (2000): 172–75, doi:10.1053/jinf.2000.0718.

4. J. M. Glanz et al., "Association between Estimated Cumulative Vaccine Antigen Exposure through the First 23 Months of Life and Non–Vaccine-Targeted Infections from 24 through 47 Months of Age," *JAMA* 319, no. 9 (2018): 906–13.

5. F. DeStefano, C. S. Price, and E. S. Weintraub, "Increasing Exposure to Antibody-Stimulating Proteins and Polysaccharides in Vaccines Is Not Associated with Risk of Autism," *Journal of Pediatrics* 163, no. 2 (2013): 561–67.

6. M. J. Smith and C. R. Woods, "On-time Vaccine Receipt in the First Year Does Not Adversely Affect Neuropsychological Outcomes," *Pediatrics* 125, no. 6 (2010): 1134–41.

7. Institute of Medicine (IOM), *Childhood Immunization Schedule and Safety: Stakeholder Concerns, Scientific Evidence, and Future Studies* (Washington, DC: National Academies Press, 2013), https://www.nap.edu/catalog/13563/the-childhood-immunization-schedule-and-safety-stakeholder-concerns-scientific-evidence.

8. J. Lighter, "We're Ignoring the Biggest Cause of the Measles Crisis," *New York Times*, September 22, 2019.

9. A. Rowhani-Rahbar et al., "Effect of Age on the Risk of Fever and Seizures

Following Immunization with Measles-Containing Vaccines in Children," *JAMA Pediatrics* 167, no. 12 (2013): 1111–17.

10. D. S. Ramsay and M. Lewis, "Developmental Change in Infant Cortisol and Behavioral Response to Inoculation," *Child Development* 65, no. 5 (1994): 1491–502, doi:10.2307/1131513.

APPENDIX D. VACCINES AND AUTISM

1. A. Kennedy et al., "Confidence about Vaccines in the United States: Understanding Parents' Perceptions," *Health Affairs (Millwood)* 30, no. 6 (2011): 1151–59, doi:10.1377/hlthaff.2011.0396.

2. A. J. Wakefield et al., "Ileal-Lymphoid-Nodular Hyperplasia, Non-Specific Colitis, and Pervasive Developmental Disorder in Children," *Lancet* 351, no. 9103 (1998): 637–41 (later retracted by the journal's editors; see note 4).

3. GOV.UK, "Confirmed Cases of Measles, Mumps and Rubella in England and Wales: 1996 to 2019," accessed December 29, 2020, https://www.gov.uk /government/publications/measles-confirmed-cases/confirmed-cases-of -measles-mumps-and-rubella-in-england-and-wales-2012-to-2013; D. K. Flaherty, "The Vaccine-Autism Connection: A Public Health Crisis Caused by Unethical Medical Practices and Fraudulent Science," *Annals of Pharmacotherapy* 45, no. 10 (2011): 1302–4, doi:10.1345/aph.1Q318.

4. Editors of the *Lancet*, "Retraction—Ileal-Lymphoid-Nodular Hyperplasia, Non-Specific Colitis, and Pervasive Developmental Disorder in Children," *Lancet* 375 no. 9713 (2010): 445, doi:10.1016/S0140-6736(10)60175-4.

5. American Academy of Pediatrics (AAP), "Joint Statement of the American Academy of Pediatrics (AAP) and the United States Public Health Service (USPHS)," *Pediatrics* 104, no. 3 (1999): 568–69.

6. T. W. Clarkson and L. Magos, "The Toxicology of Mercury and Its Chemical Compounds," *Critical Reviews in Toxicology* 36, no. 8 (2006): 609–62, doi:10.1080/10408440600845619.

7. Institute of Medicine (IOM), *Childhood Immunization Schedule and Safety: Stakeholder Concerns, Scientific Evidence, and Future Studies* (Washington, DC: National Academies Press, 2013), https://www.nap.edu/catalog/13563/the -childhood-immunization-schedule-and-safety-stakeholder-concerns-scienti fic-evidence; IOM, *Immunization Safety Review: Thimerosal-Containing Vaccines and Neurodevelopmental Disorders* (Washington, DC: National Academies Press, 2001); C. Di Pietrantonj et al., "Vaccines for Measles, Mumps, Rubella, and Varicella in Children," *Cochrane Database of Systematic Reviews*, no. 4 (2020): CD004407, doi:10.1002/14651858.CD004407.pub4; A. M. Hurley, M. Tadrous, and E. S. Miller, "Thimerosal-Containing Vaccines and Autism: A Review of Recent Epidemiologic Studies," *Journal of Pediatric Pharmacology and Therapeutics* 15, no. 3 (2010): 173.

8. L. E. Taylor, A. L. Swerdfeger, and G. D. Eslick, "Vaccines Are Not Associated with Autism: An Evidence-Based Meta-analysis of Case-Control and Cohort Studies," *Vaccine* 32, no. 29 (2014): 3623–29, doi:10.1016/j.vaccine.2014.04. 085.

9. A. Hviid et al., "Measles, Mumps, Rubella Vaccination and Autism: A Nationwide Cohort Study," *Annals of Internal Medicine*, 170, no. 8 (2019): 513–20.

10. A. Jain et al., "Autism Occurrence by MMR Vaccine Status among US Children with Older Siblings with and without Autism," *JAMA* 313, no. 15 (2015): 1534–40.

11. F. K. Satterstrom et al., "Large-Scale Exome Sequencing Study Implicates Both Developmental and Functional Changes in the Neurobiology of Autism," *Cell* 180, no. 3 (2020): 568–84.e23.

12. A. M. Persico and V. Napolioni, "Autism Genetics," *Behavioural Brain Research* 251 (2013): 95–112, doi:10.1016/j.bbr.2013.06.012.

13. R. Stoner et al., "Patches of Disorganization in the Neocortex of Children with Autism," *New England Journal of Medicine* 370, no. 13 (2014): 1209–19, doi:10.1056/NEJMoa1307491.

14. W. Jones and A. Klin, "Attention to Eyes Is Present but in Decline in 2–6-Month-Old Infants Later Diagnosed with Autism," *Nature* 504, no. 7480 (2013): 427–31, doi:10.1038/nature12715.

APPENDIX E. VACCINES AND SIDS

1. M. M. Vennemann et al., "Do Immunisations Reduce the Risk for SIDS? A Meta-analysis," *Vaccine* 25, no. 26 (2007): 4875–79, doi:10.1016/j.vaccine. 2007.02.077.

2. R. Kuhnert et al., "Reanalyses of Case-Control Studies Examining the Temporal Association between Sudden Infant Death Syndrome and Vaccination," *Vaccine* 30, no. 13 (2012): 2349–56.

3. E. M. Eriksen et al., "Lack of Association between Hepatitis B Birth Immunization and Neonatal Death: A Population-Based Study from the Vaccine Safety Datalink Project," *Pediatric Infectious Disease Journal* 23, no. 7 (2004): 656–62.

4. J. Hansen et al., "Safety of DTaP-IPV/Hib Vaccine Administered Routinely to Infants and Toddlers," *Vaccine* 34, no. 35 (2016): 4172–79.

5. L. Franck et al., "Infant Sleep after Immunization: Randomized Controlled Trial of Prophylactic Acetaminophen," *Pediatrics* 128, no. 6 (2011): 1100–1108.

APPENDIX F. ALUMINUM IN VACCINES

1. R. J. Mitkus et al., "Updated Aluminum Pharmacokinetics Following Infant Exposures through Diet and Vaccination," *Vaccine* 29, no. 51 (2011):

9538–43, doi:10.1016/j.vaccine.2011.09.124; H. Hogenesch, "Mechanism of Immunopotentiation and Safety of Aluminum Adjuvants," *Immunotherapies and Vaccines* 3 (2013): 406, doi:10.3389/fimmu.2012.00406; N. W. Baylor, W. Egan, and P. Richman, "Aluminum Salts in Vaccines: US Perspective," *Vaccine* 20, suppl. 3 (2002): S18–23, doi:10.1016/S0264-410X(02)00166-4.

2. Mitkus et al., "Updated Aluminum Pharmacokinetics."

3. M. R. Corkins and American Academy of Pediatrics (AAP) Committee on Nutrition, "Aluminum Effects in Infants and Children," *Pediatrics* 144, no. 6 (2019): e20193148; N. J. Bishop et al., "Aluminum Neurotoxicity in Preterm Infants Receiving Intravenous-Feeding Solutions," *New England Journal of Medicine* 336, no. 22 (1997): 1557–62, doi:10.1056/NEJM199705293362203.

4. R. E. Flarend et al., "In Vivo Absorption of Aluminum-Containing Vaccine Adjuvants Using 26Al," *Vaccine* 15, no. 12–13 (1997): 1314–18, doi:10.1016/S0264-410X(97)00041-8.

5. Mitkus et al., "Updated Aluminum Pharmacokinetics."

6. T. Z. Movsas et al., "Effect of Routine Vaccination on Aluminum and Essential Element Levels in Preterm Infants," *JAMA Pediatrics* 167, no. 9 (2013): 870–72.

7. M. P. Karwowski et al., "Blood and Hair Aluminum Levels, Vaccine History, and Early Infant Development: A Cross-Sectional Study," *Academic Pediatrics* 18, no. 2 (2018): 161–65.

8. P. A. Offit and C. A. Moser, "The Problem with Dr Bob's Alternative Vaccine Schedule," *Pediatrics* 123, no. 1 (2009): e164–69.

9. Mitkus et al., "Updated Aluminum Pharmacokinetics."

APPENDIX G. HOW WE KNOW BABIES NEED SO MUCH IRON

1. Joint FAO/WHO Expert Consultation on Human Vitamin and Mineral Requirements and WHO Department of Nutrition for Health and Development, *Vitamin and Mineral Requirements in Human Nutrition*, 2nd ed. (Geneva: World Health Organization, 2005).

2. K. M. Hambidge et al., "Evaluation of Meat as a First Complementary Food for Breastfed Infants: Impact on Iron Intake," *Nutrition Reviews* 69, suppl. 1 (2011): S57–63.

3. L. Davidsson et al., "Iron Bioavailability in Infants from an Infant Cereal Fortified with Ferric Pyrophosphate or Ferrous Fumarate," *American Journal of Clinical Nutrition* 71, no. 6 (2000): 1597–1602.

4. Joint FAO/WHO, *Vitamin and Mineral Requirements in Human Nutrition*.

5. K. G. Dewey and C. M. Chaparro, "Session 4: Mineral Metabolism and Body Composition Iron Status of Breast-Fed Infants," *Proceedings of the Nutrition Society* 66 (August 2007): 412–22, doi:10.1017/S002966510700568X; U. M. Saarinen and M. A. Siimes, Iron Absorption from Breast Milk, Cow's

Milk, and Iron-supplemented Formula: An Opportunistic Use of Changes in Total Body Iron Determined by Hemoglobin, Ferritin, and Body Weight in 132 Infants," *Pediatric Research* 13, no. 3 (1979): 143–47; M. Domellöf et al., "Iron Requirements of Infants and Toddlers," *Journal of Pediatric Gastroenterology and Nutrition* 58, no. 1 (2014): 119–29.

6. U. M. Saarinen and M. A. Siimes, "Iron Absorption from Infant Milk Formula and the Optimal Level of Iron Supplementation," *Acta Paediatrica* 66, no. 6 (1977): 719–22.

7. European Food Safety Authority (EFSA) Panel on Dietetic Products, Nutrition, and Allergies, "Scientific Opinion on Nutrient Requirements and Dietary Intakes of Infants and Young Children in the European Union," *European Food Safety Authority Journal* 11, no. 10 (2013): 3408, doi:10.2903/j.efsa. 2013.3408; Institute of Medicine (IOM), *Dietary Reference Intakes for Vitamin A, Vitamin K, Arsenic, Boron, Chromium, Copper, Iodine, Iron, Manganese, Molybdenum, Nickel, Silicon, Vanadium, and Zinc* (Washington, DC: National Academies Press, 2003).

8. Domellöf et al., "Iron Requirements of Infants and Toddlers."

APPENDIX H. WHY WE SHOULD WORRY ABOUT ARSENIC IN RICE CEREAL

1. P. Y. Lai et al., "Arsenic and Rice: Translating Research to Address Health Care Providers' Needs," *Journal of Pediatrics* 167, no. 4 (2015): 797–803.

2. World Health Organization (WHO), "Arsenic," International Programme on Chemical Safety, accessed January 10, 2014, http://www.who.int/ipcs /assessment/public_health/arsenic/en/.

3. G. A. Wasserman et al., "A Cross-Sectional Study of Well Water Arsenic and Child IQ in Maine Schoolchildren," *Environmental Health* 13, no. 1 (2014): 23.

4. J. Xue et al., "Probabilistic Modeling of Dietary Arsenic Exposure and Dose and Evaluation with 2003–2004 NHANES Data," *Environmental Health Perspectives* 118, no. 3 (2010): 345–50; M. Kurzius-Spencer et al., "Measured versus Modeled Dietary Arsenic and Relation to Urinary Arsenic Excretion and Total Exposure," *Journal of Exposure Science & Environmental Epidemiology* 23, no. 4 (2013): 442–49.

5. European Food Safety Authority (EFSA) Panel on Contaminants in the Food Chain, "Scientific Opinion on Arsenic in Food," *European Food Safety Authority Journal* 7, no. 10 (2009): 1351.

6. T. Shibata et al., "Risk Assessment of Arsenic in Rice Cereal and Other Dietary Sources for Infants and Toddlers in the US," *International Journal of Environmental Research and Public Health* 13, no. 5 (2016): 361.

7. M. R. Karagas et al., "Association of Rice and Rice-Product Consumption with Arsenic Exposure Early in Life," *JAMA Pediatrics* 170, no. 6 (2016): 609–16.

8. A. J. Signes-Pastor, M. Carey, and A. A. Meharg, "Inorganic Arsenic in Rice Based Products for Infants and Young Children," *Food Chemistry* 191 (January 2016): 128–34.

9. "Arsenic in Your Food," *Consumer Reports*, November 2012, https://www.consumerreports.org/cro/magazine/2012/11/arsenic-in-your-food/index.htm.

10. US Food and Drug Administration (FDA), "Arsenic in Rice and Rice Products Risk Assessment," last updated August 5, 2020, https://www.fda.gov/food/cfsan-risk-safety-assessments/arsenic-rice-and-rice-products-risk-assessment.

11. Signes-Pastor, Carey, and Meharg, "Inorganic Arsenic in Rice-Based Products"; Z. Gu, S. de Silva, and S. M. Reichman, "Arsenic Concentrations and Dietary Exposure in Rice-Based Infant Food in Australia," *International Journal of Environmental Research and Public Health* 17, no. 2 (2020): 415, doi: 10.3390/ijerph17020415.

12. Signes-Pastor, Carey, and Meharg, "Inorganic Arsenic in Rice-Based Products"; FDA, "Arsenic in Rice and Rice Products"; Gu, de Silva, and Reichman, "Arsenic Concentrations and Dietary Exposure."

13. Center for Food Safety and Applied Nutrition, "Inorganic Arsenic in Rice Cereals for Infants: Action Level Guidance for Industry," No. FDA-2016-D-1099, August 5, 2020, https://www.fda.gov/regulatory-information/search-fda-guidance-documents/guidance-industry-action-level-inorganic-arsenic-rice-cereals-infants.

14. T. Calvo, "FDA Sets Limits for Arsenic in Baby Rice Cereal," *Consumer Reports*, August 5, 2020, https://www.consumerreports.org/arsenic-in-food/fda-sets-limits-for-arsenic-in-baby-rice-cereal.

15. European Commission, "Commission Regulation (EU) 2015/1006 of 25 June 2015 Amending Regulation (EC) No 1881/2006 as Regards Maximum Levels of Inorganic Arsenic in Foodstuff," *Official Journal of the European Union* 58, L 161 (2015): 14–16.

16. FDA, "Arsenic in Rice and Rice Products."

INDEX

Page numbers in *italics* refer to figures and tables.